Primary Prevention of AIDS

Primary Prevention of Psychopathology

George W. Albee and Justin M. Joffe
General Editors

VOLUMES IN THIS SERIES:

Prevention of Delinquent Behavior, 1987
John D. Burchard and Sara N. Burchard, *Editors*
VOLUME X

Families in Transition, 1988
Lynne A. Bond and Barry M. Wagner, *Editors*
VOLUME XI

Primary Prevention and Promotion in the Schools, 1989
Lynne A. Bond and Bruce E. Compas, *Editors*
VOLUME XII

Primary Prevention of AIDS, 1989
Vickie M. Mays, George W. Albee, and Stanley F. Schneider, *Editors*
VOLUME XIII

Volumes I-IX are available from
University Press of New England
3 Lebanon Street, Hanover, New Hampshire 03755

Primary Prevention of AIDS

Psychological Approaches

**EDITORS
VICKIE M. MAYS
GEORGE W. ALBEE
STANLEY F. SCHNEIDER**

Primary Prevention of Psychopathology
Vol. XIII

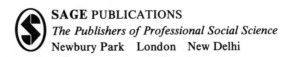

SAGE PUBLICATIONS
The Publishers of Professional Social Science
Newbury Park   London   New Delhi

Copyright © 1989 by the Vermont Conferences on the Primary Prevention of Psychopathology

For information address:

SAGE Publications, Inc.
2111 West Hillcrest Drive
Newbury Park, California 91320

SAGE Publications Ltd.
28 Banner Street
London ECIY 8QE
England

SAGE Publications India Pvt. Ltd.
M-32 Market
Greater Kailash I
New Delhi 110 048 India

Printed in the United States of America

Library of Congress Cataloging-in-Publication Data

Main entry under title:
Primary prevention of AIDS : psychological approaches / edited by
   Vickie M. Mays, George W. Albee, Stanley F. Schneider.
      p.   cm.—(Primary prevention of psychopathology ; vol 13)
   Includes papers presented at a conference held at the University
of Vermont, July 13–17, 1988.
   Includes bibliographies and index.
   ISBN 0-8039-3600-1
   1. AIDS (Disease)—Prevention—Psychological aspects. I. Mays,
Vickie M.   II. Albee, George W.   III. Schneider, Stanley F.
IV. Series: Primary prevention of psychopathology ; v. 13.
   [DNLM: 1. Acquired Immunodeficiency Syndrome—prevention &
control—congresses.   2. Acquired Immunodeficiency Syndrome—
psychology—congresses.   W3 PR945CK v. 13 / WD 308 P9525 1988]
RC454.P683   vol. 13
[RA644.A25]
616.89'05 s—dc20
[616.97'9205]
DNLM/DLC
for Library of Congress   89-10527
FIRST PRINTING, 1989   CIP

We dedicate this book to all persons who have been so deeply touched by the human immunodeficiency virus—to those living with the knowledge of their own HIV infection, to those with AIDS-related complex or the Acquired Immunodeficiency Syndrome, and to those who have died from HIV-related disease. For too long some of these individuals have had to endure the trials not only of their own disease, but also official neglect, bureaucratic denial, and discrimination, both covert and overt. Unlike other infectious diseases of recent appearance, such as Legionnaires' disease or Lyme disease, that affected people who could not be so readily labeled as unworthy of America's concern, persons affected by HIV infection, ARC, and AIDS were ignored, despite the magnitude of this particular disease. Because many HIV-affected individuals belong to groups viewed as outside the mainstream—the ethnic minority poor, gay men, intravenous drug users—America has been slow to respond to the tragedy that is AIDS. This book is dedicated to all whose lives have been so dramatically altered by this disease.

After expenses, one-half of all profits from this book will be donated directly to benefit persons living with AIDS/ARC; the remainder will go to support future conferences on primary prevention.

Vickie M. Mays
George W. Albee
Stanley F. Schneider

Contents

Preface   11

Acknowledgments   13

Part I: Introduction   15

1. Primary Prevention in Public Health: Problems and Challenges
   of Behavior Change as Prevention
   George W. Albee   17

Part II: The Faces of AIDS: What We Are Trying to Prevent   21

2. A Risk Assessment of the AIDS Epidemic
   June E. Osborn   23

3. AIDS: A Family Perspective
   G. M. "Missy" LeClaire   39

4. A Christmas Story: The Eighties
   Van R. Nelson   44

5. The Worldwide Epidemiology and Prevention of AIDS
   Stephen B. Hulley and Norman Hearst   47

6. Human Immunodeficiency Virus and Immune System
   Regulation of the Central Nervous System
   Nicholas R.S. Hall and Maureen P. O'Grady   72

Part III: Theories, Models, and Research on Health, Risk, and
   Decision Making   91

7. Using the Theory of Reasoned Action as a Framework for
   Understanding and Changing AIDS-Related Behaviors
   Martin Fishbein and Susan E. Middlestadt   93

8. The Health Belief Model: Some Implications for Behavior
   Change, with Reference to Homosexual Males
   John P. Kirscht and Jill G. Joseph   111

9. Perceived Self-Efficacy in the Exercise of Control over AIDS
   Infection
   Albert Bandura   128

10. Perceptions of Personal Susceptibility to Harm
   Neil D. Weinstein   142
11. Making Decisions about AIDS
   Baruch Fischhoff   168

Part IV: Prevention in Targeted Populations   207
   Gay Men

12. Are There Psychological Costs Associated with Changes in
   Behavior to Reduce AIDS Risk?
   **Jill G. Joseph, Ronald C. Kessler, Camille B. Wortman, John
   P. Kirscht, Margalit Tal, Susan Caumartin, Suzann Eshleman,
   and Michael Eller**   209
13. Group Intervention to Reduce AIDS Risk Behaviors in Gay
   Men: Applications of Behavioral Principles
   **Jeffrey A. Kelly, Janet S. St. Lawrence, Ted L. Brasfield, and
   Harold V. Hood**   225
14. Implications of the AIDS Risk-Reduction Model for the Gay
   Community: The Importance of Perceived Sexual Enjoyment
   and Help-Seeking Behaviors
   **Joseph A. Catania, Thomas J. Coates, Susan M. Kegeles,
   Maria Ekstrand, Joseph R. Guydish, and Larry L. Bye**   242
   Commentary
   Stephen F. Morin   262

   Ethnic Minorities and Women

15. AIDS Prevention in Black Populations: Methods of a Safer
   Kind
   Vickie M. Mays   264
16. Pulling Coyote's Tale: Native American Sexuality and AIDS
   Terry Tafoya   280
17. AIDS Prevention Models in Asian-American Communities
   Bart Aoki, Chiang Peng Ngin, Bertha Mo, and Davis Y. Ja   290
18. Women and HIV Infection: Issues in Prevention and Behavior
   Change
   Susan D. Cochran   309
   Commentary
   Juan Ramos   328

   Intravenous Drug Users

19. Mexican-American Intravenous Drug Users' Needle-Sharing
   Practices: Implications for AIDS Prevention
   Alberto G. Mata, Jr. and Jaime S. Jorquez   329
   Commentary
   Edward S. Morales   345

Part V: An Agenda for Psychological Training and Research   349

20. An AIDS Research and Training Agenda for Psychology
    Stanley F. Schneider   351
21. Mental Health Practitioners and Their Roles in the AIDS
    Crisis
    Kathleen Sheridan   358
22. Components of a Comprehensive Strategy for Reducing the
    Risk of AIDS in Adolescents
    June A. Flora and Carl E. Thoresen   374
23. The National Institute on Alcohol Abuse and Alcoholism's
    AIDS-Related Activities
    Daniela Seminara   390
24. Overview of the AIDS Program of the National Institute on
    Drug Abuse
    Charles R. Schuster   392
25. The National Institute of Mental Health
    Lewis L. Judd   397

Name Index   400
Subject Index   409
Contributors   417

Preface

The focus of the Board of Social and Ethical Responsibility (BSERP) of the American Psychological Association is on those psychological issues affecting the public interest. Historically, the BSERP has been the arm of psychology's professional group that has been concerned with psychological issues such as domestic violence and the psychological testing of minority and culturally different children, especially those whose first language is not English or who have sensory and/or motor handicaps. Issues affecting women in society, factors disrupting children and families, and the special problems of persons with handicaps are the special responsibility of committees of the BSERP. The Board has worked closely with the Board of Ethnic Minority Affairs in developing a position opposed to the death penalty and opposed to the use of psychological counseling, assessment, and treatment aimed at making persons competent for execution. The BSERP has published a number of pamphlets on topics of general public interest, such as child care, choosing a therapist, and the threat of nuclear destruction.

At a retreat meeting of the Board in November 1987, several psychological issues arose as pressing concerns. These included acquired immunodeficiency syndrome, the problems of the homeless and the elderly, the death penalty, and the treatment of incarcerated women. While each issue presents the profession of psychology with a call to action, AIDS, like no other subject, presents a variety of social and ethical issues affecting all the committees that the Board of Social and Ethical Responsibility represents: the Committees on Women in Psychology; Gay and Lesbian Concerns; Children, Youth and Family; and Disabilities and Handicaps. AIDS, like no other illness, carries with it several potentially discriminatory psychological burdens: It is associated with stigmatized groups, it is often sexually transmitted, and it is a terminal disease that can be physically disfiguring. The Board voted unanimously to make the growing problem of AIDS its first priority for 1988.

11

In discussing the issues surrounding HIV infection and AIDS, we wanted to contribute in those arenas that represented the strength of psychology; namely concerning ourselves with AIDS as a behaviorally transmitted disease that could be prevented. At that meeting, the Board voted to organize a conference on psychological and educational approaches to the prevention of AIDS in collaboration with the Vermont Conference on the Primary Prevention of Psychopathology (VCPPP). The Vermont Conference was established in 1975 as a nonprofit educational foundation that would hold an annual conference on some aspect of primary prevention, with an annual published volume reflecting the content of papers presented at the conference. Simultaneously, the Office of Prevention of the National Institute of Mental Health, under the leadership of Dr. Juan Ramos and Mr. Armand Checker, was increasingly concerned with the growing AIDS epidemic and the need for greater attention to the role that psychologically based prevention and intervention efforts could play in stopping the transmission of the human immunodeficiency virus.

The conference was held July 13–17, 1988, at the University of Vermont. Funding was provided by NIMH, with additional funding provided by the Public Interest Directorate of the American Psychological Association, with the assistance and consultation of James Jones, interim director of that Directorate. Because this was the first national conference on psychological and educational approaches to the primary prevention of AIDS, invited participants were selected with careful attention to their applied expertise on the problems involved in effecting behavior changes in the area of health maintenance, together with their special knowledge of the rapidly evolving research base on HIV infection and AIDS. The chapters in this volume provide the reader with a detailed understanding of the epidemiology of the disease, the modes of its transmission, and populations targeted for special prevention efforts. The point to be understood at the outset, however, is that transmission can be reduced or eliminated through behavior change.

George W. Albee, *Chair, Board of Social and Ethical Responsibility*
Vickie M. Mays, *Chair-Elect, Board of Social and Ethical Responsibility*
Stanley F. Schneider, *National Institute of Mental Health*

Acknowledgments

Without the loyal and dedicated staff of the Black C.A.R.E. Project, Noel Miller and Farrell Webb, who stayed late many nights and saw us through the maze of incompatible word-processing programs, file transfers, and sundry other technical feats, it would have been impossible to complete this book. They are also thanked for their patience and advice. Acknowledgments are also due for the support provided to Vickie Mays, who, while working on this book, held a National Institute of Mental Health Grant (1 R01 MH 42584–02) and a National Research Service Award (T32 HS 00007) from the National Center for Health Services Research and Health Care Technology Assessment awarded to the RAND Corporation.

A number of people at the National Institute of Mental Health who helped to make both the conference and the book a reality by assisting us in obtaining funds and offering their guidance and help in obtaining a list of outstanding participants also deserve acknowledgment. Armand Checker, who served as the project officer for our contract, was always available, wise, and fair in his recommendations. Thanks also go to Dr. Juan Ramos, director of the Office of Prevention and Special Populations, who has been continuously helpful, and Drs. Fred Altman and Sheldon Cohen, for their valued advice. Special acknowledgment also goes to Dr. Fred Altman, for helping facilitate the transfer of book material on BITNET from the National Institute of Mental Health to UCLA. Very special thanks are due to Walter Sloboda and Dr. Leonard Mitmick, for always being there when we needed them. We are also grateful to Dr. James M. Jones, interim director of the Public Interest Directorate of the American Psychological Association, for his assistance in identifying speakers and arranging for additional financial support.

The Vermont Conference on Primary Prevention of Psychopathology is a nonprofit educational foundation incorporated in the state of Vermont. Its Board members provided continuous support and guidance. They include Lynne A. Bond, Ph.D., dean of the Graduate College at the University of Vermont; Marc Kessler, Ph.D., associate professor of psychology and treasurer of VCPPP; John Burchard, Ph.D., professor of psychology; Justin M. Joffe, Ph.D., professor of psychology on leave in London, England; and Barbara York, a historian and our Washington, D.C., representative, who is employed at the Smithsonian Institution.

Special recognition is due to Melissa Perry, who worked for many months on all the complex details of advertising and organizing a major national conference. Ms. Perry was dedicated to primary prevention throughout her last couple of years as an undergraduate at the University of Vermont. As a result of her experience with the conference, she is now pursuing advanced degrees at the Johns Hopkins University School of Public Hygiene, where she plans to obtain further experience in dealing with the epidemic of AIDS.

Jean Kiedaisch, Ph.D., of the University of Vermont's English Department, was of great assistance in helping to organize a particularly difficult chapter. Special acknowledgment goes also to Dr. Marc Kessler for helping facilitate the transfer of book material on BITNET and other computerized storage and retrieval systems. This made possible a rapid exchange of materials between the University of Vermont and UCLA. We appreciate the assistance of Samantha Austin, who was always ready to work late or through lunch hours to help get the manuscript in order and out on time. The editors gratefully acknowledge the contributions of all of the authors, who share in a commitment to AIDS prevention.

Finally, thanks go to all of those individuals who have been touched in some way by the AIDS epidemic, as each of them is, in truth, our collaborator. It is our hope that we have shared your stories and experiences in ways that befit the courage that you have shown us.

1

Primary Prevention in Public Health: Problems and Challenges of Behavior Change as Prevention

George W. Albee

Throughout human history, plagues have had devastating effects on human life, killing large numbers of people unexpectedly, in disparate parts of the world. These plagues nearly always have involved an infectious agent that might be transmitted accidentally or randomly through direct personal contact with contaminated food or water or through some intermediate host, such as rats, lice, or mosquitoes. The AIDS epidemic, like past plagues, kills people. Like past plagues, it also results from the transmission of an infectious agent. But AIDS is also a very different kind of epidemic in important ways. Human immunodeficiency virus infects, but it does not show its effects overtly for many years, allowing the virus to infect again silently, without human awareness. AIDS also stigmatizes, not simply because of the disease itself, but because of the behaviors with which it is so strongly associated.

Acquired Immune Deficiency Syndrome has been studied intensively for less than a decade. Its viral agent, HIV, and the mode of its transmission have only recently come to be understood. The transmission of HIV is now known to be the result of the exchange of specific bodily fluids—blood, semen, and vaginal secretions—under conditions that are potentially preventable and controllable through education and modification of behavior. In other words, AIDS is the first epidemic in human history in which we have learned so quickly that the identified noxious agent can be kept from spreading by specific behavioral changes.

The virus that causes AIDS is transmitted in several ways: by transfusions of blood or blood products where a donor is infected; by the needles, syringes, and paraphernalia used to inject drugs

17

when these are shared among intravenous drug users so that the blood of an infected person infects another; by mothers prenatally or postnatally by breast-feeding their offspring; and by unprotected sexual intercourse where bodily fluids (i.e., semen, secretions, or blood) containing the virus enter the bloodstream of an uninfected person. In the case of the sexual transmission of HIV, anal intercourse appears to be a higher-risk activity than vaginal intercourse, because of the greater likelihood that fluids containing the virus will pass directly into the bloodstream due to the greater susceptibility of rectal mucosa to tearing.

Although, in this country, the sexual transmission of AIDS to date has most frequently occurred during male homosexual sexual activity in which high-risk contact with blood or semen has occurred, clearly heterosexual transmission does happen. This is evidenced by the epidemiology of the disease. In this country, both men and women have been HIV infected through heterosexual sexual activity. In certain other countries and cultures, both sexes are nearly equally affected.

The field of public health has traditionally taught us much of what we need to know to prevent plagues effectively. First of all, it is well established that no mass disorder afflicting humankind has ever been eliminated by attempts at treating only infected individuals. Incidence (the number of new cases in a time period) can be reduced only through successful primary prevention. Primary prevention means proactive steps to reduce or eliminate the undesirable condition in unaffected populations. Primary prevention nearly always involves the reduction of risk to populations or to large groups at high risk.

There are some specific and logical approaches in public health methodology useful in the prevention of widespread disease and disorders. Basically, three strategies exist. The first is to identify the noxious agent and then to take steps to neutralize it, kill it, or otherwise render it impotent. Many water-borne diseases, for example, are controlled by ensuring a water supply free of microorganisms or other contaminants, often by treating drinking water with chemicals that eliminate the disease-causing organisms or by forbidding the contamination of the water supply with dangerous substances.

The second approach involves strengthening the resistance of the host. By making the host resistant to the noxious agent, the transmission of the disease may be prevented. Familiar examples here include inoculation—such as against polio, measles, and smallpox—which builds up the host's antibodies through the injection of inactive or weakened disease-causing organisms. Vitamins and other substances may also strengthen the body's resistance to disease.

The third public health approach to prevention of the spread of disease involves attempts to prevent transmission of the noxious agent to the host. A good example here is the success that has been achieved against the mosquitoes that carried the noxious agents causing malaria or yellow fever from an infected person to a noninfected person. By killing the mosquitoes, transmission was halted. Any method that prevents a noxious agent from reaching the host effectively reduces the incidence of the disease.

In the case of AIDS, with its significant behavioral components, traditional public health approaches are not enough. For AIDS, the noxious agent is known. It is a retrovirus, usually designated as HIV. The prospects for finding a mechanism for killing this virus within the body are currently very slim. While there is increasing hope that virologists may find treatment methods that suppress the reproduction of the virus, and while this could have the effect of prolonging the life of the person infected, this treatment by itself would not reduce the extent of the epidemic. We already have effective treatment for other venereal diseases, such as syphilis and gonorrhea, but successful treatment has not eradicated these diseases.

The prospects for strengthening the resistance of the host—that is, developing a vaccine that will protect uninfected persons—also seem slim, according to virologists. At least, such a vaccine is many years down the road.

The strategy of prevention of HIV transmission through education and the modification of behaviors is clearly the most hopeful approach to the prevention of AIDS. Educating persons with information that leads to changed behaviors that reduce or eliminate high-risk, unprotected sexual encounters constitutes effective prevention. Safer sexual practices, particularly if one partner has been infected, reduce the likelihood of transmission. Educating intravenous drug users about the use of clean needles and techniques for sterilizing needles and injection paraphernalia can reduce this form of transmission between IV drug users and thereby reduce the infection of IV drug users' sexual partners and many of the babies born within this social network.

As is clear from this brief discussion, the problems of informing the public, particularly among some specific groups for whom our outreach strategies have been less effective, are enormous, but the problems of getting these groups to change their behavior in ways that will reduce transmission are even more of a challenge. Many of the chapters in this volume review research relevant to efforts at changing health-related behaviors. The challenge to psychologists and educators is enormous, but effective efforts at behavior change may be the only hope of containing this devastating epidemic.

PART II

The Faces of AIDS: What We Are Trying to Prevent

This section attempts to provide the reader with an understanding of the complexity of what it is we are trying to prevent. Some readers may know several persons or at least one person with AIDS, or may be directly affected by the disease. Yet there are many others reading this book whom AIDS has not touched personally. We thought it important to give AIDS a face, not merely its numbers and the target groups, but the human side of how it affects individuals, their families, and our society. In the opening chapter, June Osborn, trained as both a pediatrician and a virologist, provides an excellent overview of the impact of the AIDS epidemic. This is followed by two firsthand accounts of people directly affected by AIDS. The first is the story of a young gay man who must return home for assistance with his health care. The story illustrates what happens in a context of love, ignorance about AIDS, and life-style conflicts. The second is the account of a wife who discovered, shortly after her marriage, that her husband was developing AIDS symptoms. Her commitment and struggle to make his remaining life easier make personal and real the problems of daily support of a person living with AIDS, particularly outside an AIDS epicenter. Both of these first-person accounts illustrate the human tragedies that lie behind the statistics of the epidemic.

This section also provides the reader with a detailed picture of the magnitude of the disorder both in the United States and worldwide (Hulley and Hearst) and an in-depth look at the HIV virus and its effects on the immune system (Hall and O'Grady).

Dr. Osborn touches on many of the major themes that must be heard more widely. She makes it clear that the disease reminds us forcefully of the worldwide interdependence of people. The dependence of the Moslem world and of Japan on imported blood and blood fractions resulted in the spread of infection in those countries. The appearance of the disease in more than 100 countries of the world threatens freedom of international travel and commerce as countries belatedly try to throw up emergency barriers to reduce the

21

threat to their populations. And many current public pronounce-
ments provide major examples of denial in operation. The seriousness of the growing epidemic was denied for a long time; currently we
are hearing reassurances about the unlikelihood of heterosexual transmission becoming a major vector of infection. Dr. Osborn's frank
discussion of the "irreversible beachhead," as well as warnings of the
homophobic undertones inherent in discussions of AIDS, should be
required reading for everyone concerned with the epidemic.

Professors Hulley and Hearst clarify the epidemiology of AIDS
geographically (with cautions about problems of underreporting), by
age (it strikes the young adult primarily during the most productive
time of life), by sex, race, targeted populations, and so on. They
remind us again that the disease is transmitted by behavior that touches on powerful human satisfactions, but behavior that may be modifiable with education and knowledge.

For some there are thoughts that the real answer to this epidemic
lies in the development of a vaccine. Too often, manuscripts about
AIDS begin with "until a vaccine is developed, education is the primary method of prevention of HIV infection." The reality is that in
spite of available vaccines for the likes of hepatitis B and measles, we
are in the midst of a measles epidemic. Drs. Hall and O'Grady give us
a glimpse of the difficulties inherent in vaccine development for the
AIDS virus through their discussion of the effect of the virus on the
immune system.

2

A Risk Assessment of the AIDS Epidemic

June E. Osborn

There is an ancient Chinese curse—reserved, I presume, for special enemies—"May you live in interesting times." We seem to have been well and truly cursed, for the times are monumentally interesting. Within our own generation, a virus new to humankind developed the capacity for spreading among humans by means of sexual inter- course, blood exchange, or birth to an infected mother. While these modes of transmission were (and are) sharply limited, they converged propitiously with the cofactors of frenetic travel, urbanization, and social disruption that characterize the human family in the late twenti- eth century, and so the new virus thrived. In only the last two decades, after a presumed interval of relative endemicity in isolated popula- tions, it began its horrific pandemic march, spreading with surprising efficiency in just a few years to virtually every country on the face of the earth.

This virus is an awesome enemy, but it is not unbeatable, for it is not contagious like influenza or measles or polio, which spread by uncon- trollable environmental means. Indeed, therein lies the only good news, for it is strictly dependent on intimate, consensual human activi- ties for its transmission. That behavioral aspect of its propagation makes avoidance a feasible strategy and cessation of the epidemic a real possibility in countries where the safety of the blood supply can be secured. The behaviors at issue—drug use and sexual intercourse— are so intractable and/or fundamental to human society, and so over- laid with totem and taboo, that the task of education and behavior modification appears overwhelming. But we must undertake that task regardless, for it is very clear that the virus has established an irrevers- ible beachhead in our world and will be an indelible part of the terrain henceforth. Respect for this new pathogen and knowledge of its features will be a prerequisite of the healthy survival of our children and their children's children.

The virus now has a name—the human immunodeficiency virus or, more familiarly, HIV—which it acquired, of course, only belatedly, when scientists uncovered its tracks several years into its subversive march. That name replaces earlier ones, by agreement of an international committee; and in due course we will probably also drop some of the early clinical terminology (perhaps not AIDS, but certainly ARC, lymphadenopathy syndrome, and the like) that developed before tools were at hand to track the virus directly. It will make more coherent sense in the long haul to speak simply of stages of HIV infection and disease, such as asymptomatic, mild, or lethal; but for now it is best to stick to familiar terms. As you know, of the clinical consequences of HIV infection, the most definitive and dramatic is the lethal complex of diseases we have been calling the acquired immunodeficiency syndrome, or AIDS.

The problem has come on us rapidly. The first report of a cluster involved fewer than a dozen men in the summer of 1981, and yet new cases of AIDS are now being reported to the Centers for Disease Control at the rate of 100 a day, and that rate will continue to accelerate. There have already been over 68,000 persons diagnosed with AIDS in the United States, of whom more than half have died. In 1986 it was projected by the Institute of Medicine/National Academy of Sciences committee on AIDS that there would be 270,000 cumulative cases by 1991. Sadly, experience to date has validated the curves used for those estimates, and both the IOM and the USPHS updated their assessments recently and projected that there will have been over 400,000 young adults diagnosed with AIDS by the end of 1993.

Much of this discussion will be devoted to these figures, their breakdown, and their meaning for public health strategies. I will not have much time to delve into specific issues of health care and economic impact; but to a certain extent the sheer predictable magnitude of the problem will allow you to extrapolate for yourselves. In order to appreciate some of the complex issues invoked by this horrifying prospect, it is useful to have a working concept of how the virus wreaks such havoc, as well as an understanding of how we have arrived at our present, rather advanced state of knowledge about its epidemiology, pathogenesis, and molecular biology, and why it is that no cure or vaccine is expected during the next five or ten years.

Pathogenesis: Why Vaccines and Cures Are So Problematic

A few details of pathogenesis are worth noting. Within a matter of weeks after HIV infects a person, detectable antibodies to the virus appear in blood; while these antibodies do not play a protective role as they do in more familiar virus infections, they are useful as markers of continued virus presence and allow one to follow events associated with persistence of the virus. Except for those antibodies, there is no evidence of harm to the infected host during a latency interval of several years. But then, like a quietly malevolent guest, the human immunodeficiency virus gradually activates; and once roused from its dormancy it inexorably subverts both immune and nervous system functions, resulting in a dreadful array of infections and tumors, fevers and dementia, and a wasting of both body and spirit over months of clinical decline.

The exact means whereby the virus destroys immune cells and neurons is under intense study at present. It is of more than passing interest, for any effort at vaccine or improvement in therapy will be dependent on a rather sophisticated understanding of the balance between virus and host. Since HIV intertwines its genetic message with that of the cell at the very outset, it is difficult even to conceive of effective therapies that will not maim or at least wound the host en route to killing the virus; and since there is thus far no suggestion that natural immune responses serve to protect an infected person from virus damage, the usual strategy for development of vaccines—which is to imitate nature—is not available as a blueprint for progress in provoking immunity through immunization. Indeed, there is reason to be concerned that some facets of the naturally occurring immunologic reaction to HIV may be harmful or may even mediate the ultimate onset of clinical illness, so caution in vaccine development is dictated by genuine concerns.

Whatever the stimuli that disturb the virus-host balance, once progression has reached a stage that qualifies for the label AIDS, the outcome is invariably fatal—and often unpeaceful, as undertakers recoil and families react to previously covert facets of their loved ones' lives that have been laid brutally bare by epidemiologic inference. (It is perhaps not so hard to understand why a frightened public clings to the fancy that mosquitoes might yet prove a tenable excuse for infection, when the consequences of behavioral revelation are so harsh.) The disease called AIDS represents the final denouement of a story of inexorable destruction of those cells and tissues most critical to both survival and creativity. In a very real sense it is a "fate worse than death."

The Global Picture: Minor Variations on a Dominant Theme

This terrible new disease was first recognized when it occurred in clusters in the United States in 1981. In retrospect, sporadic cases had been seen in the 1970s in the United States, in the Caribbean, and in Brazil. The rest of the world was quick to follow, with epidemic onset staggered by only two or three years in most of the remainder of the Western Hemisphere as well as in Europe and Australia. In general, the initial pattern of spread in these countries reflected the special transmission efficiency of homosexual anal receptive intercourse and the relative insularity of defined homosexual and drug-using communities; but there was also clear evidence that heterosexual intercourse could spread the virus, and the Caribbean pattern—like the African, which I will discuss shortly—was predominantly heterosexual from the beginning. The contribution of intravenous drug use varied widely from country to country, but in some venues such as Italy, Spain, and of course in the United States (in New York and New Jersey), that mode of blood-borne spread via shared drug-injection apparatus quickly began to dominate the pattern.

In industrialized countries other than our own, the slight delay allowed governments to learn from the American experience, to adopt blood-screening programs early in their own epidemics and to initiate national educational campaigns quickly, which in many instances offer at least some hope of influencing the epidemic curve in a relatively few years. Blood screening came belatedly for other countries, such as the Moslem world, where religious implications of blood donation had fostered a dependence on imported blood that was provided primarily by the United States and Brazil prior to 1985. Similarly, reliance on exporters for antihemophilic factors accelerated introduction of HIV into specific subpopulations of countries such as Japan. A price was paid for global interdependence, but it is almost certain that it merely accelerated the inevitable; that same interdependence may serve us handsomely as we respond as a global community to the common enemy.

By contrast with Europe and Australia, epidemic onset in Africa seems to have been either simultaneous with or only slightly later than that in the United States, but conditions were ripe for an epidemic explosion of catastrophic proportions that is now under way in at least a dozen countries in central and east Africa. The move to urbaniza-tion had been nothing short of phenomenal in the years since 1950, and cultural restraints gave way to a plethora of sexual expression fostering both prostitution and sexually transmitted disease patho-gens; hidden among them was the virus of AIDS. In Africa there is no question that HIV is spread primarily by heterosexual intercourse; among other effects, it is causing disproportionate decimation of the upper and middle classes of men to whom the mantle of leadership was to have been passed.

Horrifying glimpses of the future in the affected parts of Africa can be gleaned from scattered serologic surveys of pregnant women or of blood donors—warning that the stage is already set for the wipe-out of very measurable percentages of the young adult population and of children. It has been soberly predicted that as a result of the intractable public health dilemmas posed by cultural barriers, illiter-acy, and unsecured blood supplies, negative population growth may return to those areas as a direct result of AIDS (although sufficient perturbation of agriculture and economic structure through specific losses in those working groups may hasten the effect). I don't know where help will come from, either, for the annual per capita health care expenditure in those countries is less than the cost of a single blood screening test.

At least for the moment, the Eastern Hemisphere is more fortu-nate. The virus invaded Asia just later enough that only the first few clinical cases are now surfacing in most of those populous countries. This has given the opportunity to sound a warning, although the recognition recently that HIV had spread suddenly and dramatically in drug users in Thailand serves as a reminder that warnings alone do not suffice if they are too narrowly focused or if they are not heeded. Thailand had focused its response on education about sexual modes of spread per se and had not attended to the threat from drug use; nor had it fully secured its blood supply.

Global perspectives are important, but the most striking fact is that the United States is at the epicenter of this explosion and, with the exception of parts of Africa and perhaps Brazil, is likely to remain so for years to come. The updated estimate of numbers of infected per-sons in the United States is 1.4 million; the average incubation interval is now thought to be 7–10 years; and the possibility that most if not all infected persons will progress to AIDS seems to become more of a certainty with each passing year of experience. While it has been said that no country in the industrialized world was less well positioned to deal with the sudden health care burden this will impose, we are at least affluent enough to try—and we have a very special responsibility to try to lead in the science that must be pursued in haste.

The Contribution of Basic Science

Most of this chapter deals with truly horrendous news; so it is worth pausing briefly to celebrate some victories to maintain a sense of balance. Since the disease AIDS was recognized only seven years ago, with virus discovery following less than three years later, it is a dramatic fact that we know more about the epidemiology, virology, and molecular genetics of HIV than about any other human pathogen. There are gaps in our knowledge, of course, but the broad outlines are vivid, and their clarity not only points the way to a focused, activist agenda for prevention, control, and care, but should make us glad as well at the wisdom of investment in basic research that fortuitously was conducted during those silent decades of virus incubation.

The timeliness of progress leaves one breathless—without that slight head start, we would now be facing a nameless, amorphous enemy, overwhelmed with dread and completely impotent to predict or prepare for the future. In contemplating that coincidence of timing, it is important to comment on the font of basic science information that was ready at hand as the crisis hit. I think it should serve as an antidote to the common misperception that basic research is somehow frivolous and its results irrelevant; rather, it would be wise to recognize that basic results are those for which the relevance is not yet evident.

In any event, with what we now know of HIV and its ways, we could actually interrupt its spread and blunt its awesome demographic potential—at least in industrialized nations—were it not for the difficult terrain it has chosen for battle: that of sexual behavior, procreation, and illicit drug use. That, of course, is the societal territory where we are at our most inept and awkward. Unhappily, the elegant advance of biomedical science and molecular genetics has not been matched by comparable progress in behavioral sciences, for their funding has been problematic and in some areas their very existence has been under threat in recent years.

We are condemned to citing "Kinsey, 1949," when estimating frequencies of variation in sexual behavior. Even "1949" is misleadingly modern, for Kinsey began collecting his samples more than 50 years ago. I do believe things have changed—or maybe they haven't. We must attend to that; the fact that AIDS is basically a sexually transmitted disease means that we must understand sexual behavior well; and yet there is a startling scarcity of information concerning homosexuality, bisexuality, variations in heterosexual practices, and the like, on which much of our prognostication should be based. Only a few clues exist in the sparse literature of human sexuality concerning bisexual behavior, and yet one could contend that it exceeds drug use in importance as a vehicle of future spread beyond "recognized risk groups." I am sad to say that even now there persists a deep reluctance to acknowledge this gap in our fundamental information about human behavior and move to close it.

The U.S. Epidemic: Current Status and Projections

Having laid out the broad outlines of the global AIDS problem and the virus's biology, I want to narrow my focus to the United States. First, let me talk about AIDS cases—but as I do so, keep in mind that they represent a snapshot of epidemic events that occurred as many as 10 years ago. As another caveat, note that there may be some underreporting of AIDS cases, and perhaps more so with increasing time. Branding someone with that diagnosis carries such an overlay of social turbulence and jeopardy that compassionate physicians may sometimes decide to use a diagnostic euphemism to avoid setting off such turbulence; having AIDS listed as cause of death guarantees an unpeaceful demise, and in fact one of the most awful facts of the epidemic is that, for fear of social reprisals, thousands of families already are having to grieve in secret.

In cities like New York, where well-meaning, compassionate laws have been passed expressly forbidding hospital discharge of AIDS patients if they have nowhere to go, one kind of reaction has been the withholding of the diagnosis for pragmatic reasons; indeed, the *New York Times* recently estimated that practice to be so frequent that 10–20% of the shelter population now is composed of AIDS patients. So, there may be some nonrandom errors even in such definitive numbers as the AIDS case count; but you should know that, unlike HIV seropositivity, about which there is considerable argument, reporting of actual AIDS cases is required by law in every state, so these data are relatively firm and complete.

Nonetheless, the numbers reported to CDC are increasing by 100 a day. So far the figures show a distribution that has not varied greatly since the onset of the epidemic: 92% are male, and the category of gay/bisexual men accounts for just over 70% of the total if one includes the 8% who use intravenous drugs as well. While the early brunt of the epidemic was borne by homosexual men—notably in the gay communities in San Francisco, Los Angeles, and New York—their self-generated educational programs have resulted in the past year in dramatic reductions in rates of virus spread. While this does not mean the trouble is over, it does provide a compelling illustration that education can be a potent weapon even in groups with deeply entrenched patterns of risky behavior. The remarkable fact that no new seroconversions occurred in a large study group in San Francisco last year is a welcome antidote to the chronic pessimism that usually pervades discussion of the efficacy of health educational interventions.

In a more troublesome context, however, it is interesting to note that a man falls into that gay/bisexual risk category if he has had three or more same-sex encounters in a lifetime; so it is difficult to be sure that some heterosexual spread is not hidden under this heading. It is certainly the case that this group includes a large pool of difficult-to-identify, closeted men who "cover" their sexual orientation with the trappings of marriage and family and are important potential spreaders to the so-called heterosexual community. The impact of bisexuality will be very central to the future of the epidemic, and it may prove to be one of the most difficult behaviors to amend, since bisexual men actually may not even recognize their risk if we persist in talking about homosexuals as if the risk were to the group rather than to the behavior of male-male sex.

The next large risk category of AIDS cases is made up of intravenous drug users—17% have that as the sole risk factor, but when the overlap with gay and bisexual men is noted, fully 25% of the epidemic could be explained by that behavior. Nowhere in the epidemic picture is prevention more feasible or more desperately important—IV drug use presents the broadest avenue to the virus's future. Directly or indirectly, it constitutes the source of the virus for 80% of women and 90% of children with AIDS, and theirs are the most rapidly growing numbers of AIDS diagnoses of all. Furthermore, drug injection with sharing of needles contributes substantially to the shocking disproportion of Black and Hispanic minority groups caught up in the epidemic.

The numbers of persons estimated to be addicted to intravenous heroin in the United States are usually given in ranges—never lower than 500,000 but perhaps over 750,000. That's quite a spread! But the number who inject drugs recreationally at least once a month is even more vague—I have heard estimates ranging from 750,000 to over

3,000,000. And as heroin—rather than injection—gets a reputation for danger in association with AIDS, there is a nightmarish trend for users to shift to IV cocaine, which is a far more demanding master, dictating injections at ever-narrowing intervals. News from the front is really awful in the war on drugs. And I don't think "Just say no—or else!" quite meets the challenge.

It may startle you to hear that the potential for interruption of HIV transmission is at its most promising in this difficult population, but the data are very convincing on this point. First, there is a vast difference from city to city in the extent to which IV drug users are infected thus far. In New York and New Jersey, well over 50% now carry HIV and the absolute majority of AIDS cases now come from that group. Some cities, such as Chicago, Detroit, and San Francisco, have seen the percentage of infected users climb rapidly in the past year or so, while still others such as Los Angeles have thus far escaped this facet of the epidemic almost entirely, with less than 2% infected on repeated measurements over several years.

Clearly there is potential for explosive spread, and since it is needle sharing, not drug use per se, that is the important risk behavior for HIV transmission, there are some obvious strategies that offer hope of containment quite quickly. Such strategies—the most prominent being needle exchange programs—are the topic of hot debate, but data supporting their efficacy are accumulating rapidly, and this is one area in which there is striking opportunity to reduce the size of the future caseload. In this context too there is some recent optimistic news, for the precipitous rate of increase of HIV infection among intravenous drug users in New York has at last leveled off in the face of concerted efforts at education about clean needles and risk reduction.

Of course drug treatment—available on demand for all addicts—is or should be the cornerstone of preventive efforts, and as you know it was the first and most urgent matter to capture Admiral Watkins's attention as the Presidential Commission began its series of statements. I have yet to find a major city in the United States in which the wait for drug treatment, once one is on the list, is shorter than one month. More characteristically, addicts seeking help are told they will be called back in 3–6 months. What a horror! Waiting lists have a special significance in this context, for, as Dr. Robert Newman has commented wryly, drug addicts are, of course, notorious for their ability to defer gratification. I don't mean to pretend that this is an easy area for resolution, but our current paucity of treatment, coupled with our superficial efforts at alerting addicts to the hazards of AIDS, seems to me to be like shouting "Fire!" ie at some length from the summary talk in Stockholm delivered last week by Justice Michael Kirby of Australia, who is president of the Court of Appeals of the Supreme Court of New South Wales. As he introduced the topic of drugs and AIDS, he referred to drug users and then commented as follows: "You will note that I call them 'drug users.' Lawyers develop ears attuned to words with value judgments. There is no place in science, or in stemming an international epidemic, for value-loaded words like 'intravenous drug abusers.' Let us drop that phrase once and for all. The business we are in—or should be in—is saving lives and protecting communities and individuals from a lethal virus. Calling a major cohort (which may become a main vector of this virus to previously untouched heterosexual people) 'abusers' is the surest way to scramble the message to them and to reinforce obstacles in the path of vital preventive strategies. Nor is 'drug addict' right. The risk of infection may be run by occasional recreational drug users too. So let us get back to value neutral scientific language, as befits scientists."

Justice Kirby goes on to discuss the variety of laws pertaining to needle exchange in other countries (many of which have installed such programs recently) and then comments that "in the United States, still the epicenter, similar laws permit the supply of cleaning bleach but deny the possibly life saving exchange of sterile needles. This is a sensitive subject for politicians. But change must come quickly. Sadly it may take AIDS finally to force drugs out of the courtrooms and prisons into the public health issue they really are. But many will die first. Rare political courage will be required."

Besides the major risk behaviors already discussed, there are persons with AIDS who represent sad vestiges of the first days of the epidemic: hemophiliacs, recipients of HIV-contaminated blood, and persons of Haitian descent whose prominence in the early months probably simply represented their clustering as recent immigrants in New York and Miami. As discussed earlier, the Caribbean basin seems to have been an early site of HIV invasion of the Western Hemisphere and, indeed, it turns out that other Caribbean countries have a higher per capita rate of AIDS cases than does Haiti. Trouble continues for the Haitians, whose dire poverty continues to serve as an incubator for risk behaviors; but the blood-related risks associated with medical/

surgical therapy have been brought under secure control by rigorous blood-screening programs.

Given the long incubation period of AIDS, the hemophiliacs are on the dismal upslope of the AIDS curve now, and there will continue to be transfusion-related cases of the disease that had their origin in the prescreening era. Much less understandably, there will be an ongoing crisis of blood supply as long as an underinformed public continues to make the false association between HIV infection and the donation of blood. Public education is truly vital. I will not dwell on transfusion-associated risk here, since that has been and will be the focus of some carefully constructed discussions by OTA and other groups.

In discussing heterosexual spread of HIV there are a number of pitfalls, both of concept and of language, that are worth avoiding. Discussing the frightening specter of AIDS's emergence in "the general population" or some such phrase is a reliably inflammatory provocation of hardworking gay groups, who have felt—with considerable justification—that the social reaction to the epidemic was retarded by homophobia. From the other side, people who have dedicated their careers to liberating sexual behavior (among heterosexuals), such as the now-famous Dr. Gould of *Cosmopolitan* magazine, reject the assertion (and the evidence) that heterosexual spread can even occur in the context of so-called normal vaginal intercourse, and call for a return to monkey-business-as-usual for "straights."

In the midst of all this fuss, Masters and Johnson tossed in their anecdotal and poorly documented entry, asserting that AIDS would "run rampant" in the heterosexual community and urging a new world of chastity. Not content with the careless damage thus done to the carefully developed epidemiologic discourse, they went further and reopened the firmly closed issues of spread by toilet seats, mosquitoes, and the like, abandoning even the pretext of data in favor of uninformed opinion. If I may be forgiven a brief gasp of self-pity, it took fully 48 hours after their dramatic press conference before my phone stopped ringing and I was able to return to normal function, for the hardworking members of the print and electronic media had learned their lessons well enough to be aware of the danger of such unsubstantiated stuff, and yet they needed reassurance to convert that batch of pseudonews into well-digested commentary.

Where does the proper emphasis lie? I think part of the problem lies in the phrase "running rampant," which is used by otherwise thoughtful people as if it had some meaning. I suppose something is running rampant if you are in its path, and it is not running rampant if you want to minimize your sense of risk. In point of fact, since we are a couple of years ahead of our industrialized allies in epidemic experience, it is the case that while the percentage of AIDS cases firmly attributable to heterosexual intercourse is small, the absolute number of such cases is greater than most other countries have total cases of AIDS. I guess I'll just let you decide whether that is rampant enough to justify our attention. But I don't want anyone persuading my kids "not to worry"!

There has never been any question that heterosexual spread can occur; within the first few dozen AIDS cases were the sexual partners of both male and female intravenous drug users who themselves did not use drugs. And, as noted earlier, heterosexual intercourse is the dominant mode of spread of the epidemic in large parts of the world. Contrary to occasional suggestions, Americans are not a different species.

To summarize this important issue, the question may be best separated into two parts. The first is, "Does heterosexual intercourse spread HIV?" and the answer is an unequivocal "Yes!" The second is, "How efficiently?" and the answer to that is still coming in. The public health and medical implications seem clear: The co-occurrence of other sexually transmitted diseases, multiple sexual partners, sex with persons of unknown background, and the like present genuine risk of infection with HIV and will be increasingly important in upcoming years. Proper condom use can reduce risk very significantly and needs to be advocated and supported when realistic appraisal of the situation makes monogamy or chastity unlikely—as will be the case much of the time.

Asymptomatic HIV Infection: The Shadow of the Future

We have been talking primarily about AIDS case numbers thus far, but those give an epidemic picture that is 5–10 years out of date. Let me turn to more current snapshots of the epidemic, provided by serologic screening for HIV antibodies in various U.S. populations. While these data are still fragmentary and may be unrepresentative to a certain extent, they have a considerable internal consistency and seem to carry a strong warning that worse is yet to come, and that the preceding discussion about heterosexual spread may be more important than one would wish. Two years ago the U.S. military reported the initial results obtained from screening several hundred thousand volunteers; nationwide the rate of infection (as reflected by antibody positivity in sera) was 1.6 per 1,000 among men and 0.6 per 1,000 among women—an alarming shift from the 11:1 male-to-female ratio of AIDS cases.

When data from recruits in the New York City area were analyzed, the news was even worse—the rates were 1.6 per 100 for men and 1.3 per 100 for women. Lest one doubt the validity of these numbers, they were indirectly supported by the results of a study done last winter in which umbilical cord blood from every baby born in New York over a two-month period was tested for HIV antibodies, and 1 in every 61 babies tested positive. While only about half of those infants will themselves turn out to be infected, the presence of those antibodies means unequivocally that their mothers harbored the virus of AIDS.

Subsequent military data have suggested a steady state at levels described two years ago; but that conclusion must be viewed with some skepticism, since the word traveled quickly that seropositive volunteers would be rejected and returned abruptly to their communities without counseling or care, and left to figure out for themselves what to say to family and friends who had just seen them off. So, well-meaning counselors began to suggest informally that would-be recruits get tested first if they thought they had any risk behavior in their backgrounds. I suspect that the presumed steady state is more apparent than real.

In Stockholm the first results were presented from a different kind of survey: testing of anonymous collections of blood from several so-called sentinel hospitals in cities located away from the most concentrated AIDS centers of the United States. Since these studies involved blinded sera, a breakdown to yield demographic details could not be ascertained; but the results suggested that the military's rate of roughly 1.5 per 1,000 nationally might be low by a factor of 3 or 4 even in the so-called heartland. Epidemiologists have been noting for some time now that there is a steady diffusion of AIDS cases away from the initial epicenters and away from risk groups; no state is untouched by the epidemic, and Michigan, for example, which is technically a low-incidence state, has had reported cases from the great majority of its counties.

Clearly we have trouble coming! We need more such survey data to know just how big the trouble is; but the data must be worth having and the present public mood of hostile fear would surely lead persons at risk to go underground if comprehensive screening were attempted. When the CDC first tried to initiate city surveys based on careful sampling, with due attention to oversampling of important groups, and so on, they ran into a 33% refusal rate. I didn't find that so surprising, for in the present hostile atmosphere, I think I'd consider it a kind of IQ test if someone rang my doorbell and said, "Hello, I'm from the government and I'd like to take a sample of your blood to test for AIDS!" Smart people know that life is not kind to HIV seropositives right now. It is that consideration, among others, that prompted Admiral Watkins to place effective antidiscrimination legislation at the top of the list of urgent needs in the report from the Presidential Commission.

Survey data about seropositives are only one kind of gap in the information we need for intelligent public health planning. As noted earlier, we need to know the size of the groups at primary risk, and that involves politically unattractive studies about sexual behavior, habitual and intermittent intravenous drug use, and the like. There are studies under way that should help our understanding of factors that influence the efficiency of HIV spread by various sexual means. And of course there is a great need for fundamental data about the costs of health care and how they would be influenced by diversification of health care options. It makes intuitive sense that substitution of long-term care options for tertiary hospital care might be cost-effective, but the permutations of that kind of plan will vary greatly from one community to another, and development of good data bases could help to optimize the options. Home care, coordinated outpatient care with case management, hospice care—all of these variations may ease the fiscal and hospital bed crises as we approach half a million total cases over the next five years.

I am not expert in these matters, but it strikes me that we have no reason to doubt the order of magnitude of the projected numbers, and there are enough reliable projections at hand to approximate health care personnel needs; this should be done formally as part of strategic planning. I know that even preliminary estimates show the preexisting nursing shortage to be a potential catastrophe in these equations, and studies of the severity of such deficits and their impact should not be leisurely.

In short, there is plenty of work to be done. The scope of the epidemic for the next 5–10 years will be massive, of that we are sure, for the long latency period of HIV infection before AIDS begins guarantees that much of the next decade's trouble is already incubating. That means we have a dual agenda, both components of which are equally urgent. The price of prior failure to prevent will seem to overwhelm our human and fiscal resources, and yet ongoing efforts at prevention must not be downgraded out of discouragement or set aside in the face of desperate need to care for the sick and dying.

There is one particularly grim specter I should mention in order to lend weight to the need for ongoing prevention activities: Right now, as I have mentioned, voluntary and consensual sexual and drug-injecting behavior can be identified clearly as the means of spreading the virus of HIV. Numbers and kinds of sexual partners count, and persons at risk can recognize their own hazard and react responsibly if we provide them with the wherewithal to do so—confidential or anonymous opportunities for counseling and testing, ways of intervening with addictive drug-using behavior, and the like. But if we delay our educational response and allow the epidemic to diffuse, there could come a time ten years or so from now when risk will be too unpredictable to allow for that strategy. The spouses of ostensibly risk-free individuals will themselves be at risk—and yet no one will have suspected. This is what Surgeon General Koop was trying to get at when he said, long ago, that in choosing a sexual partner one was becoming partners with his or her prior partners for several years preceding.

There are risks I have not talked so much about today, since I have tried to focus on numbers for the sake of the audience. But I would like to take one more opportunity to quote Justice Kirby's Stockholm talk, for he identified some qualitative societal dangers that motivate me even more strongly than the awful numerical exercises I have been doing for you. He pointed out the threat to international travel that looms with panicky governmental restrictions, and, indeed, the richness that ready commerce between countries and continents has brought to our lives is at considerable risk. There are fundamental human activities such as cultural and social exchange and qualities such as creativity that thrive on diversity—and they could be profoundly threatened by international fear and isolation.

Furthermore, he said, "One common feature [among nations] to be watched most carefully is the new danger to so-called 'marginalized people.' Governments, under pressure to be seen to be doing something to contain the epidemic, may impose ineffective laws on voiceless, powerless groups. Prisoners. Drug users. Migrant workers." As he spoke, the warning reminded me of Hubert Humphrey's admonition in his last speech in 1977 that "the moral test of government is how it treats those who are in the dawn of life, the children; those who are in the twilight of life, the aged; and those who are in the shadows of life, the sick, the needy and the handicapped." AIDS has brought to large numbers of our citizens a new kind of disadvantage and dread, and the humanity of our response will say more about us than any assertion of moral rectitude can ever do.

This brings up the question of human rights and public health. I dispensed with most of the aspects of that discussion with my cursory summary comments that casual contact does not pose a risk of transmitting HIV; the purported conflict between human rights and social good is spurious in this case, for human rights and public health march hand in hand on the AIDS issue, as Jonathan Mann constantly stresses. Turning back to Justice Kirby one last time, "Each is needed to reinforce the effectiveness of the other. No one has a human right to spread a deadly virus. But a society protecting itself from that virus will respect the person who carries the burden of the knowledge of HIV infection. Unless it does so, that society will destroy all effective chance of modifying that person's behaviour to help contain the spread of the virus. As Admiral Watkins revealed last week to the United States [please note, these are Justice Kirby's words, not mine] effective antidiscrimination protection is, paradoxically, the sine qua non of an effective HIV containment policy."

To that I say, "Amen."

3

AIDS: A Family Perspective

G. M. "Missy" LeClaire

In the beginning there was pure confusion. What could be wrong? Why is he so sick? What about the weight loss, the night sweats, the fatigue, the personality changes? How about the awful infection in his mouth? At least we have health insurance. Surely we are covered for any possible health crisis.

Then the diagnosis came—HTLV-III+. So what does that mean? Hodgkins disease? Leukemia? AIDS? AIDS!! What is AIDS? He isn't gay. He isn't an IV drug user. Sure he is a merchant marine and had traveled around the world. He had even been to Africa. And, yes, he had been in an automobile accident and had received blood transfusions to save his life. But AIDS? This doesn't happen to regular people. We've only been married for six months. What happens now?

These are only some of the thoughts and questions that go through the minds of family members of someone diagnosed with acquired immune deficiency syndrome. The turmoil is never ending.

My husband, Jim, was finally diagnosed with AIDS in late June of 1986. Earlier, in April, after months of illness, he required unrelated emergency surgery to repair urethral damage from the automobile accident he had. While hospitalized in a small community hospital, the care he received was inappropriate to say the least. Food trays were left outside the room, his bed was never changed by hospital staff, he was rarely (if ever) touched by hospital staff (with or without gloves), he was never washed by staff, and so on. All of this without a diagnosis.

After his release from this hospital, we ended up in the emergency room time after time for one problem after another. In the meantime,

Reprinted from *AIDS and Long-Term Care: A New Dimension* edited by Donna Lind Infeld and Richard Southby. Copyright 1989 by National Health Publishing. Used with permission of the publisher.

I had made arrangements to take him to a teaching hospital with an AIDS unit. We made the four-hour trip with him lying in the backseat of the car with a catheter full of blood. Upon arrival at the teaching hospital, I felt as if we had arrived in heaven. Here were people who understood and were not afraid of Jim or his illness.

The trauma we had been through took its toll. Jim had an extreme distrust of medical professionals. He couldn't understand why he had been treated so poorly at the first hospital. At the new hospital, he couldn't understand why he was constantly being asked if he had ever had a homosexual experience or used IV drugs. He just wanted to get well and go home.

Jim's denial process was so strong that he had to be told the diagnosis twice within two weeks; he then spent four days with the bed covers pulled up and over his head. He was 26 years old, newly wed, with great career possibilities—he had a great life ahead of him, or so he thought. He felt stigmatized by a disease so often associated with gay men and drug addicts. To think that he would never have a child of his own, captain his own merchant sailing vessel, or even purchase a home was devastating and demoralizing, to say the least. Add to that the fear that he may have infected his wife, along with all the fears and prejudices that go along with his elementary knowledge of AIDS, and, believe me, you have an emotionally and physically dysfunctional human being.

Jim never suffered the typical opportunistic infections. Upon release from his first AIDS-related hospitalization, we relocated to the Washington metropolitan area so that we could be closer to proper medical and community support. Jim did well, initially. He gained weight, added color, tackled the candida with diet and medications and was also able to monitor his depression through medications. This slight relief lasted from July until October of 1986.

The second week of October all hell broke loose. Jim turned from being a moody and sometimes agitated man into a volatile monster. He was sullen, angry, violent, frightened, and despondent all at one time; and then within a few minutes he was laughing and loving. He was akin to Dr. Jekyll and Mr. Hyde. He would refuse to take medications, drink alcohol, and write "goodbye" notes. It was like living deep within the twilight zone with a husband I no longer knew.

After constant calls to his physicians and psychiatrists, I finally arranged a visit for him at the outpatient clinic. When he was approached about entering the hospital for psychological and neurological tests, he went on a tangent and bolted from the hospital. He was found in the parking lot of this large inner-city hospital. He told the doctors that he was going to go live in the woods, where he knew he would be happy and could die peacefully.

A four-week stay in two different psychiatric institutions followed this altercation. The first psychiatric hospital accepted him with complete knowledge of his AIDS diagnosis. However, I soon realized that the staff and administration had little or no knowledge of AIDS or AIDS dementia complex. I was called on a daily basis to answer such questions as how I laundered his clothing or washed his dishes. Jim's primary psychiatrist also asked me what they should do if he became violent.

After a few days of this kind of communication, I started the search for a hospital that would accommodate him in a more humane and compassionate manner. I found another hospital that handled Jim and AIDS in a much more professional manner. But again, there was still very little up-to-date knowledge of the neurological ravages of AIDS. I was told by the doctor that Jimmy was depressed because he had AIDS, and his irrational behavior was caused by authority problems that stemmed from childhood disagreements with his mother. Furthermore, I was told that he needed two or three years of intense psychotherapy to overcome all of this. This recommendation was given to a man with a life expectancy of less than a year. Jim did make some strides in improving his outlook and seemed intent on having quality time with me. These changes were brought on by therapy, group support, and antidepressants.

After much discussion with the staff at the center, I decided to take Jim home. Treatment would continue on an outpatient basis with a Washington psychiatrist whose specialty is the various psychological and neurological disorders associated with AIDS. I couldn't foresee vast improvements, and insurance funds were being depleted. I also felt that he should be allowed to enjoy whatever time he had left at home. While in the hospital he gained 30 pounds and was very close to his normal weight.

He came home to a warm reception by me and my parents at Thanksgiving time. All was well. He seemed to be able to keep his "quality" resolutions and was well enough to make a trip north to upstate New York to visit his family. He was able to heal old wounds with his mother and was received with love by all. We even took a side trip to Montreal, a kind of second honeymoon. It was a marvelous trip. He tired easily, but was cheery and seemingly healthy.

Two weeks later, on Christmas day, Jim arose at home to open gifts with the family. He was so fatigued that he went to bed after breakfast and never made it to Christmas dinner. He was rarely out of bed after

Christmas; the only time he left the house was for visits to the psychiatrist's office. By the end of January, he was despondent and had no short-term memory at all. Whether this was due to medication or physical/neurological problems wasn't certain, but I knew he was failing. His doctor suggested a hospital stay, and this time he was more than willing to go.

The seven days in the hospital were a nightmare. He was a terrible patient. He was agitated and aggravated by everything and everyone. Nurses had a hard time being understanding of this seemingly healthy-looking young man who was so difficult to deal with. He would ask questions over and over. He would forget he had received medications and ask for them again. He would forget he had eaten and wonder if he was ever going to be fed. He had a new primary physician, and neither knew the other. This doctor was an excellent physician, well versed in the complex health issues of AIDS; however, his personality was a bit gruff and abrupt. Finally, the test results were in. I was told (in Jim's presence) to "line up a hospice service." When I asked why, the doctor coldly replied, "Because he's got less than six months."

Jim was diagnosed with dementia. How long had I suspected? Would an earlier dementia diagnosis have made a difference? Jim was also diagnosed with mao-cerbaic avium intracellulare (MAI), a tuberculean type of infection that enters the bone marrow and ravages the body. The only treatments available for MAI are experimental and painful.

As we left the hospital, Jim asked that he never have to return. "I'd like to die at home, if you can handle it," he said. I promised to keep him with me at home if I could manage, regardless of personal or monetary cost. As the weeks wore on, I regretted my decision many times.

This was extremely difficult work. At first, Jim was capable of getting up and around. He could walk to the bathroom, feed himself, and look after his own personal care. Jim also finally seemed at peace with himself and the world. He was a loving husband, a thankful man, happy to be with someone who loved and cared for him—what a delightful change!

Physically, he became progressively worse. In a matter of weeks, Jim became totally bedridden and required 24-hour care. He became more and more demented and wasn't able to eat. He lost nearly 100 pounds. Between the dementia and the narcotics he was given for pain control, Jimmy was "in another world" most of the time—fortunately. The MAI infection caused him to have extended fevers from 104 to 106 degrees. I thought people died immediately when their fever went that high. The fevers were preceded by chills that would actually raise his body off the bed and were followed by sweats that would soak through the bed sheets. This would happen between five and seven times a day—every day.

My main sources of help and support were my mother and dad; they kept food on the table, sheets washed, and my spirits up. I had contracted the services of a local hospice to care for Jim on an at-home basis. However, as it turned out, the hospice staff was more of a support system for me than for Jim. There was very little anyone could do for him beyond what I was doing already, except control his pain. I was taught to give him pain injections every two hours around the clock. Prior training had taught me how to change our bed with him in it, how to protect against bedsores, how to rub him down with alcohol to reduce fevers, and how to give him a bed bath. Where I found the strength and know-how to fight all the other battles and crises came from love of my man, faith in God, and faith in myself.

On April 19, 1987, Jimmy slipped into unconsciousness. He died at home in my arms on April 22. I was glad it was over—for both of us.

4

A Christmas Story: The Eighties

Van R. Nelson

This story really began Christmas of 1986. A 37-year-old Black man named Ernest took ill and was admitted to the hospital under internal medicine service and spent Christmas confined to his hospital bed. For nearly two months, this young man remained at a very low ebb physically. Being the social person he is known to be, his friends of course were there for him and continued to support him emotionally through this rough time.

For approximately three months (March-May) no one knew actually how sick he really was. His replies to inquiries into his health were consistently vague. Often he would say, "Well I'm getting along," then change the subject to something else. Family and friends alike were kept distanced from any concise information by one simple statement—"I've been a little ill."

During this same period he tried to resume his professional career full steam, maintain his alternate post as director of music and organist/director for various churches, and keep some semblance of a limited social life. However, he had secrets, secrets he knew were somehow justified.

I have discovered that degeneration takes many forms. Slowly Ernest would begin to degenerate, but this manifested itself first in the areas of his life that were most important to him—his professional, religious, and social lives. First, due to his declining health he had to resign his job. He then found that he could no longer fulfill his rigid rehearsal and church schedule. During one of his bouts of illness his mom came to his aid. This was the start of the worst kind of degeneration—isolation. Being his next of kin, she discovered that he was not only sick but that Ernest had AIDS. From that point on, Ernest's life became a tragedy of ignorance and error.

His mom began to do all of the things that she felt were right for him. We who love Ernest have watched his life take a downward spiral, changing gradually into different but declining stages; it has

44

now evolved into a stark nightmare not only for him but for us all. As mothers have a tendency to do, his mom thought that with plenty of TLC, rest, and a proper, balanced diet Ernest could witness a change in his condition. She was bizarre. She first weaned him off health foods and herbal teas, which he had been on for years, and off his vegetarian diet, because neither was "doing him any good." She consistently restricted his friends from visiting or calling because "he needs his rest." She also was known to verbalize her personal feelings—"I'm so embarrassed."

His mom has also refused anything that may tend to educate her about the disease. She doesn't utter even the word (AIDS), as if it in itself were a curse. She walks away from any conversation about AIDS issues, and turns to other channels whenever there is television coverage.

Well, here it is Christmas again. Ernest is back in the hospital. For the second consecutive hospital confinement in recent months, his mom has restricted phone service to him under the pretext that "he needs rest." This time visitors are also restricted. Why? Because she doesn't want anyone to see him and it is her way of protecting him from those who wish only to see. She refuses permission for the pastoral staff of his church to give him communion and is steadfast against visiting nurses or caregivers to administer to his medical needs when he's at home. Why? Because this would mean others would discover Ernest has AIDS. She declines information or assistance from wellwishers, friends, and family members. She refuses all services from local social service agencies and she screens all calls. Outside of intimate family members, no one can visit him at the hospital. She has taken on the total responsibility for his care and well-being. Last week she told me that she will continue without help, as difficult as it may be for her, being in the sunset years of her life, and is assured that God will bless her for her endeavors.

She stated to a mutual friend a day or so ago that her son was incapacitated due to "a gay plague." Also, that his friends were around only to take advantage of his kindness and generosity—and she is around now "to put a stop to all of that."

This crisis of love, health, and community is a world crisis, not a "gay plague."

Additionally, in May she was quite angry with her son for sharing the real facts of his condition with me. One of her many responses to him concerning that issue was, "How could you tell Van? You know we have to keep this thing quiet."

So, in a modern big city, Ernest is now in a state of denial, isolation, and uncertain care—dying. As bad as all this is, I will not judge their reasons. But where is the true spirit of compassion?

I have learned and shared an inordinate amount of information on this health crisis with everyone I come in contact with, including Ernest and his mother. I have personally experienced and have knowledge of many unkindnesses in regard to the AIDS/ARC afflicted, and these experiences helped me decide to form the Association for People Living with AIDS (APLWA), so that people can know that there is life after diagnosis, that having the AIDS virus is of itself not the end. Promoting positiveness and fostering self-help and self-determination in the minority communities (the people who are the last to be informed, the last to get help) have been my goals for some time.

This situation is especially hard for me because I, through APLWA, have earnestly and diligently worked to eradicate this type of ignorance and isolation within the Black community. Now I realize that I was preparing myself to face the unkindness, isolation, and stigmatization my family bestowed on my brother Ernest.

AIDS is a health crisis, not a moral issue. For some months APLWA has tried to persuade people of color to understand the crisis within our community and to open their hearts and minds to love and knowledge with support for their brethren. It pains me to know that with all my knowledge, I am helpless to give Ernest some warmth and happiness this Christmas.

Today, December 23, 1987, as I concluded this article, Ernest died. My plea for the future is that no one ever again should die embarrassed, alone, and afraid that his life has been judged by others to be wrong. Merry Christmas, 1987.

5

The Worldwide Epidemiology and Prevention of AIDS

Stephen B. Hulley
Norman Hearst

Since the first description of AIDS in 1981, the disease has emerged as an epidemic that will have an unprecedented effect on the world. The impact is partly due to the number of people involved. With cases reported from nearly every country, the World Health Organization (WHO) estimates 250,000 AIDS cases worldwide in this decade, and 5–10 million people infected with the human immunodeficiency virus, which causes the disease (Mann & Chin, 1988). The impact of the epidemic goes beyond these numbers, however. Other health problems, such as malnutrition, malaria, and cigarette smoking, kill more people but have less effect. What is it about AIDS that makes it such a serious threat?

The element of surprise and fear of the unknown are part of the problem. A new infection spreads deeply into our populations years before the disease it causes is even recognized, and creates an epidemic with future directions that are a matter of guesswork and analogy (Brandt, 1988; Cutler & Arnold, 1988; Yankauer, 1988). The most important factor, however, is the diabolical combination of nasty features of this virus. AIDS is incurable and uniformly fatal, striking in the prime years of life with a lingering illness after a lengthy silent incubation period during which it is insidiously contagious. As a result of these features, AIDS will influence not only the health of the public, but also the political, economic, and social circumstances of every country of the world (Piot et al., 1988). And it will do so in ways that we cannot predict.

While we await development of a vaccine or of satisfactory antiviral drugs, our only advantage in addressing the epidemic is that AIDS is a preventable disease. HIV is in fact not very contagious, and it is spread by behaviors that are modifiable. This report will set the stage for discussions of behavioral interventions to prevent HIV infection by presenting our current understanding of its epidemiology. We will begin by reviewing the distributions of AIDS in various populations. We will then consider the epidemiology of the underlying HIV infection and review evidence on the risk behaviors for transmission and on prognosis. We will conclude by formulating practical implications for health professionals in their efforts to prevent the spread of HIV infection among their patients, and by suggesting a worldwide research agenda for epidemiologists and behavioral scientists.

Definition of AIDS

In the United States, AIDS is reported to the local health department and eventually to the Centers for Disease Control when a patient has a reliably diagnosed disease that signals an underlying deficiency in the immune system not due to immunosuppressive drugs or other immunosuppressive illnesses like cancer. Pneumocystis carinii pneumonia, virtually unheard of before 1980, is the most common presenting disease. The CDC definition for AIDS, which does not require knowing the results of an HIV antibody test, was formally established in 1982 and subsequently expanded to include additional opportunistic infections and cancers of lymph tissue in people who test positive for HIV antibodies (CDC, 1987a). In many countries, AIDS is classified by the WHO criteria for AIDS, which are similar to those of the CDC but have less stringent requirements for laboratory diagnosis of opportunistic infections (Colebunders et al., 1987).

How AIDS Is Distributed in the Population

The standard approaches to describing the epidemiology of a disease are to consider first its temporal distributions, then its geographic distributions, and finally how it is distributed among various kinds of people (i.e., in groups classified by age, race, sex, and other personal characteristics). We will do this first for AIDS itself, and then for the invisible antecedent infection with HIV.

Temporal Distribution

The AIDS epidemic has grown at a steadily increasing rate in its first six years, and the total number of reported cases in the United States by mid-1988 had reached 70,000 (CDC, 1988). Figure 5.1 shows the epidemic curve, in cases per quarter, with projections

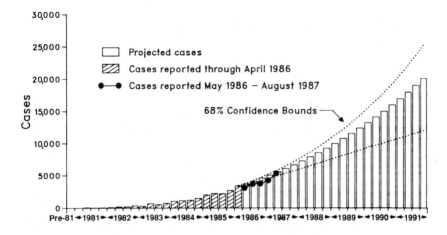

Figure 5.1 Quarterly Number of AIDS Cases in the United States Reported to CDC Through 1987 and Projected by CDC Through 1991
SOURCE: Curran et al. (1988). Reprinted by permission.

through 1991. The epidemic curve for worldwide AIDS appears to have a pattern similar to that in the United States, with a slope that also grows steeper each year (Piot et al., 1988). Although the disease was first recognized in 1981, rare individual cases from the previous decade have now been diagnosed retrospectively in several parts of the world (Piot et al., 1988).

Almost all of the early AIDS cases have died, the median survival after diagnosis of AIDS being about one year (a little longer for those presenting with Kaposi's sarcoma) (Bacchetti, Osmond, & Chaisson, 1988). This reflects experience before there was any effective treatment for AIDS, and the advent of AZT and other drugs may alter these statistics favorably.

Geographic Distribution

AIDS has been reported in 138 of the 162 countries in the world (Mann & Chin, 1988). Three-quarters of these countries report fewer than 100 cases, indicating that in many regions the epidemic is just beginning (Mann, 1987). The countries reporting the largest numbers are listed in Table 5.1, which presents counts through January 1988 (and which are thus slightly lower than other counts in this report). The pattern and mode of spread of the epidemic, as we shall discuss, differ considerably from one country to another.

TABLE 5.1

Distribution of Reported Cases of
AIDS in the World, by Country

	N	%
Americas	55,354	75
United States	48,139	
Brazil	2,325	
Canada	1,423	
Haiti	912	
Mexico	713	
All others	1,842	
Europe	8,839	12
France	2,523	
F.R. Germany	1,588	
United Kingdom	1,170	
Italy	1,104	
Spain	624	
All others	1,830	
Africa	8,620	12
Uganda	2,369	
Tanzania	1,608	
Kenya	964	
Rwanda	705	
Burundi	569	
All others	2,413	
Western Pacific	824	1
East Mediterranean	78	<<1
Southeast Asia	24	<<1
Total	73,747	100

SOURCE: Reported to WHO through January
1988 (WHO, 1988).

By far the largest number of the world's reported cases—65%—
come from the United States (Table 5.1). However, the actual percentage of cases in the United States is not nearly this high. Differences in
reporting procedures indicate that the numbers for many of the countries in Table 5.1 are a serious underestimate of the true incidence,
and WHO estimates that the true number of cases of AIDS worldwide
by mid-1988 was 250,000—two and a half times the reported 100,000
(Mann & Chin, 1988). Underreporting is a much smaller problem in
the United States (Curran et al., 1988), where the number of unre-
ported cases probably does not exceed 20% of the total.

TABLE 5.2

Distribution of AIDS Cases in the United States by Standard Metropolitan
Statistical Area of Residence

| | AIDS Cases | | Adult Population | Rate |
	N	%	(millions)	per 1,000
New York, NY	15,654	22	9.1	1.7
San Francisco, CA	5,965	8	3.2	1.9
Los Angeles, CA	5,355	8	7.5	.7
Houston, TX	2,238	3	2.9	.8
Newark, NJ	2,112	3	2.0	1.1
Washington, DC	2,094	3	3.0	.7
Chicago, IL	1,829	3	7.1	.3
Miami, FL	1,784	3	1.6	1.1
All others	33,671	48	132.2	.2
Total	70,702	100	168.6	.4

SOURCE: Reported to CDC through August 15, 1988 (CDC, 1988).

Within the United States, the AIDS epidemic is most serious in a
half dozen urban epicenters, and more than half of the AIDS cases
have occurred in eight major cities (Table 5.2). About a quarter of the
AIDS cases have been reported from New York and Newark, and the
next largest epicenters are San Francisco and Los Angeles. The prevalence of AIDS cases in New York and San Francisco in this six-year
period is about 1.8 per 1,000 adults in the population, and in several
of the other major epicenters it is about 1.0 per 1,000. These figures
represent greater metropolitan areas including suburbs, and the
prevalence in the inner cities is considerably higher. However, the
epidemic is not limited to these cities. Indications of the degree to
which the epidemic has spread are the facts that AIDS has been reported from every one of the 50 states, and that three-quarters of the
states have reported more than 100 cases (CDC, 1988).

Distribution by Age

One of the most poignant and tragic aspects of this epidemic is
that AIDS has predominantly afflicted patients in the early decades
of adulthood. The great predominance of cases around the world
have occurred between the ages of 20 and 50 (Figure 5.2). The highest rates of AIDS are generally seen in the 30–39 year age decade,
reflecting HIV infection acquired in the 20s and 30s. In the United
States nearly half of the AIDS cases occur in 30–39-year-olds, one-

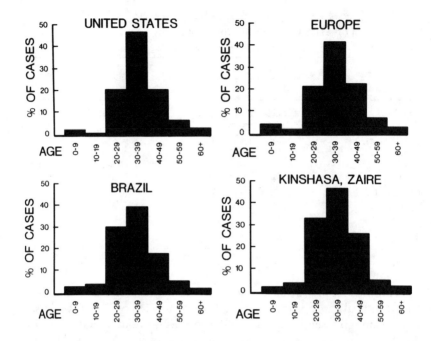

Figure 5.2 Age Distribution of AIDS Cases in Four Regions of the World
SOURCE: Liskin (1986). Reprinted by permission.

fifth occur in 20–29-year-olds, one-fifth in 40–49-year-olds, one-tenth in those 50 and over, and one-fiftieth in those under 20 (CDC, 1988).

Because the disease usually affects people in the prime years of life, AIDS has become the leading cause of premature mortality in New York and San Francisco and a prominent cause of premature mortality in the rest of the United States. The very low rate of AIDS in preteens in all countries (including Africa) is one of the strongest pieces of evidence demonstrating that AIDS infection is not spread by mosquitoes or other insects.

Distribution by Sex

In the United States, Europe, and other countries where the disease has spread chiefly in the gay men and intravenous drug user (IVDU) populations, AIDS has afflicted far more men than women (the male:female ratio is more than 10:1 in the United States; see Table 5.3). In Haiti and some of the countries in central Africa, where the

TABLE 5.3
Distribution of AIDS in the United States, by Race and Sex

Race	% of AIDS Cases			U.S. Population	
	Men	Women	Children < 15 Years	≥15 Years	<15 Years
White	62	28	19	81	73
Black	23	51	58	11	15
Latin	14	21	22	6	9
Other	<1	<1	<1	2	3
Total	100	100	100	100	100

SOURCE: CDC (1986).

disease has spread chiefly through heterosexual intercourse (Piot et al., 1988; Study Group of AIDS in Haitian-Americans, 1987), the rate of AIDS is roughly equal in the two sexes.

Distribution by Race

In the United States the prevalence of AIDS is two and a half times higher in Black and Latin populations than among Caucasians. On the other hand, the prevalence of AIDS among Asians is substantially lower than that in Caucasians. The disproportionate involvement of the Black and Latin populations is due partly to the large numbers of cases reported in IVDUs, which reflects high rates of infection in minority IVDUs. However, it is a little-known fact that half the Black and Latin AIDS cases occur in homosexual men who are members of these ethnic groups (CDC, 1986).

The disproportionate involvement of the Black and Latin minority groups in the epidemic is strikingly accentuated in women and infants. Two-thirds of all AIDS cases in women have occurred in Blacks and Latins, and four-fifths of all AIDS cases in infants have been in Blacks and Latins (Table 5.3). These striking epidemiological facts, and their social and medical implications, are important factors to consider in developing the research and public health agenda (Mays & Cochran, 1987).

Distribution by Risk Groups

Epidemiologic studies have revealed the transmission patterns of infection with HIV, and have led to the identification of certain high-risk groups: homosexual men, intravenous drug users, blood product recipients, heterosexual partners of infected individuals, and newborn infants of infected women. The proportion of AIDS cases occur-

TABLE 5.4

Distribution of AIDS in the United States by Risk Group (in percentages)

	% of AIDS Cases			
Risk Group	Men (N = 63,873)	Women (N = 5,704)	Children < 13 Years (N = 1,125)	Total (N = 70,702)
Homosexual contact with HIV	68	—	—	62
IV drug users	16	52	—	19
Homosexual and IV drug users	8	—	—	7
Transfusion recipient	2	11	13	3
Heterosexual contact with HIV	2	29	—	4
Mother with HIV	—	—	78	1
Hemophiliac	1	—	6	1
Undetermined[a]	4	8	3	3
Total	100	100	100	100

SOURCE: CDC (1988).
a. Some of the undetermined cases appear to be heterosexually acquired (Castro, 1988).

ring in each of these groups is different in men and women, and in different countries.

In the United States men show the overall pattern set out in Table 5.4—more than two-thirds of the AIDS cases are in homosexual or bisexual men, and most of the rest are in IVDUs (16%) or in men who are both homosexual and IVDUs (8%). However, there is considerable heterogeneity in the pattern among states. For example, IVDUs account for nearly half the AIDS cases in New Jersey, but only 3% of the AIDS cases in California (Allen & Curran, 1988).

In the United States, only 2% of men with AIDS have acquired the disease through heterosexual contact with an HIV-infected woman. Women show a very different pattern (Guinan & Hardy, 1987). Half of the female AIDS cases are in IVDUs, and nearly a third are attributed to heterosexual contact with an HIV-infected man. Thus a corollary of the tenfold greater number of AIDS cases in men than women is the fact that women are at higher risk of heterosexually acquired AIDS than men. This fact, which has important implications for prevention strategies (Wofsy, 1987), is not clear from the CDC counts, which in mid-1988 showed 1,661 cases of heterosexually acquired AIDS in women and 1,259 in men (CDC, 1988). However, these figures include AIDS in persons from countries such as Haiti, where heterosexual transmission has predominated to yield roughly equal numbers of men and women with AIDS; the risk of acquiring AIDS heterosexually is 3.5 times higher in women than in men (1,407 versus 405) if only native-born individuals who can identify a heterosexual partner who was the likely source of their infection are included (CDC, 1988).

Children with AIDS in the United States are numerically a very small part of the epidemic (just over 1%). They represent a very poignant aspect of the public health problem, particularly as most cases occur in disadvantaged minority populations. Many such children become orphans, moreover, because their fathers are unknown and their mothers have died of AIDS.

The distribution of AIDS cases among different risk groups varies among countries, depending on the local prevalence of these risk behaviors and on the presence of cofactors for transmission. The most striking difference is in Haiti and several central African countries, where homosexual intercourse among men and IV drug use appear to be rare or absent but the epidemic has spread widely through heterosexual transmission. One explanation for the rapid heterosexual spread in these countries is the high prevalence of other venereal diseases, such as chancroid and chlamydia, that cause chronic genital lesions and may provide a portal of entry for HIV (Piot et al., 1988). The degree to which cultural patterns such as multiple sexual partners also play a role remains to be determined.

How HIV Is Distributed in the Population

The identification of HIV as the cause of AIDS has created an interest in the distribution and determinants of the underlying infection itself. HIV infection is accompanied by the development of antibodies that are used to detect the presence of HIV infection. The standard approach is to begin with a screening test, typically an ELISA, and to confirm results that are repeatedly positive by ELISA with a more specific test such as the Western Blot. This approach has remarkable sensitivity and specificity, and the frequency of false positive and false negative tests is very low (Eisenstaedt & Getzen, 1988).

The prevalence of antibodies to HIV infection in various population groups of the United States or in the countries of the world is not known with certainty, since we do not have seroepidemiologic studies of entire populations to provide estimates of the sort that are available for AIDS itself. There are, however, many studies of samples of various populations from which we can draw inferences about the whole.

CDC (1987b) has summarized 140 studies in the United States that have examined this question in homosexual men and in IV drug users. Many of these studies are small and/or unpublished, and only one (the Men's Health Study; Winkelstein et al., 1987) is a probability sample of the population of interest. However, the findings are reasonably consistent despite different sources of bias. The prevalence of HIV infection among homosexual men is usually in the range of 20–55%. (The population-based Men's Health Study found 48.5% in San Francisco.) The prevalence among IVDUs is somewhat lower, usually in the range of 0–20%. Higher estimates have been observed among IVDUs in some northeastern cities, however, particularly New York and Newark, where the seroprevalence has reached 50–60% (CDC, 1987b).

Several studies have addressed the issue of the prevalence of HIV infection in the United States as a whole. One of the largest and most important is the study of seroprevalence in military recruits (Burke et al., 1987). The overall seroprevalence of more than a million recruits seen between October 1985 and September 1987, adjusted to reflect the age, sex, and race distribution of U.S. adults aged 17–59, was 0.14% (CDC, 1987b). Preliminary data indicate that the majority of those found seropositive belong to the known high-risk groups that have been described (in Table 5.4). The prevalence of HIV seropositivity in the United States among people who do not know themselves to be in a high-risk group, based on this study and on blood donors and other sources, is estimated to be 0.01–0.02%—that is, 1 or 2 in 10,000 (CDC, 1987b; Hearst & Hulley, 1988).

The geographic distribution of HIV infection in military recruits is illustrated in Figure 5.3. Those states reporting the highest rates of AIDS cases (shown in the bottom panel) are the same states that have the highest rates of HIV infection in their military recruits (top panel). A similar pattern emerges from a geographic analysis of blood donors (CDC, 1987b). These military recruit rates are strongly biased by the selection factors that pertain to volunteering for the Army—lower socioeconomic groups are overrepresented, and admitted homosexual men and IVDUs are excluded. However, the recruit statistics produce estimates on the same order of magnitude as those resulting from less biased sampling approaches. For example, the HIV seroprevalence for Massachusetts recruits (mostly men) was .13 per 1,000, whereas the

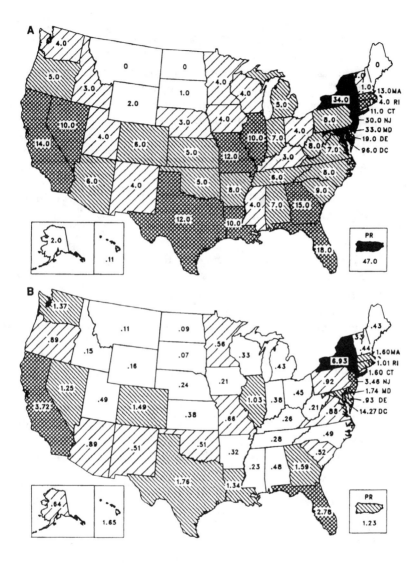

Figure 5.3 HIV Seroprevalence in U.S. Military Recruits, November 1985–September 1987, by State (upper panel); Cumulative Incidence of AIDS Through November 1987, by State (lower panel)
SOURCE: Centers for Disease Control (1986b).

HIV seroprevalence of all Massachusetts women giving birth in the first half of 1987 was .21 per 1,000 (Hoff et al., 1988).

These and other studies have examined the race and sex distributions of HIV infection. As would be anticipated, given the distributions of AIDS noted earlier, HIV infection is much more prevalent in Blacks than in Whites (Curran et al., 1988; Mays & Cochran, 1987). What is unexpected, and an ominous harbinger of the direction in which the AIDS epidemic may be heading, is the fact that Blacks have a higher prevalence than Whites even within risk group (i.e., within gay populations and within IVDUs; see CDC, 1987a, 1987b; Chaisson, Moss, & Onishi, 1987). As expected, HIV seroprevalence is higher in men than in women; the magnitude of the disproportion—about 5:1 in both military recruits and blood donors, after adjusting for age and race—is difficult to interpret, given possible sex differences in the selection biases that influence who chooses to volunteer for military service and for giving blood.

Public Health Implications of the HIV Rates

The CDC (1987b) has recently reaffirmed its estimate that the number of seropositive adults in the United States is 1–1.5 million. This figure is extrapolated from estimates of the size and seroprevalence of each of the high-risk groups—gay or bisexual men, IVDUs, hemophiliacs, and heterosexuals—as shown in Table 5.5. The estimate yields an overall prevalence among the 169 million adults in the United States on the order of 0.6–0.9%.

These estimates are summarized, with others developed earlier in this report, in the global iceberg metaphor in Figure 5.4. The number of cases of AIDS thus far is 250,000 worldwide, 70,000 in the United States. The number infected is 5–10 million worldwide, 1–1.5 million in the United States. Many of these infected individuals, perhaps 2–3 times the number with AIDS itself, already have some symptoms and signs of HIV illness (AIDS-related complex, or ARC). Most, however, are still asymptomatic, and most of these do not know they are infected or that they may be spreading the disease to their loved ones.

One important question is, What is the outlook for these HIV-infected individuals who do not yet have AIDS, the great invisible part of the iceberg? Unfortunately, recent evidence reveals the prognosis to be unfavorable. Studies of long-term cohorts of seropositive patients have discovered that most people with antibody—evidence that they have at one time been infected with HIV—are still infected and will eventually develop ARC and AIDS (Curran et al., 1988; Moss et al., 1988). Data from several studies suggest a median time from infec-

TABLE 5.5

New CDC Estimate of Number Infected with HIV in the United States, 1987

Population	Estimated Size	Approximate Seroprevalence (%)	Number Infected
Homosexual			
exclusively	2,500,000	20–25	500,000–625,000
occasional	2,500,000–7,500,000	5	125,000–375,000
IV drug use			
regular	900,000	25	225,000
occasional	200,000	5	10,000
Hemophilia A	12,400	70	8,700
Hemophilia B	3,100	35	1,100
Heterosexuals (no known risk)	142,000,000	.021	30,000
Subtotal			900,000–1,270,000
Heterosexual contacts of above (5–10% of total infections)			45,000–127,000
Total			945,000–1,400,000

SOURCE: CDC (1987b).

tion to the development of symptoms or signs of HIV illness of about five years, and a median time to the development of AIDS that is about eight years in adults (Figure 5.5) and two years in babies (Curran et al., 1988).

It is possible that experimental approaches to treating seropositive patients, for example with AZT, will alter these grim statistics favorably. In the meantime, a major task for all health care providers must be primary prevention: counseling seropositive patients on behaviors that will prevent the spread of the infection to uninfected individuals, and counseling seronegative patients (the great majority) on steps to minimize the risk of becoming infected.

Behavioral Risk Factors for the Spread of HIV Infection

The risk groups that have been identified by epidemiologic studies indicate that AIDS is spread through certain body fluids, notably blood, semen, and vaginal secretions. Studies of homosexual men have identified receptive anal intercourse and other sexual activities

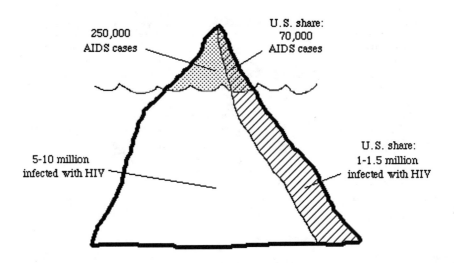

250,000
AIDS cases

U.S. share:
70,000
AIDS cases

5-10 million
infected with HIV

U.S. share:
1-1.5 million
infected with HIV

Figure 5.4 HIV Disease in the World, Summer 1988
NOTE: This iceberg illustrates that the estimated number of people infected with HIV, most of whom do not know it or have any symptoms, is more than 15 times larger than the number who have AIDS.

that promote contact between semen and traumatized anal tissue (thereby creating a portal of entry for HIV) as high-risk behaviors (Polk et al., 1987; Winkelstein et al., 1987). These studies also show the number of sex partners to be strongly associated with the prevalence of HIV infection. An important consideration here is the high normative number of sex partners in homosexual populations, with 24% of the men reporting more than 50 partners in the past two years in the Men's Health Study, and an additional 39% reporting 10–49 partners (Winkelstein et al., 1987). It is unlikely that the high prevalence of HIV infection in this group—estimated at 48.5%—would otherwise have developed, given the low infectivity of this virus (see below).

Epidemiologic studies have established the fact that HIV can be spread by vaginal as well as anal intercourse, and there are a number of factors that influence this spread (Hearst & Hulley, 1988). The infectivity of HIV during vaginal intercourse—the likelihood of infection per episode of unprotected intercourse—can be remarkably low, on the order of 1 in 500. This risk, which probably varies from one

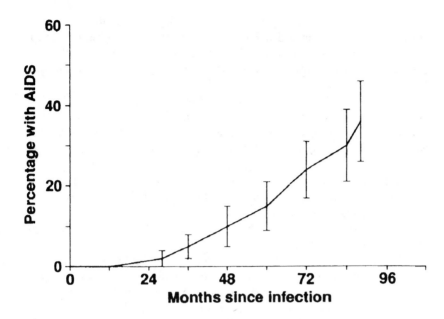

Figure 5.5 Survival Curve Showing Proportion of Men Developing AIDS by Estimated Duration of Infection in the San Francisco City Clinic Cohort
SOURCE: Curran et al. (1988). Reprinted by permission.

individual to another (Peterman, Stoneburner, Allen, Jaffe, & Curran, 1988), is estimated from discordant partner studies in the United States; a woman who is the regular sexual partner of an infected man and has frequent unprotected vaginal intercourse, sometimes for years, has a cumulative likelihood of becoming infected that is surprisingly low—only about 20% (Padian, Marquis, & Francisc, 1987; Peterman et al., 1988). Infectivity appears to be much higher in Africa (Piot et al., 1988), where, for reasons discussed below, the likelihood that both partners in a long-term couple will be infected may be as high as 60%.

Infectivity is probably higher for anal intercourse, and higher in the late stages when AIDS has developed (and perhaps briefly during the acute illness shortly after infection). In Africa, infectivity may be higher among those who are uncircumcised (perhaps because of the propensity for mucosal lesions under the foreskin); it is clearly higher in the presence of genital ulcers and other lesions, which are quite prevalent in Africa (Piot et al., 1988). Inguinal lesions may also help explain the high rate of HIV seropositivity in patients seen in sexually transmitted disease clinics in the United States—5% in one recent study, many of whom did not identify themselves as being in a high-risk group (Quinn et al., 1988). It appears that the likelihood of infection during intercourse is greater when a seropositive person inserts his penis into a seronegative person than vice versa.

The likelihood of becoming infected is reduced by the use of latex condoms. (Natural condoms made of animal tissues are not suitable, because they can leak virus particles through minute openings.) The protection conveyed by condoms can probably be increased by also using spermicidal cream, since the active ingredient (nonoxynol-9) kills HIV. However, it is important to recognize that family planning data and preliminary studies of AIDS infection in HIV-discordant couples suggest that condoms and spermicide are not fully safe, and may have a cumulative failure rate as high as 10% per year of usage (Hearst & Hulley, 1988).

The risk of acquiring HIV infection in the United States through heterosexual intercourse is estimated for various risk groups in a previous report that is summarized in Table 5.6. Because of the low infectivity of HIV, the risk per encounter with an individual who is not in a high-risk group is extremely low—about 1 in 5 million even without condoms. Choosing a high-risk partner increases this risk by almost four orders of magnitude, and using a condom reduces that risk by only one order of magnitude. Thus the most important determinant of the probability that an individual will become infected is not whether or not the individual uses a condom; it is the risk status of his or her sexual partner (Hearst & Hulley, 1988).

As to the spread of HIV infection through contact with an infected person's blood, the probability of infection after transfusion with blood from an infected person is extremely high, on the order of 90% (Curran et al., 1988). The process of needle sharing among IVDUs also carries a substantial probability of infection, because addicts draw blood back into the syringe to make sure they are in a vein before injecting the drug, and enough blood often remains in the syringe to infect the next user. Accidental exposure of health care workers to infected blood by needle stick or exposure of chapped or abraded skin, on the other hand, fortunately carries a much smaller inoculum and surprisingly low risk of infection—less than 1 in 100 (Gerberding et al., 1987).

Perinatal HIV spread from mother to child may occur while the baby is still in the uterus, during the delivery, or during breast-feeding. The relative frequency of each of these avenues is not known. (Transmission in utero and by breast-feeding are both firmly

TABLE 5.6

Risk of HIV Infection for Heterosexual Intercourse in the United States

Risk Category of Partner	Assumptions			Estimated Risk of Infection	
	Prevalence of HIV Infection	Infectivity[a]	Condom/Spermicide Failure Rate	1 Sexual Encounter[b]	500 Sexual Encounters[c]
HIV serostatus unknown					
not in any high-risk group					
using condoms	0.0001	0.002	0.1	1 in 50 000 000	1 in 110 000
not using condoms	0.0001	0.002	...	1 in 5 000 000	1 in 16 000
high-risk groups[d]					
using condoms	0.05 to 0.5	0.002	0.1	1 in 100 000 to 1 in 10 000	1 in 210 to 1 in 21
not using condoms	0.05 to 0.5	0.002	...	1 in 10 000 to 1 in 1000	1 in 32 to 1 in 3
HIV seronegative					
no history of high-risk behavior[e]					
using condoms	0.000001	0.002	0.1	1 in 5 000 000 000	1 in 11 000 000
not using condoms	0.000001	0.002	...	1 in 500 000 000	1 in 1 600 000
continuing high-risk behavior[e]					
using condoms	0.01	0.002	0.1	1 in 500 000	1 in 1100
not using condoms	0.01	0.002	...	1 in 50 000	1 in 160
HIV seropositive					
using condoms	1.0	0.002	0.1	1 in 5000	1 in 11
not using condoms	1.0	0.002	...	1 in 500	2 in 3

SOURCE: Hearst (1987). Reprinted by permission.

a. The value 0.002 represents an upper limit on the probability that an infected male will transmit HIV to an uninfected female during one episode of penile-vaginal intercourse with ejaculation. Female-to-male infectivity may be lower, and infectivity for anal intercourse or intercourse when genital ulcers are present may be higher. The value is a group mean and may vary among individuals.

b. The risk of infection for one encounter is the product of the values in columns 2 through 4 of the table (assumptions).

c. The risk of infection for 500 encounters is column $2 \times [1 - (1 - \text{column } 3 \times \text{column } 4)^{500}]$.

d. High-risk groups with prevalences of HIV infection at the higher end of the range given include homosexual or bisexual men and intravenous drug users from major metropolitan areas, and hemophiliacs. Groups with prevalences at the lower end of the range include homosexual and bisexual men or intravenous drug users from other parts of the country, female prostitutes, heterosexuals from countries where heterosexual spread of HIV is common (including Haiti and central Africa), and recipients of multiple blood transfusions between 1983 and 1985 from areas with a high prevalence of HIV infection.

e. High-risk behavior consists of sexual intercourse or needle sharing with a member of one of the high-risk groups.

established avenues, but their frequency is difficult to research because HIV infection cannot be diagnosed reliably until an infant is more than a year old—all babies of infected mothers carry maternal antibodies to HIV for many months, whether or not they are infected; see Curran et al., 1988; Piot et al., 1988.) The overall probability that a mother infected with HIV will spread the infection to a newborn infant is about 50% (Curran et al., 1988; Piot et al., 1988).

Epidemiologic studies have also provided important information on the ways in which HIV infection is not spread. Setting aside spread through the vagina, urethra, anus, and other mucous membranes, it is a fortunate fact that this virus requires a needle puncture, ulcer, or wound of some sort in order to pass through the skin. It does not enter the body across skin that is intact, and thus is not transmitted by touching, hand shaking, sharing eating utensils, sneezing, or living in the same household (Curran et al., 1988; Friedland & Klein, 1987). Although the virus is present in saliva, its concentration is low, and the epidemiologic evidence does not show that it can be transmitted by kissing with exchange of saliva, or even by biting.

Preventing the Spread of HIV

It is essential that all health professionals understand the epidemiology of AIDS, because HIV infection will be increasingly common in the patients they see, and because the epidemiologic facts provide a rational basis for strategies to prevent the further spread of the epidemic. Intervention on high-risk behaviors is the only prevention strategy at present, and it is potentially a very effective one if people adopt the low-risk behaviors set out in Table 5.7.

The strategies for preventing the sexual spread of HIV are described in more detail in other chapters in this volume and elsewhere (e.g., Francis & Chin, 1987; Hearst & Hulley, 1988; U.S. Surgeon General, 1988). In countries like the United States, where AIDS is still relatively uncommon, the most important advice for the 99% of the population who are not infected is to choose a partner who is at low risk of carrying the HIV antibody. This would mean getting to know each prospective partner very well before having sex with that person, and it seems likely that the modal heterosexual culture will evolve over the next decade toward more prolonged courtships and toward monogamy. If this advice is ignored, the likelihood of getting the HIV infection from vaginal intercourse with a person whose risk status is

TABLE 5.7

Behaviors That Will Reduce the Risk of Becoming Infected with HIV

(1) To prevent the sexual spread of HIV (decreasing priority order):
  (a) Avoid sexual intercourse, even with condoms, if partner is HIV positive.
  (b) Choose a partner who has no high-risk behaviors, past or present.
  (c) Test for HIV antibodies when there is doubt about HIV status.
  (d) Employ measures that reduce risk when there is doubt:
  • use condoms and spermicidal cream,
  • avoid anal intercourse,
  • avoid sexual intercourse if genital lesions are present.

(2) To prevent HIV spread by IV drug abusers (decreasing priority order):
  (a) Stop use of IV drugs.
  (b) Stop sharing needles.
  (c) Use bleach to sterilize needles.

(3) To prevent HIV spread by medical use of blood products:
  (a) Encourage high-risk donors to defer themselves.
  (b) Screen donated blood for HIV antibodies.
  (c) Sterilize clotting factors.
  (d) Avoid unnecessary transfusions.

(4) To prevent perinatal spread of HIV:
  (a) Test prospective mothers for HIV antibody and, if positive, advise against pregnancy or to consider abortion.
  (b) HIV positive mothers should avoid breast-feeding if feasible (see text).

(5) To prevent accidental infection of health care providers:
  (a) Treat every patient as an infected person, that is, use latex gloves and be careful when exposure to blood or other body fluids is a possibility.

partly unknown can be reduced (but not eliminated) by using condoms and spermicides.

Having sex with someone who is a prostitute or an IV drug user is generally not advisable, since these individuals are not likely to stop their high-risk behaviors permanently. Having sex with someone who belongs to any of the other risk groups in Table 5.4—a homosexual or bisexual man, a hemophiliac or transfusion recipient, a person with a history of sexually transmitted disease or many casual partners—is a choice that should be individualized once an HIV antibody test 3–6 months after stopping these high-risk behaviors is available.

Having sex with someone who is not in one of these risk groups and has had only a few largely monogamous heterosexual relationships in the last 10 years is reasonably safe, the chance of acquiring the HIV infection being about 1 in 5 million per episode of sex, even without condoms (Table 5.6). Should this evolve into a steady relationship, however, an HIV antibody test is advisable, because the risk cumulates to 1 in 16,000 after several years (an amount of time that would usually pass in a person infected with HIV before any symptoms developed). This risk seems unacceptable, not because of its magnitude—we take risks of this size every day when we drive on the freeway (Hearst & Hulley, 1988)—but because of the especially nasty characteristics of AIDS. Even at the initial encounter or while awaiting the results of the antibody tests, many people will want to use condoms with spermicide to reduce this minute but scary risk further.

Having sex with someone who has not had sexual intercourse with anyone else (and does not belong to another risk group) is of course completely safe. But there is the possibility that that person has had a secret affair, either in the past or in the present. Again, the risk for one sexual encounter is really very low, even without condoms and spermicidal cream, but, again, this risk cumulates in a steady sexual relationship or a marriage. Because the infection may be entirely without symptoms during these years, we are entering an era when people having extramarital affairs should protect their loved ones by either abandoning the affairs or having HIV tests every few months. In many places such tests are widely available at health departments, and are confidential and free of charge.

Individuals who are already infected can also use condoms with spermicidal cream when having sex with uninfected individuals, but these contraceptives probably convey only one order of magnitude of protection when used in a long-term relationship. (Condoms lubricated with spermicidal cream are always preferred over condoms alone, since the spermicide may provide some protection in the event of condom rupture.) A safer recommendation for discordant couples (one infected, the other not) is to limit sexual activity to mutual masturbation, making sure the ejaculate does not enter a body cavity or touch skin that has a rash or wound. For couples in which both people are infected with HIV, safe sex precautions to avoid reinfection with HIV are often recommended, even though it is not known whether reinfection of a person who is already HIV positive increases that individual's risk of progression to AIDS.

Strategies for preventing HIV spread by IV drug users, which are also described in other chapters in this volume, include attention to two issues. First is the advice on preventing heterosexual spread noted above, and second are the outreach and treatment programs to get IVDUs to stop using IV drugs, or in any event to stop sharing needles, or as a last resort to clean their needles with bleach between users. These goals are extremely difficult to achieve in this self-destructive, noncompliant, and inaccessible population. They are, however, extremely important for the health of these patients and of the public at large; IVDUs are a major avenue through which HIV infection spreads to the general heterosexual population (Moss, 1987).

The strategies shown in Table 5.7 for preventing HIV infection from occurring by blood transfusion have been highly effective, but not perfect. In early 1988 there were already 298 cases of AIDS associated with blood transfused in the United States in 1986 (Eisenstaedt & Getzen, 1988), and this number will rise as more of the infections from that year finish their incubation period and cause AIDS. The risk—1 in 33,000 transfusions—is ascribed to using blood from individuals who did not admit to being in a high-risk group and who were newly infected, without, as yet, HIV antibodies that could be detected when the blood was screened. This risk may decline as the principles in Table 5.7 are followed more closely, and with improved techniques for detecting HIV infection.

The strategies for preventing perinatal spread of HIV are to encourage all women who plan to become pregnant to be tested for HIV. Those who are positive should be advised to avoid pregnancy; if they do become pregnant, they should consider abortion. If they decide to have the baby, they should avoid breast-feeding (except, perhaps, in countries where supplies of baby formula are inadequate and malnutrition is likely to be a competing cause of mortality).

The strategies for preventing accidental infection of health care providers are more important than the numbers infected thus far—a few dozen at most—would suggest. Each instance represents an individual tragedy on the order, say, of a fire fighter killed in the line of duty. But the larger problem is the reaction of the medical community; many health care workers have become reluctant to provide care for patients who may have AIDS (Link, Feingold, Charap, Freeman, & Shelov, 1988). The solution—an imperfect one—is to make every effort to reduce this occupational hazard by taking great care and using protective apparel such as latex gloves and eyeglasses for procedures that involve the handling of body fluids. This should be done for all patients even in countries like the United States, where the prevalence of HIV infection is still under 1%. This level of risk is not trivial, and many HIV-infected individuals do not know that they are seropositive, or, in some cases, that they are in a high-risk group.

The Research Agenda

There are two main components of the research agenda here. First, there is a need for epidemiologists and behavioral scientists to learn more about the distributions and determinants of various risk behaviors and their antecedents in the population. How often, for example, do people in various age, sex, race, and geographic segments fail to use condoms when they have sex with persons whose risk status they know little about? And what are the factors that lead them to be more likely to use condoms?

We are beginning to see research on people's knowledge and attitudes about AIDS (e.g., Becker & Joseph, 1988) and on their AIDS-related behaviors (e.g., Kegeles, Adler, & Irwin, 1988). But, as pointed out in Becker and Joseph's (1988) extensive review of psychosocial work in this area, there are surprisingly few studies on these topics in representative samples from all the populations involved: "The immediate question becomes why most individuals successfully change their behaviors while some others do not. . . . What is required are vigorous attempts to better understand the determinants of AIDS-relevant behavioral change. Such observational studies are an essential prerequisite for the development of potentially successful intervention programs."

But it is not enough to know who is practicing AIDS-risk behaviors and what the psychosocial antecedents are. Behavioral scientists and epidemiologists must work together to design and test effective interventions that will help people to change these behaviors (Coates et al., 1987). There is an urgent need for scientists, working in all the countries and cultures of the world, to discover and test an optimal combination of educational and motivational interventions individually tailored to reduce the susceptibility of these various populations to the further spread of HIV.

Summary and Conclusions

It is useful to think of the epidemic as coming upon us in three major waves (Mann & Chin, 1988). The first of these, beginning in the mid-1970s, was the invisible wave of infection with HIV. Before AIDS was even recognized as a disease, the virus had already infected large segments of some populations, notably gay men and IV drug users in the United States and Western Europe, and active heterosexuals in some areas of central Africa and Haiti. The total number infected in the United States reached 1–1.5 million several years ago; this number is probably growing rather slowly now, because of the limited size of the gay and IVDU subpopulations and the progress that has been made in AIDS prevention among homosexual men. The worldwide estimate is 5–10 million, a number that may grow more rapidly because the potential for heterosexual spread is greater.

The second wave of the epidemic was AIDS itself, which arrived in the early 1980s (the five-year delay reflecting the long incubation period of the disease). The cumulative number by mid-1988 had reached 70,000 in the United States, with three-quarters of the states reporting more than 100 cases but the largest numbers of cases still located in half a dozen major urban epicenters. The equivalent worldwide number was 250,000, with AIDS present in almost all countries but large numbers limited to a dozen countries and the majority reporting fewer than 100 cases. The AIDS epidemic has become a major public health problem in several American, European, and African countries. It is likely that most people who have been infected with HIV will develop AIDS over the next decade; if so, the cumulative number of AIDS cases will increase 10- to 15-fold!

The third wave of the epidemic, beginning in the mid-1980s, is the socioeconomic and political consequences of the disease. This wave is only partly formed and highly unpredictable, but it seems likely that there will be unprecedented fiscal and social repercussions of this new disease (Osborn, 1988). These will result, in part, from the particularly nasty characteristics of the disease—the facts that AIDS is most prevalent in young adults and is incurable and uniformly fatal, with a lingering costly illness after a lengthy silent incubation period during which it is insidiously contagious.

While awaiting the outcome of current research efforts directed at developing vaccines and drugs to prevent or cure HIV infection and AIDS, our only advantage in addressing the epidemic is that AIDS is a preventable disease. A major task for behavioral scientists is to develop, test, and popularize effective approaches to providing emotional support for those who have the disease, and to modifying behavior to prevent its spread among those who do not.

References

Allen, J. R., & Curran, J. W. (1988). Prevention of AIDS and HIV infection: Needs and priorities for epidemiologic research. *American Journal of Public Health, 78*, 381–386.

Bacchetti, P., Osmond, D., & Chaisson, R. E. (1988). Survival with AIDS in New York [letter]. *New England Journal of Medicine, 318*, 1464.

Becker, M. H., & Joseph, J. G. (1988). AIDS and behavioral change to reduce risk: A review. *American Journal of Public Health, 78*, 394–410.

Brandt, A. M. (1988). AIDS in historical perspective: Four lessons from the history of sexually transmitted diseases. *American Journal of Public Health, 78*, 367–371.

Burke, D. S., Brundage, J. F., Herbold, J. R., Berner, W., Gardner, L. I., Gunzenhauser, J. D., Voskovitch, J., & Redfield, R. R. (1987). Human immunodeficiency virus infections among civilian applicants for United States military service, October, 1985 to March, 1986. *New England Journal of Medicine, 317*, 131–136.

Centers for Disease Control. (1986). Acquired Immunodeficiency Syndrome (AIDS) among Blacks and Hispanics—United States. *Morbidity and Mortality Weekly Report, 35*, 655–666.

Centers for Disease Control. (1987a). Revision of the CDC surveillance case definition for AIDS. *Morbidity and Mortality Weekly Report, 36*(Suppl. 1S).

Centers for Disease Control. (1987b). Human immunodeficiency virus infection in the United States: A review of current knowledge. *Morbidity and Mortality Weekly Report, 36*(Suppl. S-6).

Centers for Disease Control. (1988, August 15). *AIDS weekly surveillance report—United States.* Atlanta, GA: Author.

Chaisson, R. E., Moss, A. R., & Onishi, R. (1987). Human immunodeficiency virus infection in heterosexual intravenous drug users in San Francisco. *American Journal of Public Health, 77*, 169–171.

Coates, T., Stall, R., Mandell, J., Boccelari, T., Sorensen, J., Morales, E., Morin, S., Wylie, J., & McKusick, L. (1987). AIDS: A psychosocial research agenda. *Annals of Behavioral Medicine, 9*, 21–28.

Colebunders, R., Francis, H., Izaley, L., Kabasela, K., Nzilambi, N., Van de Groen, G., Vercauteren, G., Mann, J. M., Bila, K., Kakaonde, N., Ifoto, L., Quinn, T. C., Curran, J. W., & Piot, P. (1987). Evaluation of a clinical case-definition of Acquired Immunodeficiency Syndrome in Africa. *Lancet, 1*, 492–494.

Curran, J. W., Jaffe, H. W., Hardy, A. M., Morgan, W. M., Selik, R. M., & Dondero, P. J. (1988). Epidemiology of HIV infection and AIDS in the United States. *Science, 239*, 610–616.

Cutler, J. C., & Arnold, R. C. (1988). Venereal disease control by health departments in the past: Lessons for the present. *American Journal of Public Health, 78*, 372–376.

Eisenstaedt, R. S., & Getzen, T. E. (1988). Screening blood donors for HIV antibody: Cost-benefit analysis. *American Journal of Public Health, 78*, 450–454.

Francis, D. P., & Chin, J. (1987). The prevention of Acquired Immunodeficiency Syndrome in the United States. *Journal of the American Medical Association, 257*, 1357–1366.

Friedland, G. H., & Klein, R. S. (1987). Transmission of the HIV. *New England Journal of Medicine, 317*, 1125–1135.

Gerberding, J. L., Bryant-LeBlanc, C. E., Nelson, K., Moss, A. R., Osmond, D., Chambers, H. F., Carlson, J. R., Drew, W. L., Levy, J. A., & Sande, M. A. (1987). Risk of transmitting the human immunodeficiency virus, cytomegalovirus, and hepatitis B virus to health care workers exposed to patients with AIDS and AIDS-related conditions. *Journal of Infectious Diseases, 156*, 1–8.

Guinan, M. E., & Hardy, A. (1987). Epidemiology of AIDS in women in the United States. *Journal of the American Medical Association, 257*, 2039–2042.

Hearst, N., & Hulley, S. B. (1988). Preventing the heterosexual spread of AIDS: Are we giving our patients the best advice? *Journal of the American Medical Association, 259*, 2428–2432.

Hoff, R., Berardi, V. P., Weiblen, B. J., Mahoney-Trout, L., Mitchell, M. L., & Grady, G. F. (1988). Seroprevalence of human immunodeficiency virus among childbearing women. *New England Journal of Medicine, 318*, 525–530.

Kegeles, S. M., Adler, N. E., & Irwin, C. E. (1988). Sexually active adolescents and condoms: Changes over one year in knowledge, attitudes and use. *American Journal of Public Health, 78,* 460–461.

Link, R. N., Feingold, A. R., Charap, M. H., Freeman, K., & Shelov, S. P. (1988). Concerns of medical and pediatric house officers about acquiring AIDS from their patients. *American Journal of Public Health, 78,* 455–459.

Mann, J. (1987, October 20). [Statement at an informal briefing on AIDS to the 42nd Session of the United Nations General Assembly].

Mann, J. M., & Chin, J. (1988). AIDS: A global perspective. *New England Journal of Medicine, 319,* 302–303.

Mays, V. M., & Cochran, S. D. (1987). AIDS and Black Americans: Special psychosocial issues. *Public Health Reports, 102,* 224–231.

Moss, A. R. (1987). AIDS and intravenous drug use: The real heterosexual epidemic. *British Medical Journal of Clinical Research, 294,* 389–390.

Moss, A. R., Bacchetti, P., Osmond, D., Krempf, W., Chaisson, R. E., Stites, D., & Wilber, J. (1988). Seropositivity for HIV and the development of AIDS or AIDS related condition: Three year follow-up of the San Francisco General Hospital cohort. *British Medical Journal of Clinical Research, 296,* 745–750.

Osborn, J. E. (1988). AIDS: Politics and science. *New England Journal of Medicine, 318,* 444–447.

Padian, N., Marquis, L., & Francisc, D. P. (1987). Male-to-female transmission of human immunodeficiency virus. *Journal of the American Medical Association, 258,* 788–790.

Peterman, T. A., Stoneburner, R. L., Allen, J. R., Jaffe, H. W., & Curran, J. W. (1988). Risk of human immunodeficiency virus transmission from heterosexual adults with transfusion-associated infections. *Journal of the American Medical Association, 259,* 55–58.

Piot, P., Plummer, F. A., Mhalu, F. S., Lamboray, J. L., Chin, J., & Mann, J. M. (1988). AIDS: An international perspective. *Science, 239,* 573–579.

Polk, B. F., Fox, R., Brookmeyer, R., Kanchanaraksa, S., Kaslow, R., Visscher, B., Rinaldo, C., & Phair, J. (1987). Predictors of the Acquired Immunodeficiency Syndrome developing in a cohort of seropositive homosexual men. *New England Journal of Medicine, 316,* 61–66.

Quinn, T. C., Glassner, D., Cannon, R. O., Matuszak, D. L., Dunning, R. W., Kline, R. L., Campbell, C. H., Israel, E., Fauci, A. S., & Hook, E. W. (1988). Human immunodeficiency virus infection among patients attending clinics for sexually transmitted diseases. *New England Journal of Medicine, 318,* 197–202.

Study Group of AIDS in Haitian-Americans. (1987). Risk factors for AIDS among Haitians residing in the United States. *Journal of the American Medical Association, 257,* 635–639.

U.S. Surgeon General. (1988). *Understanding AIDS* (DHHS Publication No. [CDC] HHS-88–8404). Washington, DC: Government Printing Office.

Winkelstein, W., Lyman, D. M., Padian, N., Grant, R., Samuel, M., Wiley, J. A., & Anderson, R. E. (1987). Sexual practices and risk of infection by the human immunodeficiency virus: The San Francisco Men's Health Study. *Journal of the American Medical Association, 257,* 321–325.

Wofsy, C. B. (1987). Human immunodeficiency virus infection in women. *Journal of the American Medical Association, 257,* 2074–2076.

Yankauer, A. (1988). AIDS and public health. *American Journal of Public Health, 78*(4), 364–366.

6

Human Immunodeficiency Virus and Immune System Regulation of the Central Nervous System

Nicholas R.S. Hall
Maureen P. O'Grady

Basic Concepts

Human immunodeficiency virus, as it is now called, was first described in an article that appeared in *Science* magazine in 1983 (Barre-Sinoussi et al., 1983). Scientists working at the Pasteur Institute in the laboratory of Dr. Luc Montagnier were the first to isolate the minuscule piece of biological material called a retrovirus that is sparking the scientific, sociological, and legal debates that are permeating nearly all levels of society. It is called a retrovirus because it changes the genetic composition of the cells that it enters and subsequently destroys. Initially, it was called lymphoadenopathy virus (LAV)—a name that reflected one of the symptoms that is characteristic of the AIDS syndrome. The existence of a retrovirus in AIDS victims was later confirmed by Dr. Robert Gallo and his colleagues at the National Institutes of Health (Gallo et al., 1984). However, the manner in which their findings were presented and their designation of the virus as human T-cell leukemia (lymphotropic) virus number 3 (HTLV-III) precipitated a long and bitter debate and lawsuit that has only recently been resolved.

One of the consequences was the redesignation of the retrovirus as human immunodeficiency virus, or HIV, so named because it is predisposed to attack the human immune system. This results in the im-

Authors' Note: The first author is supported by a NIMH Research Scientist Development Award (MH00648). Some of the studies described in this chapter were supported by the NIH (NS21210 and DK41025). We greatly appreciate the excellent editorial assistance provided by Mrs. Cecilia Figueredo during the preparation of this chapter.

mune system's impaired ability to protect the body from a variety of disease-causing agents. Thus AIDS is not a single disease, but a syndrome that differs from a disease in that it is a set of symptoms that reflect a disease state. In the example of HIV, life-sustaining immune system cells are rendered impotent, permitting a variety of disease-causing organisms to invade with little or no opposition. Thus the symptoms of the syndrome correlated with HIV infection are multiple diseases. Depending upon which organisms have infected the person with AIDS, the symptoms might be manifestations of any of a number of diseases, none of which is new.

Two of the most elementary cells that regulate not only the lymphocytes but also the central nervous system are the monocyte and the closely related macrophage. These cells normally play a pivotal role during the immune response. Unfortunately, they are also a primary target of HIV. Within these robust cells, the virus can remain in a latent state for years. It can also be transported within the monocytes to other tissues throughout the body, and to T cells when the immune system is activated. It is when the T cell is subsequently destroyed that the infected individual develops the acquired immunodeficiency deficiency syndrome, known by its acronym—AIDS.

Differences in the psychological makeup and life-styles of individuals may influence their susceptibility to HIV infection. If this is true, it might explain in part why certain individuals contract AIDS within a relatively short period of time following just a brief exposure to the disease, while others experience repeated exposure with impunity. While much remains to be learned about HIV, it is known that the most common means of transmission are exposure through sexual activity and exposure through the sharing of hypodermic needles—a common mode of transmission among intravenous drug users. The extent to which other forms of transmission may be important is not clear.

It was recently argued in a highly publicized book that the prevalence of the syndrome is much greater than is suspected and that one may be at risk without engaging in the high-risk behaviors of anal intercourse and intravenous drug use (Masters, Johnson, & Kolodny, 1988). At about the same time, an article appeared in *Cosmopolitan* titled "Reassuring News About AIDS" (Gould, 1988). The author presented arguments supportive of his belief that "there is almost no danger of contracting AIDS through ordinary sexual intercourse." While each of these contrasting views is more representative of the opinions of the respective authors than of conclusions based upon well-designed empirical studies, each uses the interpretation of statistics and epidemiological data to support its claim. By providing excessive publicity to such articles, the news media subsequently play a role in the transmission of AIDS. For example, a false sense of security gained from reading the *Cosmopolitan* article might result in a person unknowingly engaging in what may be high-risk behavior, while a person preoccupied with the arguments of Masters and his colleagues might develop a "pseudo-AIDS" syndrome based upon the fear of contracting AIDS.

Several cases have now been reported in which HIV-free individuals experienced depressed mood, weight loss, and malaise despite assurances that they were HIV free. In some instances, suicidal tendencies have been reported, making the fear of AIDS a potentially fatal disease (Miller, Green, Farmer, & Carroll, 1985). Thus, as is true of cancer, AIDS can be viewed as two diseases. The first is subsequent to the anxiety of knowing that one has a disease for which there is no currently available cure, and the stigma associated with this particular disease. This AIDS hex is inadvertently placed upon an HIV seropositive individual the moment a social worker or physician conveys this information. Depending upon the coping skills of the individual, the pronouncement of the diagnosis may well have the same impact upon the patient's health as would a curse proclaimed by a witch doctor. The other disease is caused by HIV and involves destruction of the immune system. While the two syndromes are closely intertwined, this chapter will focus upon the underlying molecular events and the immunologic consequences of HIV infection, with an emphasis upon how these might affect the central nervous system (CNS)-immune system axis.

Retroviruses

Molecular Structure

HIV belongs to a broad group of viruses called retroviruses. The name HIV suggests that it is a single entity, but it is important to realize that all viruses are made up of several component parts. Each plays a different role following infection of a host. One part is crucial in order for the virus to gain entry into a cell. Another determines its ability to become incorporated into the cell's genetic code. Still other components of the virus have poorly understood roles, but may provide a means by which to identify a particular strain. While each virus has some features that are unique, there are other basic characteristics that are common to all viruses that can become incorporated into the genetic composition of the host's cells. Those that have this ability are called retroviruses.

All retroviruses are composed of two identical strands of single-stranded RNA surrounded by an envelope or coat that confers on them the ability to gain entry into specific cell types. The most common form of retrovirus is the C type, which is able to reproduce through a process that culminates in budding from the membrane of the infected cell. In addition, there is a double-stranded DNA form of the virus that is referred to as the *provirus*. The provirus is formed when reverse transcriptase catalyzes the formation of DNA from the viral RNA genome. It subsequently migrates into the cell's nucleus, where it can become integrated into the genetic code. Once there, it can persist for the life of the cell, which then becomes a potential factory capable of producing more virus. This occurs when the incorporated double-stranded DNA or provirus transcribes new viral RNA genomes while the infected cell is undergoing cell division. Normally, this would occur following exposure of the lymphocyte to an antigen. It is for this reason that some investigators believe that while HIV is clearly capable of destroying an important subclass of lymphocytes, other antigens, especially viral antigens such as cytomegalovirus and herpes, may play a permissive role in triggering HIV from a latent to an active state. They would do this by stimulating the infected lymphocytes to divide.

Biological Properties

There are many different forms of retroviruses, which were first isolated from tumors. Initially, retroviruses were found to have the ability to transmit malignant disease, although many have now been described that do not have that capability. Because of this distinction, retroviruses are sometimes classified on the basis of the type of disease that they can cause—that is, malignant versus nonmalignant or nonpathogenic. Thus gibbon ape leukemia virus and feline leukemia virus are representative of retroviruses that have the ability to cause malignant disease. Others are associated with persistent and chronic disease, but not with neoplasms. These latter retroviruses are referred to as *lentiviruses*, and it is to this group that HIV belongs. Some lentiviruses are associated with pulmonary disease, while others cause arthritis and hemolytic anemias. Sheep lentivirus visna was the first virus of this type to be described after it was found to be the causative agent of a wasting syndrome detected in Icelandic sheep between 1930 and 1950 (Sigurdsson, Palsson, & Grimson, 1957). Neuropathology that results ultimately in total paralysis is the mechanism via which this particular lentivirus causes disease.

Other lentiviruses are now known to exist in both human and non-human primates and are represented by HIV and the simian form, which also has a predisposition to infect T-lymphocytes. The latter is called simian T-lymphotropic virus (STLV-III) and has been found to be pathogenic in macaque monkeys (Kanki et al., 1985). This primate retrovirus has also been found in healthy West Africans, but when isolated was initially called HTLV-IV (Kanki et al., 1986). There is good evidence, however, that it is indistinguishable from STLV-III. HIV also shares certain characteristics with the recently described feline immunodeficiency virus and equine infectious anemia virus. It is evident that while HIV has some unique features, it does have certain similarities to other lentiviruses that exist in other species, including nonhuman primates.

This may very well represent a strategy that these lentiviruses have evolved for the purpose of evading destruction by the host's immune system, since outer envelope proteins represent the most vulnerable target of neutralizing antibodies (Gonda et al., 1985; Montelaro, Parekh, Orrego, & Issel, 1984). The ability of the virus to change its configuration may well result in an antibody that might be capable of neutralizing one form of HIV to be useless in destroying other forms. It is for this same reason that flu vaccines have to be customized each year in order for the resultant antibody to be effective against the specific form of virus that is projected to be prevalent during the forthcoming season. Even if a specific antibody were produced, it probably would be unable to destroy the virus, since there is reason to believe that the extensive glycosylation of the HIV envelope may play a role in protecting the virus from potentially neutralizing antibodies (Allan et al., 1985; Kitchen et al., 1984; Robey et al., 1985). This is based upon the observation that while high titers of antibodies can be detected against the envelope proteins of several lentiviruses, those that have neutralizing ability tend to be associated with lentiviruses, such as visna virus and equine encephalitis virus, that are only moderately glycosylated (Montelaro et al., 1984; Narayan, Griffen, & Chase, 1977). Further details pertaining to some of these topics are to be found in a review by Haseltine, Sodroski, and Rosen (1987).

Since penetration of the cell membrane represents the first step in the infectious process, the envelope is a major factor that determines the type of cell susceptible to HIV infection. Indeed, there is now evidence that there does exist a physical association between the envelope protein and the CD4 molecule that serves as the cellular binding site for HIV. CD4 can, therefore, be viewed as the entry point via which the virus enters the cell. It is quite possible that as the envelope undergoes changes, so will the type of cell that is predisposed to infection (i.e., brain cells as opposed to T helper cells).

In summary, AIDS is not a disease. It is a syndrome that includes a variety of diseases, many of which are opportunistic infections that under normal conditions would be relatively harmless to the host. Which diseases are manifested and the severity of those diseases is determined by a large number of interactive factors, including the type of virus that is present. Not only can it directly impair the immune system by infecting monocytes and T helper lymphocytes, but it may also disrupt immunomodulatory neurotransmitters and neuropeptides. Similarly, altered production of neuromodulatory cytokines could be in part responsible for some of the neuropsychiatric and neurologic consequences of the disease, a topic to be discussed below.

Mechanism of Cytolysis

Cellular Targets

Once the viral DNA is incorporated into the genetic backbone of the cell, it is possible for the integrated virus to become fully expressed. Ultimately, the viral RNA and proteins will become assembled on the cell membrane, where they will constitute a virion, which is simply a complete viral particle. From the membrane the virus is released, thereby completing the cycle. This released virus then has the potential to infect other cells, thereby starting a new cycle. Furthermore, once the cell contains incorporated viral DNA, it becomes a potential factory capable of transferring the genetic code of the virus to virtually every daughter cell. For this reason, when a host becomes infected with a retrovirus, it most likely will persist for its lifetime. Under normal conditions, a T cell would undergo clonal expansion into daughter cells following exposure to an antigen. Thus the greater the exposure to antigen, the greater the probability that more virions may be produced. Given the high incidence of Epstein-Barr virus, cytomegalovirus, hepatitis B, and/or herpes simplex virus in many individuals at risk for AIDS, the required signals are clearly available. Once opportunistic infections begin, the expression of virus could be greatly amplified. One of the factors that has been found capable of triggering infected T cells is interleukin I, which is sometimes produced spontaneously by monocytic cells from HIV-infected individuals. Other cytokines may also be capable of triggering these cells (Fauci, 1988).

Consequently, despite considerable evidence that the CD4 molecule is a high-affinity receptor for HIV, other proteins that are present on the human T4 cells may be crucial for internalization of the virus. What does appear to be required is fusion of the transmembrane portion of the viral envelope with the cell membrane (Stein et al., 1987). Regardless of the precise mechanism by which the virus becomes internalized, once inside the cell, it is uncoated and, through a mechanism involving reverse transcriptase, the viral RNA is reverse transcribed to DNA. But not all of the viral DNA becomes incorporated into the host's DNA, since a substantial amount remains in the cytoplasm of the cell.

Infection and subsequent killing of T4 cells by HIV has now been reported using both in vitro and in vivo techniques. This has been demonstrated through the use of a cloned virus genome that is capable of directing the synthesis of infectious viral particles (Wong-Staal, 1987). Following transfection with this clone, normal core T cells have been found to contain complete virions characterized by a cylindrical core. Evidence that the transfected virus was actually being produced was apparent when it was observed that the percentage of infected cells increased up to 18 days, after which cell viability dropped precipitously. Since 90% of the cells that remained were T suppressor cells and not the infected T helper cells, these data provide additional evidence for the selectivity of the HIV for helper T cells. When suppressor cells were superinfected with HIV, this subset was found to be resistant to the cytopathic effects of the virus even though the virus was able to replicate in these cells. This was not subsequent to an alteration of the virus that occurred within the suppressor cells, since it was still trophic and cytopathic for helper cells (Wong-Staal, 1987).

It has been proposed that upon sensitization of the cell to an antigen, the virus becomes expressed. This possibility is supported by the observation that mitogenic stimulation, or stimulation by bacterial, viral, or alloantigens, is required to induce HIV production in vitro. It is also consistent with the observation that individuals with AIDS frequently have a substantial antigenic load, causing some to speculate that AIDS might be the consequence not of a single virus but rather a critical mass that tips the balance between health and disease. The actual destruction of the cell usually occurs at the point when the virus assembles and forms a bud on the cell membrane.

However, the precise mechanism by which this occurs has not been clearly established.

Several possible mechanisms have been proposed, some of which are discussed in further detail in a recent review article (Fauci, 1988). One is that the large amount of unincorporated viral DNA is related to the cytopathogenicity of the virus. Another possibility is that the cell membrane loses its integrity when large amounts of the virus bud off the cell surface. This could increase the permeability of the cell membrane and disrupt its normal homeostasis. It is also of interest that budding of virus from infected cells can result in the fusing of uninfected cells, resulting in a multinucleated giant cell consisting of both infected and noninfected cells (Lifson, Reyes, McGrath, Stein, & Engleman, 1986; Sodroski, Goh, Rosen, Campbell, & Haseltine, 1986). These giant cells usually undergo cytolysis within 48 hours after the fusion occurs.

There is also evidence that the tat-III gene may shorten the life span of the cell by promoting the terminal differentiation of only T helper cells through the expression of cellular genes (Zagury et al., 1986). Another possibility is that a product of one of the viral genes is capable of selectively killing the T helper cells. Autoimmune processes have also been suggested as a mechanism via which the cell might be destroyed. For example, the association of non-self-envelope proteins on the surface of the infected cell might render it sufficiently immunogenic to be recognized and destroyed by the host's immune system. This might also occur if free-viral protein were to bind to the CD4 molecule of uninfected cells (Fauci, 1988; Lyerly, Matthews, Langlois, Bolognesi, & Weinhold, 1987). Autoantibodies might also be directed against major histocompatibility complex class 2 antigens. (These are found on the surface of cells and in association with antigen, and cause the activation of T helper cells.) This latter hypothesis is based upon the observation that the CD4 molecule is able to recognize a portion of the major histocompatibility complex class 2 determinant. Thus it is possible that by virtue of the fact that it can bind to the CD4 molecule, part of the HIV shares structural similarity with the class 2 determinant. While speculative, it is conceivable that antibodies or cytotoxic cells with specificity for the HIV envelope could also cross-react with the HIV envelope proteins (Fauci, 1988).

Furthermore, there is evidence that early in the course of the AIDS syndrome, T helper cells become functionally deficient. Exposing cells to HIV without subsequent infection was found to greatly diminish their response to antigenic and mitogenic stimulation (Margolick,

Volkman, Folks, & Fauci, 1987). This impairment has also been induced following exposure to subunits of the HIV envelope that would be unable to induce infection (Mann et al., 1987). Impaired T-cell function following exposure to subunits of the outer envelope of the virus could well be due to competition with the CD4 molecule for the MHC class 2 determinant. Thus immune responses that require a signal resulting from the MHC presented antigen binding to the CD3-Ti receptor complex on T helper cells would be impaired (Fauci, 1988). In support of this hypothesis, studies have shown that mitogens that are not as dependent upon MHC interactions can, under circumstances when antigen responses are abnormal, induce mitogenesis (Lane et al., 1984).

It is possible that exposure to HIV in the absence of infection could interfere with postreceptor signal transduction. This could be due to binding of the ligand to either the CD4 receptor molecule or the antigen receptor. Because mitogen activation of lymphocytes occurs through a different mechanism than the antigen receptor pathway, it would explain why in some cases mitogen responsiveness can be normal while the response to an antigen is abnormal (Fauci, 1988; Lane et al., 1984). There is additional evidence that noncytopathic infection of cells with HIV can impair their ability to express CD4 molecules on their surface, which would prevent MHC-restricted presentation of antigen from occurring (Hoxie et al., 1986). There is also evidence for the existence of a functional defect in interleukin-2 gene expression despite normal expression of the interleukin-2 receptor gene (Fauci, 1988). Another alternative is that precursor cells might become infected, resulting in a reduced population of mature cells (Fauci, 1988).

There is also the possibility that the virus might infect and selectively delete a subset of cells that might play an essential role in the normal proliferation of the majority of T4 cells or the opposite scenario, that is, the production of a toxic substance that is directly responsible for the cytopathogenicity (Laurence & Mayer, 1984). Regardless of the precise mechanism(s) via which T-cell destruction occurs, the net result is an impaired ability of the immune response to protect the infected host against certain opportunistic infections. Because T helper cells facilitate the function of other T cells and B cells, and because lymphokines and antibody-activated complement proteins can mobilize and facilitate the entry of monocytic cells into infected areas, as well as stimulate the release of neurotransmitters and neuropeptides, the consequences ripple throughout the immune and central nervous systems.

The Impact of AIDS on the Brain and Behavior

The Role of Immunotransmitters

Mental disturbances have now been well documented in AIDS patients. These symptoms progress in severity during the course of the disease, but initially include difficulty in performing normal activities as well as apathy with respect to both work-related and social activities. Ultimately, these symptoms can include severe dementia as well as motor impairment. Under some conditions, there is also an impaired ability to perform neuropsychological tests—especially when there is pressure to complete the task within a given amount of time or when the task involves a high degree of complexity. Depression is another complication of AIDS and has to be taken into account, especially when evaluating cognitive function (see Price et al., 1988, for a review of these symptoms). Collectively, these symptoms are referred to as AIDS dementia complex. The neurologic symptoms that are characteristic of AIDS may be due in part to the release of immune system peptides that are stimulated either by HIV or by various opportunistic infections. There are now many available data revealing that products of lymphocytes and monocytes are able to act at the level of the brain and/or the pituitary gland to modulate certain neuroendocrine circuits.

Our first evidence that a product of the immune system is able to modulate a neuroendocrine circuit came from an experiment in which a thymic extract, thymosin fraction 5 (TF5), was found to stimulate the pituitary-adrenal axis in primates (Healy et al., 1983). Premenarchial monkeys (*Macaca fascicularis*), median age 22 months (range 11–27 months; n = 18) were fitted with a vest and mobile tether assembly that permitted chronic femoral vein cannulation for blood collection. This technique allowed plasma to be harvested from monkeys that were unanesthetized, freely moving, and undisturbed by personnel in an adjacent room. TF5, at doses of 10.0 and 1.0 mg/kg or normal saline were injected intravenously via the cannula at 0700 hours. Basal ACTH, beta-endorphin, and cortisol values were as follows: mean + SEM, 24.06 + 3.91 pg/ml, 37.3 + 7.65 pg/ml, and 35.3 + 3.16 mcg/dl, respectively. TF5 produced significant increases ($p <$ 0.05) in plasma ACTH, beta-endorphin, and cortisol concentrations, peak values being 46.34 + 7.05 pg/ml, 51.3 + 13.6 pg/ml, and 56.3 + 8.7 mcg/dl, respectively. These studies have been replicated using mice and rats (McGillis, Hall, Vahouny, & Goldstein, 1985).

In a subsequent study, a group of these prepubertal monkeys underwent total thymectomy. After surgical recovery, each animal underwent femoral cannulation, and concentrations of ACTH, beta-endorphin, and cortisol were compared with similarly cannulated age-matched controls. Athymic primates had significantly lower plasma ACTH and beta-endorphin values. Cortisol values also tended to be lower than in control monkeys, although this difference was not statistically significant ($p > 0.05$).

The most parsimonious interpretation of these data was that thymosins directly stimulated the adrenal fasciculata cells. We have tested this class of immunoregulatory factors for their corticogenic potential using isolated adrenal fasciculata cells (Vahouny et al., 1983). TF5 and its constituent peptides, TSN thymosin alpha 1, alpha 7, and beta 4, were tested, as were heterogeneous preparations containing interleukin 2, interferon, and other lymphokines. Partially purified interferon was also evaluated using this model. With the exception of a mild stimulatory effect of interferon, none of the above preparations was effective in stimulating either corticosterone or CAMP production. The possibility that thymosins and interferon might act synergistically with ACTH to enhance steroidogenesis was considered. However, adding the various preparations to a suboptimal concentration of ACTH did not have a potentiating effect. Consequently, it was considered unlikely that the in vivo corticogenic effect of thymosins was due to direct stimulation of the adrenal cortex. We have subsequently determined that cultured pituitary cells are capable of producing ACTH following incubation with TF5 (McGillis, Hall, & Goldstein, 1988). Furthermore, most of the activity appeared to reside within the more hydrophobic peptides.

Several experimental approaches have been pursued in order to elucidate the site of and mechanism(s) of action of thymosin-induced steroidogenesis. Our most recent has been to identify intracerebral sites where the steroidogenic effect is maximally effective following microinjection and to identify subcortical regions that contain peptides with corticogenic effects. In the first of these studies, adult male rats were chronically implanted with stainless steel guide tubes overlying the anterior extent of the hypothalamus (Hall et al., 1982). Following a two-week recovery period, they received five daily injections of either 10 mcg of TF5 or 10 mcg of kidney fraction 5. To ascertain whether any measured changes were the consequence of an intracerebral effect and not due to leakage out of the brain into the peripheral circulation, a third group received intraperitoneal injections of the same concentrations of TF5. Wet tissue weights were determined at the time of sacrifice. There were no effects of any of these treatments upon the weight of the thyroid or testes; however, a significant increase in the combined adrenal weight was associated with the intracerebral injection of TF5 ($p < 0.025$). This enlargement of the adrenals was not observed in rats that received systemic injections of TF5 or in animals that were treated with kidney fraction 5.

Data from a subsequent experiment using mice suggested that the increase in adrenal weight was probably correlated with increased corticosteroid production. Adult Swiss-Webster mice received thymosin injections via precisely measured polyethylene cannulas that extended into the lateral ventricle. When a component peptide of TF5, thymosin alpha 1, was injected using this protocol, it triggered a significant rise in serum corticosterone. A control peptide, thymosin beta 4, was ineffective in stimulating corticosterone, but was found to stimulate LH release, a phenomenon that has also been demonstrated using an in vitro model (Hall et al., 1982; Rebar, Miyake, Low, & Goldstein, 1981). We have subsequently evaluated the corticogenic effects of thymosin alpha 1 following its injection into discrete brain regions. These included the preoptic area, substantia nigra, and nucleus locus coeruleus. Although corticosterone release was stimulated by injections into all of the brain regions, the highest release occurred after thymosin alpha 1 was implanted into the nucleus locus coeruleus (unpublished observation). The amount of corticosterone released from the other brain sites was proportional to the distance from this brain stem nucleus. These data suggest a role for norepinephrine, a hypothesis supported by a report of Besedovsky et al. (1983) in which it was found that brain levels of this neurotransmitter are decreased by lymphokine administration. If thymosin alpha 1 causes a similar decrease, the change is consistent with elevated corticosteroids, since norepinephrine inhibits serotonergic and cholinergic stimulation of CRF. Thus, through disinhibition, CRF, ACTH, and corticosterone would all be expected to rise.

Particularly intriguing is the observation that the amino acid sequence of thymosin alpha 1 shares 40% homology with the p17 gag protein of the human immunodeficiency virus (Sarin, Sun, Thornton, Naylor, & Goldstein, 1986). It was also shown that an antibody against synthetic thymosin alpha 1 could neutralize HTLV-III (HIV) clone B in vitro. As a consequence of these observations, we have conducted a preliminary study to test the hypothesis that antibody to the p17 gag protein can cross-react with thymosin alpha 1 in the brain. Previous work in this laboratory has revealed the presence of this peptide in the

CNS (Hall et al., 1982). An accelerated avidin-biotin immuno-peroxidase procedure was chosen to stain a variety of tissue sections from perfused rat brain.

We have discovered that identical staining patterns for both anti-bodies exist (manuscript in preparation). A battery of control proto-cols as well as nonbrain control tissues established that this staining pattern could not be attributed to nonspecific binding of the antibody. These data suggest that certain viral antigens may be capable of acti-vating neuroendocrine circuits at a CNS-pituitary site of action. Using a different model, we have recently found that antigenic sensitization using Newcastle disease virus can alter the metabolism of brain levels of biogenic amines (Dunn, Powell, Moreshead, Gaskin, & Hall, 1987). These results are potentially important, because they suggest that the brain does indeed respond acutely to an antigenic stimulus, or to an immune system product such as interferon that is produced subse-quent to viral challenge.

Another line of research that we are actively pursuing is the effect of viral exposure and immune system peptides on the developing neuroendocrine and immune systems. We injected pregnant Swiss-Webster mice with TF5 and studied their progeny as adults (O'Grady, Hall, & Goldstein, 1987). Briefly, the results were as follows: Com-pared to the vehicle control group, female adults (3–4 months of age) whose mothers had been injected with TF5 during gestation had larger thymuses ($p < .004$), decreased ovary weights ($p < .01$), de-creased IL-2 ($p < .03$), and a decreased response to the mitogens concanavalin A ($p < .003$) and pokeweed ($p < .001$), with no change in response to PHA. The immune measures in the male offspring in the TF5 group (measured as adults) were in a similar direction but were not statistically significant ($.05 < p < .10$). The male progeny in the TF5 group had larger thymuses ($p < .01$) and larger adrenals ($p = .004$). We have just concluded a pilot study in which the experimental treatments were expanded to include interferon or an active state of immunity in response to Newcastle disease virus. In this study, Sprague-Dawley rat pups received four daily injections (s.c.) with ei-ther biologically derived rat interferon (alpha/beta) or a control sub-stance (days 1–4) or one injection of Newcastle disease virus (on day 4, s.c.). We performed behavioral, immune, and endocrine measures on these animals. Several neurobehavioral reflexes were observed that are considered to be developmental milestones reflecting maturation of the nervous system. There seemed to be no consistent differences among the groups in the negative geotaxis or cliff avoidance tests. However, animals in the interferon group and the Newcastle disease virus group showed an accelerated attainment of the acoustic startle response ($p < .05$) compared to controls, suggesting an activation of the sensory and/or motor processes mediating this response. This acoustic startle response is a complex integration of central and peripheral systems, but it is interesting to note that there have been reports of peripheral auditory nerve damage in pediatric AIDS.

The extent to which cytokines such as thymosins, interleukins, and interferons contribute to the symptoms collectively referred to as AIDS-related dementia is not clear. But the potential for such a contribution is quite great and needs to be considered whenever relevant data are being interpreted.

Summary and Conclusion

The human immunodeficiency virus has the potential to disrupt physiological processes via a number of potential mechanisms. First and foremost is its ability to infect and impair the ability of monocytes and T helper cells to function. However, infection with this virus is also correlated with impaired brain function as manifested by the symptoms that are collectively referred to as AIDS-related dementia. These symptoms may be the consequence of opportunistic infections that happen to have a predisposition for the brain or they may be due to the virus itself. In some cases it is possible that components of the virus, for example the p17 gag protein, may be capable of mimicking the effects of endogenous peptides such as thymosin alpha 1. It is also possible that excessive amounts of interleukin I and certain types of interferon may be capable of causing or exacerbating some of these symptoms, since both peptides have been reported to induce neurologic symptoms. Neuronal dysfunction consequent to AIDS could directly impair immunoregulatory pathways and, conversely, disruption of the immune system may well impair the normal functioning of neuroendocrine circuits. Changes in brain levels of biogenic amines consequent to altered production of immune system peptides also require that we consider the possibility that behavior is directly modulated by the immune system itself. While it is too early to speculate whether or not this would affect the probability of engaging in high-risk behaviors, the possibility must be considered. To date, there is no effective cure for AIDS and any effective strategy will have to take into account all of these potential mechanisms that could contribute to the symptoms that are manifested.

It is quite apparent that eradicating this disease is going to require more than a competent immune system. Sources of funding as well as attitudes toward funding will be determined largely by political factors and views expressed by those perceived to be authorities in the field. Opposing views are already resulting in confusion with respect to how to perceive this particular syndrome. The virus is being portrayed by some powerful and influential members of the scientific and political community as a runaway killer disease. Others urge caution and place the AIDS statistics into a different perspective. In a recent editorial, columnist James Kilpatrick (1988) noted that in the first seven years following the identification of AIDS, 37,481 cases had been officially reported and that, of those, approximately 13,000 were new cases that were diagnosed in 1986. The perspective was presented as follows: "In 1985, more than 19 million Americans were suffering from heart conditions, 29 million from significantly high blood pressure, 30 million from serious arthritis. In 1986, physicians reported 930,000 new cases of cancer. In 1985, roughly 771,000 persons died of heart disease, 462,000 of cancer and 46,000 in automobile accidents. What's the big deal?" The big deal is that the more we know about AIDS, the more we realize what we don't know. James Kilpatrick might be right. Government may be pouring billions of dollars into the 1980s version of the swine flu scare. On the other hand, if the projections of some epidemiologists are correct, it is not just the toll on human life that is at issue, but also the economic foundation of our entire health care system. The total pecuniary cost of AIDS is projected to be $48.8 billion in 1991 (Bloom & Carliner, 1988).

While a considerable sum of money is being allocated to study this virus, there will be numerous side benefits, many of which will probably not be evident for many years. One can cite the example of the space program, in that the real prize was not landing a man on the moon, but all of the spinoff technology that resulted from that investment. By learning about AIDS, we are learning about the immune system. When the immune system fails, we become susceptible to disease-causing organisms in all categories. Consequently, AIDS research can be viewed as a model system that will enable us to understand better both viral diseases in general and our ability to combat them. The discovery of a cure for AIDS may turn out to be no big deal considering the impact that other diseases have upon our society, but it is almost guaranteed that serendipitous discoveries along the way will benefit victims of numerous other illnesses.

It should also be a concern that AIDS research has lured a certain type of personality. Many scientists have traded their data books for stock portfolios as they have transformed their basic research laboratories into research and development facilities for newly founded companies. This has led to the perception that some data are being generated for the purpose of attracting investors instead of knowledge. Even those who have not followed this route have much to gain by conducting AIDS research in an atmosphere of public hysteria that becomes translated into research dollars. Ultimately, the health industry, the pharmaceutical companies, and the scientists investigating AIDS will benefit from increased spending for this disease. Therefore, the opinion of James Kilpatrick should be heeded as a counterpoint to what may be overly pessimistic predictions being voiced for self-serving purposes. But at the same time, we are confronted with an apparently lethal disease for which there is still no effective treatment. A publication of the San Francisco AIDS Foundation that is currently being distributed to persons living with AIDS concludes that of all the experimental protocols being tested, "the best treatment at present for the immune deficiency itself is to live as healthily as possible— eating well, getting enough rest, exercising moderately, decreasing stress, avoiding excessive alcohol and recreational drug intake. It is also very helpful to seek support from family, friends, counselors, support groups, clergy, or whatever resource is supportive to you" (Maxey & Gee, 1986). If James Kilpatrick is wrong, the $3 billion requested for appropriation toward AIDS research in 1990 may not be enough. If he is right, the investment will not have been wasted.

References

Allan, J. S., Coligan, J. E., Barin, F., McLane, M. F., Sodroski, J. G., Rosen, C. A., Haseltine, W. A., Lee, T. T., & Essex, M. (1985). Major glycoprotein antigens that induce antibodies in AIDS patients are encoded by HTLV-III. *Science, 228,* 1091–1094.

Arya, S. K., Guo, C., Josephs, S. F., & Wong-Staal, F. (1985). Trans-activator gene of human T-lymphotropic virus type III (HTLV-III). *Science, 229,* 69–73.

Barre-Sinoussi, F., Chermann, J. C., Rey, F., Nugeyre, M. T., Chamaret, S., Gruest, J., Dauguet, C., Axler-Blin, C., Vezinet-Brum, F., Rouzioux, C., Rozenbaum, W., & Montagnier, L. (1983). Isolation of a T-lymphotropic retrovirus from a patient at risk for acquired immune deficiency syndrome (AIDS). *Science, 220,* 868–870.

Besedovsky, H., Del Rey, A., Sorkin, E., Da Prada, M., Burri, R., & Honnegger, C. (1983). The immune response evokes changes in brain noradrenergic neurons. *Science, 221,* 564–566.

Bloom, D. E., & Carliner, G. (1988). The economic impact of AIDS in the United States. *Science, 239,* 604–610.

Brun-Vezinet, F., Rouzioux, C., Barre-Sinoussi, F., Klatzmann, D., Saimot, A. G., Rozenbaum, W., Christol, D., Gluckmann, J. C., Montagnier, L., & Cherman, J. C.

(1984). Detection of IgG antibodies to lymphadenopathy associated virus (LAV) by ELISA, in patients with Acquired Immuno Deficiency Syndrome or lymphadenopathy syndrome. *Lancet, 1*, 1253–1256.

Cianciolo, G. J., Kipnis, R. J., & Snyderman, R. (1984). Similarity between p15E of murine and feline viruses and p21 of HTLV. *Nature, 311*, 515.

Dafny, N., Prieto-Gomez, B., & Reyes-Vazquez, C. (1985). Does the immune system communicate with the central nervous system? Interferon modifies central nervous activity. *Journal of Neuroimmunology, 9*, 1–12.

Dayton, A. I., Sodroski, J. G., Rosen, C. A., Goh, W. C., & Haseltine, W. A. (1986). The trans-activator gene of the human T cell lymphotropic virus type III is required for replication. *Cell, 44*, 941–947.

Dunn, A. J., Powell, M. L., Moreshead, W. V., Gaskin, J. M., & Hall, N. R. (1987). Effects of Newcastle disease virus administration to mice on the metabolism of cerebral biogenic amines, plasma corticosterone, and lymphocyte proliferation. *Brain, Behavior, and Immunity, 1*, 216–230.

Fauci, A. S. (1988). The human immunodeficiency virus: Infectivity and mechanisms of pathogenesis. *Science, 239*, 617–622.

Fisher, M., Ensoli, B., Ivanhoff, L., Chamberlain, M., Petteway, S., Ratner, L., Gallo, R., & Wong-Staal, F. (1987). The sor gene of HIV-1 is required for efficient virus transmission in vitro. *Science, 237*, 888–893.

Gallo, R. C., Salahuddin, S. Z., Popovic, M., Shearer, G. M., Kaplan, M., Haynes, B. F., Palker, T. J., Redfield, R., Oleski, J., Safai, B., White, G., Foster, P., & Markham, P. D. (1984). Frequent detection and isolation of cytopathic retroviruses (HTLV-III) from patients with AIDS and at risk for AIDS. *Science, 224*, 500–503.

Gonda, M. A., Wong-Staal, F., Gallo, R. C., Clements, J. E., Narayan, O., & Gilden, R. V. (1985). Sequence homology and morphologic similarities of HTLV-III and visna virus, a pathogenic lentivirus. *Science, 227*, 173–177.

Gould, R. (1988, January). Reassuring news about AIDS. *Cosmopolitan*, pp. 146–204.

Gresser, I., Torey, M.G.F., Maury C., & Chouroulinkov I. (1975). Lethality of interferon preparations for mice. *Nature, 258*, 76–78.

Hall, N. R., McGillis, J. P., Spangelo, B. L., & Goldstein, A. L. (1985). Evidence that thymosins and other biological response modifiers can function as immunotransmitters. *Journal of Immunology, 135*, 806–811.

Hall, N. R., McGillis, J. P., Spangelo, B. L., Palaszynski, E., Moody, T. W., & Goldstein, A. L. (1982). Evidence for a neuroendocrine-thymus axis mediated by thymosin polypeptides. *Developments in Immunology, 17*, 653–660.

Harper, M. E., Marselle, L. M., Gallo, R. C., & Wong-Staal, F. (1986). Detection of lymphocytes expressing human T-lymphotropic virus type III in lymph nodes and peripheral blood from infected individual by in situ hybridization. *Proceedings of the National Academy of Sciences of the United States of America, 83*, 772–776.

Haseltine, W. A., Sodroski, J. G., & Rosen, C. A. (1987). Progress and puzzles: Molecular biology of HTLV-III. In S. Broder (Ed.), *AIDS: Modern concepts and therapeutic challenges* (pp. 53–62). New York: Marcel Dekker.

Healy, D. L., Hodgen, G. D., Schulte, H. M., Chrousos, A. L., Loriaux, D. L., Hall, N. R., & Goldstein, A. L. (1983). The thymus adrenal connection: Thymosin has corticotrophin releasing activity in primates. *Science, 222*, 1353–1355.

Hoxie, J. A., Alpers, J. D., Rackowski, J. L., Huebner, K., Haggarty, B. S., Cedarbaum, A. J., & Reed, J. C. (1986). Alterations in T4(CD4) protein and MRNA synthesis in cells infected with HIV. *Science, 234*, 1123–1127.

Kanki, P. J., Barin, F., M'Boup, S., Allan, J. S., Romet-Lemonne, J. L., Marlink, R.,

McLane, M. F., Lee, T.-H., Arbeille, B., Denis, F., & Essex, M. (1986). New human T-lymphotropic retrovirus related to simian T-lymphotropic virus type III (STLV-III AGM). *Science, 232*, 238–243.

Kanki, P. J., McLane, M. F., King, N. W., Jr., Letvin, N. L., Hunt, R. D., Sehgal, P., Daniel, M. D., Desrosiers, R. L., & Essex, M. (1985). Serologic identification and characterization of a macaque T-lymphotropic retrovirus closely related to HTLV-III. *Science, 228*, 1199–1201.

Kilpatrick, J. (1988, June). *AIDS: What's the big deal?* Universal Press Syndicate.

Kitchen, L. W., Barin, F., Sullivan, J. L., McLane, M. F., Brettler, D. B., Levine P. H., & Essex M. (1984). Aetiology of AIDS-antibodies to human T-cell leukemia virus (type III) in haemophiliacs. *Nature, 312*, 367–369.

Krueger, J., Dinarello, C., Wolff, M., Chedid, L., & Walter, J. (1984). Sleep-promoting effects of endogenous pyrogen (interleukin 1). *American Journal of Physiology, 246*, R994.

Lane, H. C., Depper, J. M., Greene, W. C., Whalen, G., Waldmann, T. A., & Fauci, A. S. (1984). Qualitative analysis of immune function in patients with the Acquired Immunodeficiency Syndrome. *New England Journal of Medicine, 313*, 79–84.

Laurence, J., & Mayer, L. (1984). Immunoregulatory lymphokines of T hybridomas from AIDS patients: Constitutive and inducible suppressor factors. *Science, 225*, 66–69.

Liciw, P. A., Cheng-Mayer, C., & Levy, J. A. (1987). Mutational analysis of the human immunodeficiency virus: The orf-B region down-regulates virus replication. *Proceedings of the National Academy of Sciences of the United States of America, 84*, 1434–1438.

Lifson, J. D., Reyes, G. R., McGrath, M. S., Stein, B. S., & Engleman, E. G. (1986). AIDS retrovirus induced cytopathology: Giant cell formation and involvement of CD4 antigen. *Science, 232*, 1123–1127.

Lyerly, H. K., Matthews, T. J., Langlois, A. J., Bolognesi, D. P., & Weinhold, K. J. (1987). Human T-cell lymphotropic virus IIIB glycoprotein (gp 120) bound to CD4 determinants on normal lymphocytes and expressed by infected cells serves as target for immune attack. *Proceedings of the National Academy of Sciences of the United States of America, 84*, 4601–4605.

Mann, D. L., Lasane, F., Popovic, M., Arthur, L. O., Robey, W. G., Blattner, W. A., & Newman, M. J. (1987). HTLV-III large envelope protein (gp 120) suppresses PHA-induced lymphocyte blastogenesis. *Journal of Immunology, 138*, 2640–2644.

Margolick, J. B., Volkman, D. J., Folks, T. M., & Fauci, A. S. (1987). Amplification of HTLV-III/LAV infection by antigen-induced activation of T-cells and direct suppression by virus of lymphocyte blastogenic responses. *Journal of Immunology, 138*, 1719–1723.

Masters, W. H., Johnson, V. E., & Kolodny, R. E. (1988) *Crisis: Heterosexual behavior in the age of AIDS.* New York: Grone.

Maxey, L., & Gee, G. (1986). *AIDS medical guide.* San Francisco: San Francisco AIDS Foundation.

McGillis, J. P., Hall, N. R., & Goldstein, A. L. (1988). Thymosin fraction 5 (TF5) stimulates secretion of adrenocorticotropic hormone (ACTH) from cultured rat pituitaries. *Life Sciences, 42*, 2259–2268.

McGillis, J. P., Hall, N. R., Vahouny, G. V., & Goldstein, A. L. (1985). Thymosin fraction 5 causes increased serum corticosterone in rodents in vivo. *Journal of Immunology, 134*, 3952–3955.

Miller, D., Green, J., Farmer, R., & Carroll, G. (1985). A "pseudo-AIDS" syndrome following from fear of AIDS. *British Journal of Psychiatry, 146*, 550–551.

Montelaro, R. C., Parekh, B., Orrego, A., & Issel, C. J. (1984). Antigenic variation during persistent infection by equine infectious anemia virus, a retrovirus. *Journal of Biological Chemistry, 259*, 10539–10544.

Narayan, O., Griffen, D., & Chase, J. (1977). Antigenic shift of visna virus in persistently infected sheep. *Science, 197*, 376–378.

O'Grady, M. P., Hall, N. R., & Goldstein, A. L. (1987). Developmental consequences of prenatal exposure to thymosin: Long-term changes in immune and endocrine parameters. *Society of Neurosciences Abstracts, 1380*.

Price, R. W., Brew, B., Sidtis, J., Rosenblum, M., Scheck, A. C., & Cleary, P. (1988). The brain in AIDS: Central nervous system HIV-1 infection and AIDS dementia complex. *Science, 239*, 586–592.

Rabson, A. B., & Martin, M. A. (1985). Molecular organization of the AIDS retrovirus. *Cell, 40*, 477–480.

Rebar, R. W., Miyake, A., Low, T.L.K., & Goldstein, A. L. (1981). Thymosin stimulates secretion of luteinizing hormone-releasing factor. *Science, 214*, 669–671.

Robey, W. G., Safai, B., Oroszlan, S., Arthur, L. O., Gonda, M. A., Gallo, R. C., & Fischinger, P. J. (1985). Characterization of envelope and core structural gene products of HTLV-III with sera from AIDS patients. *Science, 228*, 593–595.

Sarin, P. S., Sun, D. K., Thornton, A. H., Naylor, P. H., & Goldstein, A. L. (1986). Neutralization of HTLV-III/LAV replication by antiserum to thymosin. *Science, 232*, 1135–1137.

Schnittman, S. M., Lane, H. C., Higgins, S. E., Folks, T., & Fauci, A. S. (1986). Direct polyclonal activation of human B lymphocytes by the Acquired Immune Deficiency Syndrome virus. *Science, 233*, 1084–1086.

Sigurdsson, B., Palsson, P. A., & Grimson, M. (1957). Visna, a demyelinating transmissible disease of sheep. *Journal of Neuropathology and Experimental Neurology, 16*, 389–403.

Sodroski, J., Goh, W. C., Rosen, C., Campbell, K., & Haseltine, W. A. (1986). Role of the HTLV-III/LAV envelope in syncytium formation and cytopathicity. *Nature, 322*, 470–474.

Stein, B. S., Gowda, S. D., Lifson, J. D., Penhallow, R. C., Bensch, K. G., & Engleman, E. G. (1987). pH-independent HIV entry into CD4-positive T cells via virus envelope fusion to the plasma membrane. *Cell, 49*, 659–668.

Stewart, S. J., Fujimoto, J., & Levy, R. (1986). Human T-lymphocytes and monocytes bear the same Leu-3 (T4) antigen. *Journal of Immunology, 136*, 3773–3776.

Strebel, K., Daugherty, D., Clouse, K., Cohen, D., Folks, T., & Martin, M. A. (1987). The HIV "A" (sor) gene product is essential for virus infectivity. *Nature, 328*, 728–730.

Terwiliger, E., Sodroski, J. G., Rosen, C. A., & Haseltine, W. A. (1986). Effects of mutations within the 3' orf open reading frame region of human T-cell lymphotropic virus type III (HTLV III/LAV) on replication and cytopathogenicity. *Journal of Virology, 60*, 754–760.

Vahouny, G. V., Kyeyune-Nyombi, E., McGillis, J. P., Tare, N. S., Huang, K.-Y., Tombes, R., Goldstein, A. L., & Hall, N. R. (1983). Thymosin peptides and lymphokines do not directly stimulate adrenal corticosteroid production in vitro. *Journal of Immunology, 30*, 791–794.

Wong-Staal, F. (1987). Molecular biology of the HTLV family. In S. Broder (Ed.), *AIDS: Modern concepts and therapeutic challenges* (pp. 39–52). New York: Marcel Dekker.

Zagury, D., Bernard, J., Leonard, R., Cheynier, R., Feldman, M., Sarin, P. S., & Gallo, R. C. (1986). Long-term cultures of HTLV-III infected T cells: A model of cytopathology of T-cell depletion in AIDS. *Science, 231*, 850–853.

PART III

Theories, Models, and Research on Health, Risk, and Decision Making

As Dr. Osborn points out in Chapter 2, the acquired immuno-deficiency syndrome epidemic is the first in human history in which the transmission of the causative noxious agent is under voluntary control. At the same time, one of the primary behavioral activities that facilitates transmission is usually an extremely pleasurable sexual experience, frequently with a long history of positive reinforcement.

The challenge to the social and behavioral sciences is unprecedented. The magnitude of the challenge to behavioral science is sometimes trivialized as a stopgap measure, of use until basic sciences can develop an effective treatment and/or vaccine. This misconception is widely held by the general public as well as by many in decision-making positions. It ignores the public health dictum that no mass disease afflicting individuals has ever been eliminated solely through attempts at treating affected individuals. It also ignores the high probability that a successful treatment or successful vaccine is either unobtainable or far down the road. Even if a vaccine were available, there would be incredible social problems in deciding who should be vaccinated. Should society offer to vaccinate only specific groups? Should vaccination be required? Because a very large number of intravenous drug users are invisible and a very large number of gay and bisexual men are still closeted, problems of either voluntary or compulsory vaccination seem almost insurmountable. A vaccine for hepatitis B has not been effective in eliminating that disease. Effective treatment strategies for syphilis and gonorrhea have not reduced the incidence of those diseases. Clearly, the mere presence of an effective treatment or vaccine does not ensure elimination of the disease.

So it remains the urgent task of the behavioral sciences to develop effective methods of conveying information that will affect attitudes and belief systems that influence risky health-related behaviors. In some populations, behavioral change has already occurred on the basis of attitudinal change and personal experience with the death of close friends and relatives. But many other groups are less motivated, because of perceived lower risk and/or lack of information. Television and other mass media are hesitant to join in information sharing because of the public's moral perception of information about safer sex and safer injection practices. High-risk sexual activity frequently involves behaviors heretofore not openly discussed. If past behavior is the best predictor of future behavior, the history of sex education in the United States does not generate much optimism for change in sex education curriculums. The addition to sex education courses of relevant information about patterns of same-sex behavior, anal receptive intercourse, rimming, and oral-genital stimulation hardly seems likely for the fifth-grade curriculum. Yet we know that, particularly in some inner cities, children in this age group are sexually active. The challenges confronting behavioral science are awesome.

This section brings together knowledgeable people who have worked in the field of behavior change, particularly self-directed change. Self-directed change clearly is often a function of perception of risk, psychological assessment of costs and benefits, underlying beliefs about the efficacy of change, and relationships among belief, attitudes, intentions, and behavior change. We learn that behavior change in order to be effective must be geared to specific behaviors, and that broad goals and abstractions are not as clearly related to actual behavior. Many of the changes in behavior that are required mean agreement between intimate partners. Partners must choose what it is that is risky that needs to be changed. Weinstein helps us to understand how risk is perceived. Perceptions of personal vulnerability or invulnerability are key elements on the road to changing behavior. Fischhoff helps us to understand how we make decisions, how we order our hierarchy of choices. It is important to remember that in changing AIDS-related behavior it is easier if we begin with distal determinants. It is harder to "just say no" in the bedroom than when the date first begins. Several of the contributors to this section present information on those distal facets of behavior, attitudes and intentions (Kirscht & Joseph; Fishbein & Middlestadt) and self-efficacy (Bandura). The usefulness of these chapters is in how they help us begin to think about and conceptualize the determinants of the behavioral outcomes we are seeking to change.

7

Using the Theory of Reasoned Action as a Framework for Understanding and Changing AIDS-Related Behaviors

Martin Fishbein
Susan E. Middlestadt

According to the U.S. Department of Health and Human Services, the foremost public health problem in the United States is Acquired Immunodeficiency Syndrome. Transmitted primarily through the exchange of body fluids of infected sexual partners and through the use of contaminated equipment by intravenous drug users, there is a fairly general consensus that, at least at the present time, behavior change is the only way to prevent or reduce the spread of the HIV epidemic. Unfortunately, the phrase "at least at the present time" implies that a behavior change approach is merely a temporary, stopgap measure, to be used until a vaccine or cure becomes available. Such a view is shortsighted and dangerous. The availability of hepatitis B vaccine has not eliminated hepatitis, nor has the availability of contraceptive technology eliminated unwanted pregnancies.

Even if a vaccine or cure becomes available, behavioral issues will continue to be important. First, it will continue to be necessary to maintain low-risk and reduce high-risk sexual and drug-use behaviors. Second, it may be necessary to develop behavior change programs to encourage people to make use of medical remedies. In addition, there are many other behavioral questions that will require attention. For example, there are important concerns with respect to providing care for AIDS patients. Not only are we faced with a general problem of ensuring a sufficient number of doctors, nurses, and other health care personnel in the medical profession, but there is the more specific problem of maintaining adequate staff to work with AIDS patients. It will also be necessary to change a variety of behaviors (e.g., health care and sexual behaviors) among those already infected with AIDS and to change or prevent discriminatory and prejudicial behaviors of the general population with respect to persons living with AIDS.

Clearly, the number of behaviors that will have to be addressed in the long-term battle against AIDS is enormous. And we must not lose sight of the fact that we are concerned with behavior, not with populations. It is true that some segments of the population may be more prone to engage in high-risk behaviors, but it is behavior that puts an individual at risk, and not affiliation with any particular racial, religious, or sexual preference group. For this reason, prevention and care will depend upon our ability to influence specific behaviors.

In order to change or maintain any behavior, however, we must first understand the determinants of that behavior. The more that is known about the factors underlying the performance or nonperformance of a given behavior, the greater the probability that successful interventions can be developed to influence it. Despite the general pessimism that often surrounds attempts to understand and change socially relevant behaviors, we would like to argue that there is an empirically supported, systematic, social psychological theory of behavior that provides a framework for identifying and analyzing the factors underlying the performance or nonperformance of any given behavior. In addition, the theory provides guidelines for developing educational communications or other behavior change interventions.

The purpose of this chapter is to show the relevance of this theory to a wide range of AIDS-related behaviors, including the reduction of high-risk and the maintenance of low-risk sexual and drug-use behaviors. In particular, we will try to point out some of the implications of the theory for developing educational or other types of community interventions aimed at changing or maintaining behaviors in this domain.

A Theory of Reasoned Action

The theory of reasoned action (Ajzen & Fishbein, 1980; Fishbein, 1967, 1980) is based on the assumption that humans are reasonable animals who, in deciding what action to take, systematically process and utilize the information available to them. Thus, in the final analysis, changing behavior is viewed primarily as a matter of changing the cognitive structure underlying the behavior in question. According to the theory, different beliefs should underlie different behavioral deci-

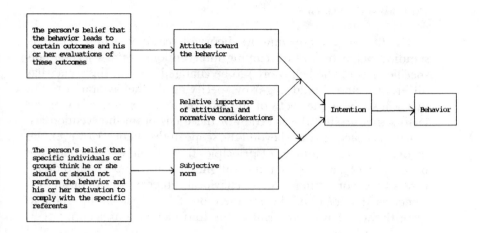

Figure 7.1 A Theory of Reasoned Action: Factors Determining a Person's Behavior
SOURCE: Ajzen and Fishbein (1980, p. 8).
NOTE: Arrows indicate the direction of influence within hypothesized relationships.

sions, and two people making the same behavioral decision could have arrived at this decision on the basis of very different sets of beliefs. It is important to recognize, however, that *although substantive specifics are expected to differ from one behavior and/or from one population to another, the theory argues that most behaviors can be understood in terms of the same small set of theoretical constructs and psychological processes.*

Since the theory has been described in detail elsewhere (e.g., Ajzen & Fishbein, 1980; Fishbein, 1980; Fishbein & Ajzen, 1975), we will provide just a brief overview of the theory as it is currently formulated. The reader is referred to Ajzen and Fishbein (1980) for a complete presentation of the theoretical constructs, the procedures to measure these constructs, and illustrations of the theory's applicability in a number of different content domains.

First introduced in 1967, the theory of reasoned action (Ajzen & Fishbein, 1980; Fishbein, 1967, 1973, 1980; Fishbein & Ajzen, 1975) is a general theory of human behavior that deals with the relations among beliefs, attitudes, intentions, and behavior. In some respects, the theory is best looked at as a series of hypotheses linking (a) behavior to intentions, (b) intentions to a weighted combination of attitudes and subjective norms, and (c) attitudes and subjective norms to behavioral and normative beliefs, respectively. These hypotheses are represented in Figure 7.1 by the arrows between adjoining columns.

The Behavioral Criterion

The first step in applying the theory of reasoned action to understanding behavior and developing interventions is the selection and specification of the behavior(s) to be changed. To put this somewhat differently, one should begin by specifying the behavioral criterion that will serve as the focus of the intervention attempt. Many of the factors that go into the selection of the focus of an intervention are practical aspects that are beyond the scope of the theory. However, the theory specifies a number of principles that, if followed, increase the probability of a successful intervention. First, it is important to designate a behavior, rather than a behavioral category, a goal, or an outcome, as the focus of the intervention. Second, it is important to identify the behavior in terms of the four elements of action, target, context, and time.

Behavior, behavioral categories, goals, and outcomes. Although the theory of reasoned action can provide insights into the performance or nonperformance of categories of behaviors as well as into goal or outcome attainment, its central focus is upon the prediction and understanding of single, directly observable behaviors that are primarily under an individual's control. Unfortunately, distinctions among different types of criteria have often been overlooked; all too often, goals, outcomes, and behavioral categories are treated as "behavioral criteria." To use this theory successfully, it is important to distinguish among an overt, observable action (i.e., a single-act behavioral criterion), an inference based on one or more such acts (i.e., a behavioral category), and an outcome that may result from the performance of one or more behaviors (i.e., a behavioral outcome).

As an illustration of these distinctions, consider the following three criteria: (a) whether or not an individual used a condom the last time he or she had sexual intercourse, (b) whether or not an individual practices "safe" sex, and (c) whether or not an individual is seropositive. Clearly, although HIV serostatus may be treated as a dependent variable in some studies, whether an individual is seropositive or seronegative is not a behavior. Serostatus is an outcome that may be related to the performance of one or more behaviors, but it could also be the result of nonbehavioral factors. For example, as mentioned above, positive serostatus could be a result of engaging in unprotected receptive anal intercourse or of sharing a needle used to inject heroin. However, positive serostatus can also be perinatally transmitted or it can be the result of a transfusion of contaminated blood or blood products. Thus one distinction between behaviors and outcomes is that there are often a number of different behavioral or nonbehavioral paths to the same goal or outcome.

Another, and perhaps more important, distinction between the attainment of goals or outcomes and the performance of a behavior concerns the notion of volitional control. Whether or not an individual reaches a goal or attains some outcome almost always depends not only upon what he or she does, but also upon a variety of other factors (i.e., people, events, circumstances) that are usually outside of the individual's control. Although behaviors also vary in the extent to which they are under an individual's control, the performance or nonperformance of most behaviors of social relevance are typically under the individual's control. For a successful intervention, it is important to select a behavior that the person can perform if he or she wants to, rather than one that depends on factors outside of the person's control.

Turning now to the second criterion, it should be recognized that engaging or not engaging in "safe" sex is also not a behavior, but a category of behaviors. There are many different behaviors that can be classified as "safe" or "unsafe" sex. It is thus possible for two people to define "unsafe" sex in very different ways. This being the case, asking a person whether he or she practices "safe" or "unsafe" sex is not very meaningful. For example, one person might assume that engaging in any type of intercourse without a condom is unsafe, while another may believe that this is true only with respect to anal intercourse. A third person may believe that condoms are necessary only when one doesn't know one's partner; and a fourth might believe that "unsafe" sex is defined as having sex with a gay male or a drug user. From the perspective of the medical community, all of these people may be engaging in high-risk sexual behaviors, yet all might report that they are practicing "safe" sex. Such ambiguity is avoided when one focuses on single, directly observable behaviors. For example, rather than asking about "safe" or "unsafe" sex, one can ask whether or not the individual used a condom the last time he or she engaged in anal, oral, and/or vaginal intercourse.

Identification of the behavior. In addition to selecting a behavior that is under volitional control rather than an outcome or a category of behaviors, it is also necessary to identify the behavior(s) of interest. A full identification of any behavior or behavioral criterion requires consideration of the four elements of action, target, context, and time. That is, every action occurs with respect to some target, in a given context, and at a given point in time. A change in any one of the four elements redefines the behavior of interest.

For example, buying condoms is a behavior different from using condoms, and starting IV cocaine use is different from stopping IV cocaine use (changes in action). Similarly, shooting cocaine is a behavior different from shooting amphetamines, and using a latex condom is different from using a nonlatex condom (changes in target). While most researchers have recognized that changes in action or target define different behaviors, there has been less recognition of the importance of variations in context and time. For example, sharing a needle or using a condom with a long-term primary partner are very different behaviors from performing these same actions with a casual acquaintance. Clearly, one may decide to perform a particular action with respect to a given target in one context but not in another. In the same way, changes in time also change the behavioral criterion under consideration. Not injecting heroin for one week is a very different behavioral criterion from not injecting heroin for one month or for one year; and measuring behavioral change one week from now is assessing a different behavioral criterion than measuring the same behavioral change one month or one year from now.

Although one may arrive at more general behavioral criteria by generalizing across one or more of the elements of action, target, context, and time, it is vital to consider whether each of these elements should be defined at a specific or general level. For example, generalizing across the action element results in a behavioral category rather than a single behavior. As indicated above, this is not recommended as the focus of an intervention unless one is willing to investigate all the actions that make up the category. In contrast, it is often useful to generalize across one or more of the other three elements. For example, it may be more useful to direct an intervention at "always using a latex condom" than at "using a latex condom in a given situation during a given time period." The final choice of a criterion should depend on both the behavioral domain in question and the population toward which the intervention will be directed.

Implications. As discussed above, the full identification of the behavioral criterion in terms of action, target, context, and time is important because changes in any of these elements change the behavior under consideration. And, more important, when one moves from one behavior to another, one also moves from one set of determinants to another. This means that the factors that lead to the initiation of some activity may be very different from those that maintain, increase, decrease, delay, or lead to the cessation of that same activity. For this reason, programs designed to increase (or prevent) the initiation of some activity will often have to be very different from those designed to maintain it, which in turn have to be very different from programs attempting to stop the performance of that activity. Thus an effective change program may be an ineffective maintenance program, and vice versa.

Even worse, the inappropriate use of a change program when a maintenance program is called for, or the inappropriate use of a maintenance program when a change program is called for, may have unwanted negative effects on the targeted behavior. Trying to prevent the initiation of sexual behavior among the sexually active, for example, or trying to reduce drug use among those who have never used drugs, can have unwanted consequences. Unfortunately, inappropriate interventions sometimes take place when attempts are made to transfer an intervention program from one population to another. All too often, programs effective for one age group (e.g., children in ninth or tenth grade) are used for another (e.g., seventh or eighth graders); programs effective in one part of the country are used in other parts of the country; or programs effective among White adolescents are used with Black or Hispanic youth. The fact that the shift from one population to another may mean a shift from a population requiring a prevention or maintenance program (e.g., sexually inexperienced or non-drug users) to one that requires a change program (e.g., sexually experienced or drug users), or vice versa, is sometimes forgotten. Clearly, in developing an effective intervention, it is vital to determine and identify fully the behavior that is most appropriate for the population of interest.

Predicting Behavior from Intentions

Once a behavior has been identified, the theory assumes that the performance or nonperformance of that behavior is primarily a function of the person's intention to perform that behavior. However, just as one must distinguish among behaviors, behavioral categories, and goals, so too must one distinguish among intentions to perform a behavior, intentions to perform a class of behaviors, and intentions to reach a goal or to attain some outcome. In addition, like behaviors, intentions are defined by the four elements of action, target, context, and time. And, for accurate prediction, intentions must correspond to the behavior(s) of interest with respect to all four elements. A final issue in predicting behavior from intentions concerns volitional control.

Intentions to reach goals and to engage in a class of behaviors. In contrast to behavioral intentions, an individual's intention to reach a certain goal or to attain a given outcome is not viewed as the immediate determinant of goal or outcome attainment. As we saw above, goal or outcome attainment is often the result of an individual's performing one or more behaviors plus a number of other factors that are beyond his or her control. Clearly, if the individual does not know what behaviors are most likely to increase (or decrease) the likelihood of achieving some goal and/or if most of the variance in goal attainment is controlled by factors outside of the individual's control, then the intention to achieve that goal will have little to do with actual goal attainment.

Similarly, an individual's intention to engage (or not engage) in a class of behaviors is not viewed as the immediate determinant of whether or not he or she performs one or more of the behaviors in that class. As we saw above, different people may define a behavioral category in different ways; hence a given behavior may not be included in an individual's definition of the category. More important, the person may not know, or may be incorrectly informed about, the behaviors that another person (e.g., a doctor or an AIDS researcher) would include in a given behavioral category (e.g., unsafe sex).

Correspondence of intention and behavior. Clearly, to change or maintain a given behavior, the behavioral intention that corresponds directly (i.e., in terms of action, target, context, and time) to the behavior of interest must be strengthened. For example, if the desired behavior is for a person to use a latex condom every time he or she has sexual intercourse, the person's intention to "use a latex condom every time I engage in sexual intercourse" must be increased, and not his or her intention to "practice safe sex," or to "use a condom," or even to "use a condom every time I engage in sexual intercourse."

Volitional control. It should be obvious, however, that even behavioral intentions do not always predict behaviors. There are many factors that can influence whether or not a measure of intention will permit accurate prediction. We have already seen how lack of correspondence affects the intention-behavior relationship. In addition, just as the individual's lack of control over outcomes serves to reduce the prediction of goal attainment, so the individual's lack of volitional control over some behavior can affect behavioral prediction. When the performance or nonperformance of some behavior is not under an individual's control—that is, when the individual cannot perform (or cannot prevent him- or herself from performing) some action, even if he or she has the desire to perform the action—intentions cannot be expected to serve as primary determinants of behavior. However, as indicated above, most behaviors of social relevance are under volitional control, and thus, under most circumstances, appropriately measured intentions are strongly related to behavior.

Implications. Many educational campaigns and interventions have been unsuccessful because they have not focused directly upon the appropriate intention. All too often, intervention programs attempt to change one or more behaviors by changing people's intentions to reach goals and/or their intentions to perform a class of behaviors. Changing a person's intention to reach a certain goal (e.g., to avoid getting AIDS, to have a long-term monogamous relationship) may have little or no effect on the likelihood that he or she will reach that goal. Similarly, changing a person's intention to engage in a class of behaviors (e.g., to practice safe sex) may have little or no effect on the likelihood that the individual will perform the particular behavior or set of behaviors that one is interested in promoting. To change any given behavior (be it specific or general), one must change the intention that corresponds exactly (in terms of target, action, context, and time) to the behavior in question. Finally, care must be taken to focus on intentions to engage in behaviors that are primarily under volitional control.

Predicting Intentions from Attitudes and Norms

According to the theory of reasoned action, a person's intention to perform any behavior is a function of the person's attitude toward performing the behavior and/or the person's subjective norm concerning his or her performance of the behavior. A person's attitude toward performing a behavior is his or her feeling of favorableness (or unfavorableness) toward performing the behavior in question. A person's subjective norm with respect to the behavior is his or her perception that important others think he or she should (or should not) perform the behavior in question. The relative importance of these two components can vary from behavior to behavior and from population to population.

The discussion to this point is summarized as follows:

$$B \approx I = f[w_1 Ab + w_2 SN] \qquad (1)$$

where B is the behavior of interest (e.g., "using a latex condom every time I engage in sexual intercourse"); I is the intention to perform that behavior (i.e., the likelihood that "I intend to use a latex condom every time I engage in sexual intercourse"); Ab is the attitude toward performing that behavior (i.e., the attitude toward "my using a latex condom every time I engage in sexual intercourse"); SN is the subjective norm concerning this behavior (i.e., the belief that "most of my important others think I should/should not use a latex condom every time I engage in sexual intercourse"); and w_1 and w_2 are the weights (or relative importances) of the attitudinal and normative components, respectively.

Implications. To change or reinforce a given intention, one must change or strengthen the attitude toward performing that behavior and/or the subjective norm with respect to that behavior. Whether one should change the attitude or subjective norm depends upon the relative importance of these two components as determinants of that behavior in that population. It is important to recognize that the relative weights of the attitudinal and normative components are expected to vary from population to population, as well as from one behavior to another. For example, young women's intentions to abstain from sex may be under attitudinal control, while this same behavior may be under normative control among young men. In addition, young women's intentions to have one and only one partner may be under normative control, while attitudinal considerations may underlie this same intention among men. If a behavior is primarily under attitudinal control, attempts to change that behavior through the use of normative pressure will not be very successful. Similarly, if the members of some group perform a given behavior because they believe that their significant others think they should perform the behavior, little will be accomplished by trying to change their attitudes toward performing that behavior.

Unfortunately, these kinds of theoretical considerations are rarely taken into account in determining intervention programs or in message development. Instead, most messages and interventions are constructed somewhat arbitrarily on the basis of intuition and what all too often turn out to be false assumptions about the determinants of the behavior one wishes to change.

The Underlying Cognitive Structure

As indicated above, the theory of reasoned action views behavior change as ultimately being a matter of changing the cognitive structure underlying that behavior. Thus a key in developing a successful intervention is determining and examining the cognitive structure of behavioral beliefs and evaluations underlying the attitude as well as the cognitive structure of normative beliefs and motivations to comply that determine the subjective norm.

Attitude and behavioral beliefs. A person's attitude toward performing a given behavior is a function of the person's salient ("top of the mind") beliefs that performing the behavior will lead to certain outcomes and the person's evaluation of these outcomes. The more the person believes that performing the behavior will lead to positive outcomes (or prevent negative outcomes), the more favorable his or her attitude. Conversely, the more the person believes that performing the behavior will lead to negative consequences (or prevent positive outcomes), the more negative the attitude.

This expectancy-value relationship between attitude and behavioral beliefs is summarized symbolically as follows:

$$Ab = f(\Sigma\, b_i e_i) \qquad (2)$$

where Ab is the person's attitude toward performance of the behavior in question (e.g., "My using a latex condom every time I engage in sexual intercourse"), b is the belief that performance of the behavior will lead to a given outcome, i (e.g., the likelihood that "my using a latex condom every time I engage in sexual intercourse will decrease my sexual pleasure"), e is the person's evaluation of outcome, i (e.g., how good or bad is "a decrease in my sexual pleasure"), and a belief × evaluation cross product is formed for each of n salient outcomes. Note that not all of the possible outcomes of performing a behavior are seen as determinants of the attitude toward the behavior. The determinants of a given attitude in a given population are only those behavioral beliefs that are salient in the population under examination. Furthermore, an individual's attitude toward a behavior is determined by the evaluative implications of the total set of salient beliefs he or she holds; attitudes are not determined by any single belief.

Subjective norm and normative beliefs. A person's subjective norm with respect to a given behavior is a function of his or her normative beliefs that particular salient individuals or groups think that he or she should (or should not) perform the behavior and the person's motivation to comply with those individuals or groups. Generally speaking, if a person believes that most referents with whom she is motivated to comply think she should perform the behavior, she will perceive social pressure to do so. Conversely, if a person believes that most referents with whom he is motivated to comply think he should not perform the behavior, he will have a subjective norm that puts perceived pressure on him to avoid performing the behavior.

The relation between subjective norm and normative beliefs is expressed mathematically as follows:

$$SN = f(\Sigma \; b_j m_j) \qquad (3)$$

where SN is the subjective norm (e.g., the person's belief that "most people who are important to me think I should/should not use a latex condom every time I engage in sexual intercourse"); b is a normative belief that referent j thinks "I should/should not perform the behavior" (e.g., the person's belief that "my parents think I should use a latex condom every time I engage in sexual intercourse"); m is the person's motivation to comply with referent j (e.g., the belief that "with respect to health matters, I want to do what my parents think I should do"); and a normative cross product is formed for each of n salient referents. Again, note that the theory designates that subjective norms are determined by the normative implications of a set of salient normative beliefs rather than by the perceived normative pressure being exerted by any one referent.

Implications. In order to change or reinforce attitudes toward performing a given behavior, one must change or reinforce salient behavioral beliefs and/or their evaluative aspects. Similarly, in order to change or reinforce a subjective norm with respect to a given behavior, one must change or reinforce salient normative beliefs and/or motivations to comply. At this level of analysis, however, there are four main points that should be considered in developing educational messages or other types of interventions.

(1) Salience. Just as one must determine whether a given behavior in a given population is under attitudinal or normative control, one must also identify the behavioral and normative beliefs that underlie the attitude or subjective norm. That is, in order to develop effective interventions, one should first determine the outcomes and referents that are salient for the behavior in the population under consideration. As indicated above, salient outcomes and referents vary from behavior to behavior and, perhaps more important, from population to population. For example, the "top of the mind" consequences a person thinks about when considering using a condom with a long-term primary partner may be very different from those that are salient when considering using a condom with a casual partner. And the outcomes and referents that are salient vis-à-vis either of these behaviors are quite likely to differ depending upon the ethnic or religious status of the population of interest. Thus in applying the theory to a new behavior or with a different population, it is imperative to conduct an elicitation survey to determine the salient outcomes and referents. Unfortunately, very few practitioners identify the behavioral

and/or normative beliefs that are salient in a population *prior* to developing a behavior change campaign.

(2) Selecting target beliefs. Once salient outcomes and referents have been identified, decisions must be made as to which of these behavioral or normative beliefs to target in an intervention. As indicated previously, these decisions should be guided by the relative weights of the attitudinal and normative components. In addition, with respect to either component, it is important to identify those beliefs that discriminate between people who do and do not intend to perform the behavior in question. For example, consider a salient outcome such as "reducing my chances of getting AIDS." It is necessary to determine whether all members of the population are homogeneous with respect to this belief (i.e., do they all believe or do they all disbelieve that "my using a latex condom every time I have sex will reduce my chances of getting AIDS"?). Or, instead, does this belief discriminate between those who do and do not intend to always use a latex condom (i.e., those who intend to always use a latex condom believe that its use will reduce their chances of getting AIDS, while those who do not intend to always use one believe that its use will not reduce their chances of getting AIDS)?

One of the main reasons communications and other forms of interventions fail is that they often do not address appropriate beliefs. For example, messages all too often provide people with information they already have or try to convince them of something they already believe. If most members of a group already believe that performing some behavior will lead to a certain consequence or outcome (e.g., that abstention is the surest way to prevent AIDS, or that sharing a needle increases the risk of AIDS), little will be accomplished by a persuasive communication that focuses upon that information. Similarly, if most members of a group or segment of the population are aware that their parents are strongly opposed to their engaging in sexual intercourse, little will be accomplished by basing an intervention upon parental pressure.

(3) Multiple determinants. Since both attitudes and subjective norms are based on sets of beliefs, a change in any one behavioral or normative belief may not be sufficient to produce a change in attitude or subjective norm. Changing one belief may have an impact on another belief, and, depending upon the direction of this effect, the impact may facilitate or inhibit change. For a successful intervention, one must change the evaluative or normative implication of the underlying cognitive structure (i.e., one must change the value of the attitudinal or normative cross products).

(4) The rule of correspondence. Just as an intention must correspond exactly to the behavior one wishes to predict, change, or understand, so too must attitudes, subjective norms, behavioral beliefs, and normative beliefs correspond with the intention. Thus to change a person's intention to use a latex condom every time he engages in intercourse, one must change that person's attitude or subjective norm with respect to "using a latex condom every time I engage in sexual intercourse"; to do this, one must change the person's beliefs about using a latex condom every time he has intercourse or his beliefs that particular others think he should use a latex condom every time he has sexual intercourse. In sum, behavior change is brought about by producing changes in the correspondent intention, which is in turn created by changing the correspondent attitude and/or subjective norm, which is, in the final analysis, produced by altering a set of correspondent beliefs.

The Role of External Variables

Note that the theory of reasoned action does not include many variables that have traditionally been studied in attempts to explain human behavior in general and preventive health behaviors in particular. We have said nothing about personality, demographic, or other more traditional psychological or sociological variables, such as attitudes toward objects or institutions (e.g., health care), perceived efficacy, and perceived risk. This is not because the theory views these variables as unimportant; rather, it reflects the fact that these types of variables are assumed to influence intentions, and hence behavior, only indirectly.

According to the theory, attitudes and subjective norms are the sole determinants of intentions. The effects of other variables on intention are assumed to be mediated by the attitude toward the behavior, the subjective norm, and/or the relative weights of these components. For example, Black and Hispanic males may differ in their intentions to "always use a condom when I engage in sex." According to the theory, this difference should be due to differences between Black and Hispanic males in (a) their beliefs about the consequences of always using a condom, (b) their evaluations of the consequences, (c) their beliefs about the normative prescriptions of relevant others, (d) their motivations to comply with these relevant others, or (e) the relative weights they place upon attitudinal and normative considerations. Indeed, one advantage of the theory is that it makes it possible to study the locus of effect of one or more external variables.

Although a complete discussion of external variables is beyond the scope of this chapter, it might be useful to consider a set of variables that have often been used to account for people's performance or nonperformance of protective health behaviors. According to the health belief model (see, e.g., Rosenstock, 1974a, 1974b; see also Kirscht & Joseph, Chapter 8, this volume), an individual will be most likely to engage in preventive health behavior if (a) she believes she is personally susceptible to the illness, (b) she believes that the occurrence of the illness would have at least moderately severe consequences and would thus affect some aspect of her life, and (c) she believes that performing the behavior in question would reduce her susceptibility to (or the severity of) the illness without involving a variety of psychological barriers (e.g., cost and inconvenience). For illustrative purposes, let us consider how these three beliefs (about susceptibility, severity, and risk reduction) are viewed from the framework of the theory of reasoned action.

Susceptibility. Susceptibility is not explicitly included within the theory of reasoned action. Instead, it is viewed as a potentially important "external" variable that may or may not have an indirect effect on behavior. In some cases, people who perceive themselves as susceptible to a disease may perceive very different consequences of performing a preventive behavior from those who do not. In other cases, however, susceptibility may be unrelated to behavioral beliefs. Similarly, if one believes one is susceptible, one may perceive more social pressure to perform a preventive behavior than if one believes one is not susceptible. But again, this may not always be the case. According to the theory of reasoned action, susceptibility will influence behavior only if (a) it influences either attitudinal or normative considerations and (b) the component influenced is an important determinant of the intention in question. This helps to explain why the relation between perceived susceptibility and performing health care behaviors varies from study to study and from one behavior to another.

Severity. Like susceptibility, severity is also viewed as an external variable that may or may not be related to any given preventive health behavior. Indeed, everything said above with respect to susceptibility could also be said about severity. For example, with respect to at least some health protective behaviors, people perceiving the disease as very severe might perceive different consequences of performing the behavior from those who perceive little severity. Unlike susceptibility, however, severity is likely to have a more direct tie to behavior in addition to an indirect one. Clearly, the more severe the disease, the greater the value one will place on avoiding that disease. In other words, perceived severity may be highly correlated with one or more outcome evaluations. Recall, however, that the importance of any outcome evaluation (as a determinant of attitude) depends upon (a) its saliency and (b) the strength of the belief that performing the behavior will lead to the outcome. For these and other reasons, one should not expect perceived severity always to be related to the likelihood that an individual will perform a given health protective behavior.

Risk reduction. For all practical purposes, this variable is included within the theory of reasoned action. That is, in the health belief model, the concept of risk reduction refers primarily to beliefs that engaging in the recommended behavior will reduce susceptibility to (or severity of) the disease. In addition, most discussions of risk reduction recognize the importance of a number of associated beliefs about barriers to performing the behavior in question (e.g., beliefs that performing the behavior is expensive or inconvenient). As we have seen, beliefs about performing the behavior in question play a central role in the theory of reasoned action. Recall, however, that according to theory of reasoned action, only those beliefs that are salient in the population under study serve as determinants of the attitude toward performing the behavior. In addition, it must be recalled that some behaviors are primarily under normative rather than attitudinal control. Thus there is no guarantee that the beliefs about performing a behavior that are identified by the health belief model will serve as important determinants of any given behavior.

Implications. Interventions based on the health belief model will often be ineffective. Although under certain circumstances any one of the variables identified by the health belief model may be directly or indirectly related to the performance of a given behavior, one cannot assume that all health beliefs are relevant for all behaviors. In particular, one should not assume that focusing an intervention on perceived susceptibility, severity, or risk will always affect the performance or nonperformance of the particular behavior (or set of behaviors) that one is attempting to change. To maximize the success of an intervention, one must first demonstrate the behavioral relevance of each of the health beliefs one is trying to change.

Concluding Remarks

To summarize, the theory of reasoned action suggests that in order to change or reinforce a given behavior in a given population effectively, we must first determine whether that behavior is under attitudinal or normative control *in that population*, and we must identify the salient beliefs underlying the attitude or subjective norm. That is, we should be aware of what the members of that population already know about performing that behavior, and we should try to identify the beliefs that discriminate between those members of that population who do and do not perform the behavior. In other words, research is needed *before* messages, educational programs, or community interventions are developed.

This does not mean that we need to wait forever before developing educational messages or other intervention programs. That is, we are not proposing large-scale, nationwide surveys. A small elicitation study based on a sample of 30 to 60 members of the population in question can provide invaluable information about the relative importance of attitudes and norms and can identify both salient outcomes of performing the behavior in question and the salient referents for that behavior. These outcomes and referents can then be used to construct a closed questionnaire to obtain the information necessary to identify the salient normative or behavioral beliefs that distinguish between those who do and those who do not intend to perform the behavior(s) of interest. Such a closed questionnaire should assess other variables that will make it possible to test one or more behavioral models fully. It is important to note that by utilizing this questionnaire both before and after the intervention, researchers can obtain all the necessary information for testing (i.e., evaluating) the effectiveness of the messages or interventions that are developed.

What we have tried to point out throughout this chapter is that there are certain types of information that are necessary for developing effective educational communications or other types of interventions. The AIDS epidemic is much too serious to allow interventions to be based upon some communicator's untested and all too often incorrect intuitions about the factors that will influence the performance or nonperformance of a given behavior in a given population.

References

Ajzen, I., & Fishbein, M. (1980). *Understanding attitudes and predicting social behavior.* Englewood Cliffs, NJ: Prentice-Hall.
Fishbein, M. (1967). Attitude and the prediction of behavior. In M. Fishbein (Ed.), *Readings in attitude theory and measurement* (pp. 477–492). New York: John Wiley.
Fishbein, M. (1973). The prediction of behavior from attitudinal variables. In C. D.

Mortensen & K. K. Sereno (Eds.), *Advances in communication research* (pp. 3–31). New York: Harper & Row.

Fishbein, M. (1980). A theory of reasoned action: Some applications and implications. In H. E. Howe & M. M. Page (Eds.), *Nebraska Symposium on Motivation, 1979* (pp. 65–116). Lincoln: University of Nebraska Press.

Fishbein, M., & Ajzen, I. (1975). *Belief, attitude, intention and behavior: An introduction to theory and research.* Reading, MA: Addison-Wesley.

Rosenstock, I. M. (1974a). Historical origins of the health belief model. *Health Education Monographs, 2,* 328–335.

Rosenstock, I. M. (1974b). The health belief model and preventive health behavior. *Health Education Monographs, 2,* 354–386.

8

The Health Belief Model: Some Implications for Behavior Change, with Reference to Homosexual Males

John P. Kirscht
Jill G. Joseph

Introduction

In the relatively brief history of research on health-related behavior, the health belief model has played a significant role. In a critical review, Leventhal, Zimmerman, and Gutmann (1984) note that "the health belief model is the cognitive model most frequently used in studies of health behavior and compliance." The model has also been widely used in the development of interventions aimed at changing health behavior. This chapter is intended to provide an overview of work with the model, along with critical remarks, to note potential applications to the prevention of AIDS, and to present some data derived from a large-scale study of homosexual men. Because several reviews of literature on health beliefs are available (e.g., Janz & Becker, 1984; Kirscht, 1988), we will attempt to illustrate the range and quality of applications, without being comprehensive.

The health belief model developed in the context of applied problems in health education rather than within academic psychology. It was an effort to understand and deal with health behaviors using a few basic dimensions. Four components constitute the essential model: personal susceptibility to a negative health condition, the per-

Authors' Note: The data presented in this chapter came from the Coping and Change Study, supported by a grant (2 RO1 MH39346) from the National Institute of Mental Health.

ceived severity of the condition, the value of a behavior or line of action (variously labeled "benefits," "efficacy," or "effectiveness"), and barriers to the action. Severity of the condition is regarded as all of the significant disutilities seen in the menace to health; barriers represent all of the major costs believed to be associated with actually taking the behavior. Susceptibility as a concept reflects likelihood in the absence of special actions; otherwise it is confounded with benefits. The latter refers to value for threat reduction.

Taken together, the belief elements produce some degree of psychological readiness to act; if the degree of readiness is above threshold, and the environmental conditions permit the action, the behavior is likely to occur or change to be initiated. Although the structure has not been well specified, most studies have treated the model as additive. Some time ago, Rosenstock (1974) wrote that a cue was necessary to initiate action; that the beliefs must become salient is an assumption that seems characteristic of cognitive models of many sorts. In addition, some health belief proponents added other elements, most notably "modifying factors" and self-efficacy beliefs. Modifiers comprised personal and social characteristics, such as age, sex, knowledge, and culture. These can be regarded as exogenous variables. While group differences in beliefs certainly occur, the beliefs themselves must be regarded as the final path to the behavior. Thus the beliefs are assumed to be causal (without excluding their being influenced by behavior) and modifiable. Given that the model deals with health threats, it appears axiomatic that threats arouse coping tendencies, whether these are thought to be adaptive or not. No one thought of the model as predicting a rational decision in a narrow sense; the elements may be far away from objective reality and heavily colored with emotion.

Applications to Health Behavior

A major portion of the work on the model has related to medically oriented preventive and screening behaviors. The beliefs studied have concerned specific disease conditions, such as heart disease or influenza. Much of this research has been reviewed elsewhere (Janz & Becker, 1984; Rosenstock, 1974). While a number of the studies have been retrospective, there are supportive findings from prospective research. Haefner and Kirscht (1970) showed that, following exposure to educational films on heart disease, cancer, and TB, beliefs about the threats and the benefits of acting were increased and were associated with subsequent voluntary checkups. In a prospective study of the swine flu program, Cummings, Jette,

Brock, and Haefner (1979) found that each measure of health beliefs, including susceptibility, severity, benefits of vaccination, and barriers to taking the shot, was related to the action. Intention, however, was the best predictor of behavior, but the beliefs were important predictors of intention in a path model. These same data were used by Brock (1984) to examine relationships over time. Beliefs were most stable for those who did not obtain the shot, as might be expected; susceptibility to swine flu was significantly reduced for the shot-takers. At the same time, the behavior predicted later beliefs better than earlier beliefs predicted behavior.

As part of a study of influenza vaccination in Seattle, Carter, Beach, Inui, Kirscht, and Prodzinski (1986) gathered health belief information from a large group of chronically ill patients, for all of whom flu shots were recommended. In regression analyses, measures of susceptibility, severity, and benefits were significant predictors for both intention (R^2 = .5) and behavior (R^2 = .25). Benefits were by far the best predictor. Largely the same sorts of results were obtained for acceptance of hepatitis B vaccine among hospital workers (Bodenheimer, Fulton, & Kramer, 1986), a program that was affected, in part, by fear about AIDS.

Programs that screen for disease have been studied extensively in terms of the model. A recent study by King (1982) on hypertension found that susceptibility and benefits (but not severity) predicted attendance at screening; intention was the best predictor and was, in turn, related to perceptions of severity and benefits. In contrast, Pirie et al. (1986) report that none of the health beliefs was related to participation in a cardiovascular screening program offered on a community wide basis. Of the several studies on breast self-examination (BSE), results have been inconsistent, although belief in benefits and barriers have been associated with both attendance at instruction (Grady, Kegeles, Lund, Wolk, & Farber, 1983) and practice of the behavior (Calnan & Moss, 1984; Hallal, 1982; Howe, 1981). Susceptibility is sometimes associated with BSE (e.g., Hallal, 1982). In a study of women in Detroit, Ronis and Harel (1986) note that benefits of detection should be related to the perceived threat of the condition, given action or inaction. Their results yielded direct effects of benefits and costs on BSE and indirect effects of severity. Susceptibility had direct effects only, however, and did not interact with severity.

Extension of the health belief model to both illness and sick-role behavior (Becker, 1974) has yielded mixed findings; these will be largely passed over here, as they have been reviewed in detail by Janz and Becker (1984). Use of medical care for symptoms has been related to health beliefs by Leavitt (1979), Berkanovic, Telesky, and Reeder (1981), and Tanner, Cockerham, and Spaeth (1983). Symptom-specific beliefs appear to be predictive of seeking care. Yet, in the many studies concerning compliance with medical treatment, the results are not overly persuasive. In a prospective study on hemodialysis patients, certainly faced with a life-threatening illness, Cummings, Becker, Kirscht, and Levin (1982) found that beliefs regarding benefits and barriers were modestly associated with compliance measures, particularly those involving self-report: "The assumption . . . that an individual decides to comply, or not comply, with a treatment regimen based on beliefs . . . was generally not supported by these data" (p. 578). Kirscht (1988) argues that many aspects of regimens, especially in chronic disease, are strongly habitual, and that different parts of regimens are largely unrelated (e.g., education and appointment keeping).

Many behaviors of great interest to health researchers involve personal habits and characteristics that relate to risk of future disease and do not require medical interventions. Health promotion and disease prevention emphasize control of smoking, diet, use of alcohol, exercise, and safety practices.

In two widely cited studies of preventive health behavior, health beliefs were associated with multicomponent behavioral indexes (retrospectively), but vulnerability was negative in one and nonlinear in the other (Harris & Guten, 1979; Langlie, 1977). Both studies also found only low levels of relationships among the different behaviors studied. Several studies of smoking cessation have utilized health belief variables. Higher levels of vulnerability to health problems have been associated with smoking cessation both retrospectively (Weinberger, Greene, Mamlin, & Jerin, 1981) and prospectively (Kirscht, Janz, & Becker, 1989). In the latter study, the health beliefs, including the benefits of quitting, barriers, perceiving a health problem from smoking, and susceptibility, predicted intention to quit, which, in turn, related to subsequent quitting. On the other hand, Strecher, Becker, Kirscht, Eraker, and Graham-Tomasi (1985) found only an interaction between perceived benefits and barriers to predict change in smoking, with high benefits and lower barriers yielding the most change. In a cohort study of Michigan adults (Kirscht, Brock, & Hawthorne, 1987), beliefs concerning the health value of not smoking did not predict cessation over a two-year period, but did relate to initiation (actually, resumption) of smoking.

Related Work

Health risk appraisal (HRA) has been widely used in connection with programs of health promotion. In its educational aspect, HRA feedback is designed to persuade the individual that those behaviors contributing to elevated risk should be modified, thereby decreasing the risk. It appears to be assumed that risk perceptions will follow analytic feedback that is based on epidemiological evidence. Thus HRA is based on assumptions about health beliefs. Unfortunately, the educational components of the procedure have not been well evaluated. In a study of telephone company employees, we compared groups that received or did not receive feedback and found little difference in subsequent behavior change. Perceptions of susceptibility and of barriers to change were, however, quite consistent with the appraisal (those at higher risk of heart disease saw themselves at higher risk; those not exercising claimed more barriers to activity). In following the participants over six months, we obtained information on attempts to change behaviors. For exercise, weight control, and BSE, there were sufficient numbers of people needing to change. In path models, beliefs regarding benefits and barriers for each of the behaviors were significant predictors of intentions to change, and intent predicted attempts to change prospectively. For exercise, susceptibility to heart disease was also a predictor.

Protection-motivation theory (Rogers, 1983) is closely related to the health belief model and has developed somewhat more explicit hypotheses regarding reactions to threats, as well as providing closer linkages to the literature on attitude change. In the original statement of the theory, protection motivation was a function of the noxiousness of a threat (= severity), the conditional probability that the negative event would happen (susceptibility), and the perceived effectiveness of a coping response (benefits). Revisions to the original formulation incorporated the notion of self-efficacy, that is, belief regarding ability to take the action, and the interplay of adaptive and maladaptive responses. Protection motivation is now a function of threat appraisal and coping appraisal. Actions entailing risk are increased by virtue of associated rewards (e.g., enjoyment of smoking) and decreased by perception of severity of and vulnerability to the associated threat. Actions to decrease risk are strengthened by response efficacy and self-efficacy, and are diminished by response costs. According to Rogers, the level of protection motivation is expected to predict intention to take an action. In this formulation, a more complex set of components is explicitly recognized, and competing action tendencies are encompassed, including ego-defensive ones. Research utilizing this theory has generated some positive findings. Maddux and Rogers (1983), in a study of smokers, found main effects on intentions to quit of benefits, self-efficacy, and vulnerability, but also a three-way interaction among these. Very recently, Wurtele and Maddux (1987) reported generally similar findings in a study of exercise, with vulnerability and self-efficacy showing main effects on intentions, and the same three-way interaction. An interpretation of the interaction is that if self-efficacy is sufficiently high, higher levels of intention to act are generated, even if susceptibility and benefits are not high, reflecting a "precautionary" strategy. These studies, and a recent one on BSE (Rippctoc & Rogers, 1987), illustrate the links of the theory with persuasive communications.

From all this, it can be seen that the health belief model presents a mixed picture as an explanatory framework for health-related behavior. Rarely has there been a confirmation of the full model; more often, different elements are predictive of behavior. Interventions have been designed around the health beliefs in a number of instances (e.g., Carter et al., 1986; Janz et al., 1987). Health beliefs were not the only considerations involved in the development of messages, but they did provide an organizing framework (with, apparently, mixed success). In fact, the health belief model may have significant value as a heuristic device in the development of interventions. Such applications can consider the nature of existing beliefs and what aspects need the most attention.

AIDS-Related Behavior

What, if any, is the potential utility of the health belief model in relation to AIDS, particularly with reference to the behaviors regarded as carrying increased risk for HIV infection? In a very stimulating discussion of why people take actions against health risks, Cleary (1987) points out that our rather simple models have trouble dealing with the very real complexity of behavior, and, particularly in the case of AIDS, cognitive models of health behavior may not encompass the key factors involved or the affective meanings of the relevant concepts and behaviors. Yet, the health belief model is an approach to examining health threats, and AIDS is a threat of monumental proportions. The health belief model does call attention to personal vulnerability and to expectancies held by people as to what actions are implicated in the threat. Further, it points to the value imputed to behavior change of various sorts and, ideally at least, recognizes that there are personal, social, and environmental costs to behavior change. An aspect of health beliefs that has received little attention is the role of uncertainty itself, as an attribute of perceptions of the threat and perceptions of various actions to take. In the realm of AIDS, there seem to be vast areas of uncertainty that are not characteristic of many other health threats, and these undoubtedly affect the health beliefs.

In searching for application of the health belief model to the problem of behavior related to HIV infection, we find rather little in the literature, with a notable exception that will be discussed. Becker and Joseph (1988) provide a very thorough review of the research on behavioral change and on studies of knowledge and attitudes concerning AIDS. Even though, as they note, it is generally assumed that knowledge and attitudes are prerequisites of planned behavior change, few studies thus far have examined such factors. That behavior changes have occurred is apparent from a number of studies. Becker and Joseph conclude that "in some populations of homosexual/bisexual men, this may be the most rapid and profound response to a health threat which has ever been documented" (p. 407). It also should be pointed out that the behavior changes are not simple, but involve an array of different practices that may well be related to diverse predictive factors. At any rate, it is the past, present, and future behavior change that we are trying to understand, as a basis for possible interventions.

The research in Chicago on a cohort of homosexual men by Joseph and her colleagues serves as the focus for discussion of health beliefs and behavior (Joseph, et al., 1987). Nearly 1,000 men were enrolled in the study in 1984–85. After responding to an extensive, self-administered questionnaire at baseline, the participants were asked to complete follow-up instruments at intervals of approximately six months. In addition to detailed assessment of behavior, an array of health belief and sociodemographic items were included. From the former set, indexes of health belief concepts were constructed (see Emmons et al., 1986, for the major indexes). A key measure was that of perceived risk, derived from two questions on "what are your chances of getting AIDS." It should be noted that these items were stated in terms of unconditional probabilities, based on whatever set of factors the individual took into account. In a cross-sectional analysis of the baseline data, the beliefs were examined in relation to reported changes in behavior, including any behavioral change, reduction in number of partners, and avoidance of anonymous partners and of receptive anal intercourse. In logistic regressions, there was a consistent relationship of "knowledge" to behavior change. For the most part, the items in that index can be regarded as beliefs about factors contributing to infection. A general efficacy measure related to behav-

ior change, except for avoiding anonymous contacts. Barriers, as assessed by difficulty controlling impulses, related to not avoiding
anonymous partners. Perceived risk results were very mixed: positive
relationships to any reported change and reducing the number of
partners, but negative to avoiding anonymous partners, and no relationship to receptive anal practices.

Behavior change between the first and second data collection was
the focus of a second report (Joseph, et al., 1987). In these analyses,
perceived risk was the major belief construct studied; a number of
outcomes were examined, including dichotomous measures of behaviors (monogamy, avoiding receptive anal intercourse, and so on) and
analytic measures of numbers of partners, number anonymous, and
number of receptive anal exposures. The findings for the perceived
risk measure defy simple description. At the correlational level, risk
generally related negatively to outcomes for the dichotomous measures, but positively for the analytic measures. For the latter, this
meant that higher levels of risk were associated with more positive
behavior changes. All relationships, however, disappeared when the
initial behavior was introduced into multiple regression analyses, except for the number of anonymous partners, where the regression
coefficient for risk turned significantly negative. No relationship of
the risk measure was found with subsequent health belief scores. In
conclusion, the investigators state, "It appears that baseline behavior
influences both a sense of risk and subsequent behavioral changes" (p.
247). This at least raises the problem of the role of perceived susceptibility in understanding change in behavior.

Further Analyses of the Chicago Data

A wealth of data are available from the Coping and Change Study
conducted in Chicago, including a number of belief measures and
detailed behavioral assessments, providing an excellent opportunity
to explore factors related to changes over time. As documented in
Joseph, et al. (1987), profound changes have occurred in the patterns
of behavior. In addition, the validity of the reported behavior patterns
has been assessed by relating a risk index to seroconversion rates; a
linear relationship was found.

Analyses of health belief predictors of behavior were undertaken to
examine the repeatability of the previously reported results at a later
time, and to assess other health belief measures in relation to behavior
change. Data from the second and third data collections were used for

these purposes. By the third wave (Time 3), data from some 760 participants were available.

A quite complex set of behaviors was tapped in the questionnaire, with detailed accounting of different practices ranging from celibacy to sex with anonymous partners. To simplify the situation, we selected three areas of behavior for the analyses: (a) the number of different male partners in the preceding month, (b) the number of different anonymous partners in the last month, and (c) participation in receptive anal intercourse in the last month. The measures also included reports of (a) efforts to limit the number of partners, (b) whether anonymous partners and receptive anal intercourse were avoided because of concerns about AIDS in the preceding month, and (c) whether condoms were used in receptive anal intercourse. Thus there were analytic measures for numbers of partners, anonymous partners, and receptive anal intercourse and categorical measures of change in three areas, plus condom use. In addition, the summary risk index, a four-category variable, was used.

Measures of health beliefs were derived from various items in the questionnaire. The index of susceptibility (risk perception) reported in Emmons et al. (1986) was used; it is derived from two items on perceived risk of AIDS. Indicators of perceived severity of the condition were constructed from six items concerning whether worry about AIDS interfered with different aspects of life. This index is closely related to measures of negative feeling states deriving from the health threat, and represents reactions to cognitions about AIDS, rather than the more usual cognitive measures of severity. Several indicators of the benefits of change were utilized. An overall benefits item asked how much more the risk of AIDS could be reduced if the respondent did everything possible. Second, those who reported any behavior change to reduce risk (83% of the Time 2 sample) were asked how much they reduced the chance of AIDS ("risk reduction"). In addition, items concerning beliefs about the contribution of specific behaviors (receptive anal intercourse, sex with anonymous partners, and so on) to the chance of developing AIDS were used as indirect measures of the potential benefit of changing the practice. An overall index was derived by taking the mean of the seven items ("knowledge"). With respect to barriers on costs of changes, there was a limited amount in the questionnaire. One general indicator was an item dealing with how stressful it had been to maintain any changes in behavior.

The measures used in the analyses are summarized in Table 8.1. An examination of the associations among the belief measures revealed generally modest relationships. Risk perceptions were associ-

TABLE 8.1

Behavior and Belief Measures

	Level
Behaviors at Time 3	
Number of partners, past month (mean)	3.40 (3.84)[a]
Number of anonymous partners (mean)	1.21 (2.76)[a]
Number of anal exposures (mean)	2.04 (4.86)
Risk Index (1–4 scale)	2.47
Effort to reduce number of partners (%)	90.6
Avoided receptive anal intercourse, past month (%)	55.1
Avoided anonymous sex, past month (%)	64.1
Beliefs at Time 2	
Risk perceptions (mean, two items, 1–5)	2.52
Worry about AIDS (mean, six items, 0–1)	.26
Stress of change (one item, 1–5)	2.40
Knowledge (mean, six items, 1–3)	2.39
Benefits of change (one item, 1–3)	1.97
Risk reduction (one item, 1–5)	3.38
Beliefs about contribution to AIDS (1–3)	
Receptive anal intercourse	2.63
Anonymous partners	2.48

a. Of those with one or more partners.

ated with worry, stress of changing, and benefits of change. There was a fairly strong negative relationship (−.38) with risk reduction, as would be expected. Worry was strongly (.51) related to stress of change. Risk reduction showed a small positive association with both stress and knowledge, but negative with benefits of change. The beliefs about how much behaviors contribute to risk of AIDS were positively (but very modestly) related to stress, worry, and benefits, but unrelated to risk perceptions. Those who engaged in a given behavior, it might be noted, rated the contribution of that behavior to vulnerability to AIDS as significantly less. Generally, then, the belief measures were, with a few exceptions, tapping different content dimensions.

As a first step in relating the belief measures to behavior change, correlations of beliefs to the Time 3 behavioral measures were examined. As might be expected, the number of different partners reported at Time 3 and the number of anonymous partners were closely related (r = .87) and were associated with the same beliefs: positively with risk perceptions and benefits of change, negatively to knowledge, specific contributors to risk, and risk reduction. That risk perceptions related to higher levels of the behaviors during the subsequent six months is consistent with the unexpected but previously reported findings (Joseph, Montgomery, et al., 1987) for an earlier time period. It is somewhat surprising, however, that the item on the benefits of change also related positively to the risky behaviors. Worry and the reported stress of change yielded no relationships to these analytic variables. Risk index at Time 3, the summary measure of behavioral risk, yielded patterns of relationships that were similar to those for number of partners and number of anonymous partners, except for a negative relationship to worry and no relationship to risk perception.

Efforts to reduce the number of partners in the past month, as reported at Time 3, were associated with worry, stress of change, knowledge index, specific contributors to increased risk, and risk reduction. Such efforts were unrelated to risk perceptions and benefits of change. Having no anonymous partners in the past month, also a categorical variable, and including only those who were involved with anonymous partners in the past (or present) was positively related to worry, knowledge, and risk reduction, and negatively related to risk perception; the specific belief concerning how much anonymous partners contribute was also positively correlated with recent avoidance. Thus reported behavior changes generally covaried with health beliefs as expected, with the exception of risk perception.

By contrast, the belief measures employed were virtually unrelated to reported receptive anal intercourse (number of exposures in past month) or avoiding the practice in the past month, or use of condoms in connection with the behavior. A single exception was the association of two specific beliefs about contributors to risk: avoidance in the past month was associated with believing the practice was more of a contributor to susceptibility, and believing anonymous partners were less of a contributor.

In regression analysis, the beliefs yielded patterns of relationship to the outcome measures that were similar to correlational analysis (See Table 2). For number of partners at Time 3, number of anonymous partners, and the risk index, risk perceptions and benefits showed significant positive coefficients, while knowledge and risk reduction yielded negative coefficients. In addition, worry was significantly positive for anonymous partners and risk index, as were beliefs in specific behavioral contributors. When Time 2 behavior measures are introduced into the regressions, many of the coefficients for beliefs become insignificant. Beliefs are no longer predictive of number of partners or risk index score. For anonymous partners, on the other hand, risk perceptions, benefits, worry, and risk reduction remain significant. All predictors of avoidance of anonymous partners remain significant, except for knowledge, when the Time 2 avoidance measure is intro-

TABLE 8.2

Regressions of Behaviors (Quantitative) on Belief Measures: Standardized Coefficients

Belief (Time 2)	Number of Partners	Number of Anonymous Partners	Risk Index
		Behavior (Time 3)	
Risk perception	.190*	.199*a	.102*
Worry	−.062	−.071*a	−.146*
Stress of change	−.030	−.028	−.014
Knowledge	−.162*	−.131*	−.077*
Benefits of change	.182*	.209*a	−.074*
R^2 (beliefs)	.102	.108	.042
N	648	655	675
Risk reduction	.163*	.153*a	.146*
Specific contributions	−.071	−.132*	−.080*

a. Significant coefficient after Time 2 behavior added.
*$p < .05$.

duced as a predictor. This approach to the predictiveness of beliefs is stringent in that it asks what the beliefs can account for after removing the variation in behavior associated with prior behavior (or level of behavior reported previously). This assumes that all of the relationships between beliefs and behavioral levels at the time beliefs are assessed can be attributed to behavior. On the other hand, the approach does provide a test that is definitely prospective.

Discussion

This exercise in predicting behavior change via health belief measures presents a very mixed picture. From the perspective of a model for understanding change, however, there was no real instance in which the set of elements together give a coherent picture of what is happening. Perhaps the best possibility of the model prospectively was in relation to reported efforts at reducing the number of partners. Even here, though, the measure "stress of attempting to change," intended as an indicator of barriers, functioned more as willingness or intent to continue trying. Effort at change is an appropriate dependent variable, since it indicates a trial. As Ajzen (1985) has discussed recently, where uncertainties exist regarding performance of the behavior, whether due to ability, resources, or the environment, the relation of beliefs to outcomes is also more uncertain, and the attempt

TABLE 8.3

Regressions of Categorical Behaviors on Belief Measures: Standardized
Coefficients

	Behavior (Time 3)	
Belief (Time 2)	Avoid Anonymous Partners	Effort to Reduce Number of Partners
Risk perception	−.179*[a]	.006
Worry	.147*[a]	.103*
Stress of change	−.014	.171*
Knowledge	.086*[a]	.101*
Benefits of change	−.172*[a]	.055
R^2 (beliefs)	.087	.078
N	622	592
Risk reduction	.145*[a]	.117*[a]
Specific contributions	.064	.072

a. Significant coefficient after Time 2 behavior added.
* $p < .05$.

becomes a more appropriate variable. Yet prior effort to reduce partners removed much of the covariance of beliefs with Time 3 effort.

Even though the behaviors are highly related, differences in pre-
dictability were found between changing the number of partners and
changing the number of anonymous partners. Worry and risk reduction related positively, and risk perception and benefits of change
related negatively to the latter but not the former. Even more striking is the nearly total lack of relationship of beliefs to any change
relating to receptive anal practices. Are there differences in the role
of personal decisions about the different behaviors? Are some under
greater personal control, or, conversely, more subject to environmental or situational influences?

Both risk perceptions and the benefits of behavior change were
consistently related to subsequent higher levels of potentially risky
behavior. Even taking into account the initial levels of behavior, these
perceptions were significant predictors of the number of anonymous
partners, not avoiding anonymous partners, greater likelihood of stay-
ing in the higher risk category (risk index), and less ability to maintain
a change in behavior. It is unusual to find that beliefs regarding the
effectiveness of behavior change are negatively associated with subsequent change. Analysis of variance of the quantitative behavior scores,
including the risk index, classified by level of belief in the benefits of
behavior change, yielded significant F-values; with increasing belief,

there was a stepwise increase in number of partners, number of anonymous partners, and risk score.

Measures of risk reduction suggest beliefs in the benefits of changing behavior, although they are more closely related to risk perceptions. If we take the results for the risk-reduction beliefs and put them together with the fact that efforts at reducing number of partners is substantially related to past efforts (.44), and avoidance of anonymous partners and of receptive anal contacts relate to past success at avoidance, there emerges a somewhat consistent picture. Perceived success at change is seen as reducing risk, which, in turn, facilitates future behavior change. Some of the data also suggest that lack of success may play a negative role in further change. This sounds familiar in terms of self-efficacy and problems of relapse (Bandura, 1982; Marlatt & Gordon, 1985). Self-efficacy has been a point of contention for the health belief model; some writers strongly suggest incorporating the notion into the model (Strecher, DeVellis, Becker, & Rosenstock, 1986).

What are the implications of these results for behavior change, if any? Meanings of the perception of risk or vulnerability to health threats can follow several paths. They reflect many different facets of the problem, including the past, the future, communication and information, self-protection and despair. In the context of AIDS and sexual behavior, very specific risk perceptions need to be investigated. Similarly, beliefs about the benefits of change may carry negative information, and a much clearer understanding of the costs that are incurred in behavior change is required, including short-term and long-term costs to both self and others. As with other areas of change in risky habits, information on the specifics of change and its maintenance is needed.

Similar considerations apply to attempts to modify behaviors. Their results are not so much at issue as is the interpretation made by those who try. What is the meaning of failure or success? It appears that success, as seen by the individual, is an important component in relation to beliefs that will sustain the effort. Again, the importance of reductions in cost and rewards for maintenance of behavior change comes to the fore. From the data we have examined thus far, we are impressed with the dynamic and complex nature of the processes involved in behavior change. In this situation, the health belief model has useful features, but it requires synthesis with other frameworks for change.

References

Ajzen, I. (1985). From intentions to actions: A theory of planned behavior. In J. Kuhl & J. Beckmann (Eds.), *Action control: From cognition to behavior* (pp. 12–39). New York: Springer-Verlag.

Bandura, A. (1982). Self-efficacy mechanism in human agency. *American Psychologist, 37*, 122–147.

Becker, M. (Ed.). (1974). The health belief model and personal health behavior. Thorofare, NJ: Charles B. Slack.

Becker, M., & Joseph, J. (1988). AIDS and behavioral change to reduce risk. *American Journal of Public Health, 78*, 394–410.

Berkanovic, E., Telesky, M., & Reeder, S. (1981). Structural and social psychological factors in the decision to seek medical care for symptoms. *Medical Care, 19*, 693–709.

Bodenheimer, H., Fulton, J., & Kramer, P. (1986). Acceptance of hepatitis B vaccine among hospital workers. *American Journal of Public Health, 76*, 252–255.

Brock, B. (1984). *Factors influencing intentions and behavior toward swine flu vaccine.* Unpublished doctoral dissertation, University of Michigan.

Calnan, M., & Moss, S. (1984). The health belief model and compliance with education given at a class in breast self-examination. *Journal of Health and Social Behavior, 25*, 198–210.

Carter, W., Beach, L., Inui, T., Kirscht, J., & Prodzinski, J. (1986). Developing and testing a decision model for predicting influenza vaccination compliance. *Health Services Research, 20*(6, Pt. II), 897–932.

Cleary, P. (1987). Why people take precautions against health risks. In N. Weinstein (Ed.), *Taking care: Understanding and encouraging self-protective behavior.* Cambridge: Cambridge University Press.

Cummings, K., Becker, M., Kirscht, J., & Levin, N. (1982). Psychosocial factors affecting adherence to medical regimens in a group of hemodialysis patients. *Medical Care 20*, 567–580.

Cummings, K., Jette, A., Brock, B., & Haefner, D. (1979). Psychosocial determinants of immunization behavior in a swine influenza campaign. *Medical Care, 17*, 639–649.

Emmons, C., Joseph, J., Kessler, R., Wortman, C., Montgomery, S., & Ostrow, D. (1986). Psychosocial predictors of reported behavior change in homosexual men at risk for AIDS. *Health Education Quarterly, 13*, 331–345.

Grady, K., Kegeles, S., Lund, A., Wolk, C., & Farber, N. (1983). Who volunteers for a breast self-examination program? Evaluating the bases for self-selection. *Health Education Quarterly, 10*, 79–94.

Haefner, D., & Kirscht, J. (1970). Motivational and behavioral effects of modifying health beliefs. *Public Health Reports, 85*, 478–484.

Hallal, J. (1982). The relationship of health beliefs, health locus of control, and self-concept to the practice of breast-self-examination in adult women. *Nursing Research, 31*, 137–142.

Harris, D., & Guten, S. (1979). Health protective behavior: An exploratory study. *Journal of Health and Social Behavior, 20*, 17–29.

Howe, H. (1981). Social factors associated with breast self-examination among high risk women. *American Journal of Public Health, 71*, 251–255.

Janz, N., & Becker, M. (1984). The health belief model: A decade later. *Health Education Quarterly, 11*, 1–47.

Janz, N., Becker, M., Kirscht, J., Eraker, S., Billi, J., & Woolliscroft, J. (1987). Evaluation of a minimal-contact smoking cessation intervention in an outpatient setting. *American Journal of Public Health, 77*, 805–809.

Joseph, J., Montgomery, S., Emmons, C., Kirscht, J., Kessler, R., Ostrow, D., Wortman, C., O'Brien, K., Eller, M., & Eshleman, S. (1987). Perceived risk of AIDS: Assessing the behavioral and psychosocial consequences in a cohort of gay men. *Journal of Applied Social Psychology, 17*, 231–250.

Joseph, J., Ostrow, D., Montgomery, S., Kessler, R., Phair, J., & Chmiel, J. (1987, June). *Behavioral risk reduction in a cohort of homosexual men at risk for AIDS: A two-year longitudinal study.* Paper presented at the Third International Conference on AIDS, Washington, DC.

King, J. (1982). The impact of patients' perceptions of high blood pressure on attendance at screening. *Social Science and Medicine, 16*, 1079–1091.

Kirscht, J. (1988). The health belief model and predictions of health actions. In D. Gochman (Ed.), *Health behavior: Emerging research perspectives* (pp. 27–41). New York: Plenum.

Kirscht, J., Brock, B., & Hawthorne, V. (1987). Cigarette smoking and changes in smoking among a cohort of Michigan adults, 1980–82. *American Journal of Public Health, 77*, 501–502.

Kirscht, J., Janz, N., & Becker, M. (1989). Psychosocial predictors of change in cigarette smoking. *Journal of Applied Social Psychology, 19*, 298–308.

Langlie, J. (1977). Social networks, health beliefs, and preventive health behavior. *Journal of Health and Social Behavior, 18*, 244–260.

Leavitt, F. (1979). The health belief model and utilization of ambulatory care services. *Social Science and Medicine, 13A*, 105–112.

Leventhal, H., Zimmerman, R., & Gutmann, M. (1984). Compliance: A self-regulation perspective. In D. Gentry (Ed.), *Handbook of behavioral medicine* (pp. 369–436). New York: Guilford.

Maddux, J., & Rogers, R. (1983). Protection motivation and self-efficacy: A revised theory of fear appeals and attitude change. *Journal of Experimental Social Psychology, 19*, 469–479.

Marlatt, A., & Gordon, J. (Eds.). (1985). *Relapse prevention.* New York: Guilford.

Pirie, P., Elias, W., Wackman, D., Jacobs, D., Murray, D., Mittelmark, M., Luepker, R., & Blackburn, H. (1986). Characteristics of participants and nonparticipants in a community cardiovascular risk factor screening: The Minnesota Heart Health Program. *American Journal of Preventive Medicine, 2*, 20–25.

Rippetoe, P., & Rogers, R. (1987). Effects of components of protection motivation theory on adaptive and maladaptive coping with a health threat. *Journal of Personality and Social Psychology, 52*, 596–604.

Rogers, R. (1983). Cognitive and physiological processes in fear appeals and attitude change: A revised theory of protection motivation. In J. Cacioppo & R. Petty (Eds.), *Social psychophysiology: A sourcebook* (pp. 153–176). New York: Guilford.

Ronis, D., & Harel, Y. (1986). *Health beliefs and breast examination behaviors: Analyses of linear structural relations.* Unpublished manuscript.

Rosenstock, I. (1974). Historical origins of the health belief model. *Health Education Monographs, 2*, 328–335.

Strecher, V., Becker, M., Kirscht, J., Eraker, S., & Graham-Tomasi, R. (1985). Psychosocial aspects of changes in cigarette-smoking behavior. *Patient Education and Counseling, 7*, 249–262.

Strecher, V., DeVellis, B., Becker, M., & Rosenstock, I. (1986). The role of self-efficacy in achieving health behavior change. *Health Education Quarterly, 13*, 73–92.

Tanner, J., Cockerham, W., & Spaeth, J. (1983). Predicting physician utilization. *Medical Care, 21*, 360–369.

Weinberger, M., Greene, J., Mamlin, J., & Jerin, M. (1981). Health beliefs and smoking behavior. *American Journal of Public Health, 71*, 1253–1255.

Wurtele, S., & Maddux, J. (1987). Relative contributions of protection motivation theory components in predicting exercise intentions and behavior. *Health Psychology, 6*, 453–466.

9

Perceived Self-Efficacy in the Exercise of Control over AIDS Infection

Albert Bandura

Prevention of infection with the AIDS virus requires people to exercise influence over their own motivation and behavior. Social efforts designed to control the spread of AIDS have centered mainly on informing the public on how the human immunodeficiency virus (HIV) is transmitted and how to safeguard against such infection. It is widely assumed that if people are adequately informed about the AIDS threat they will take appropriate self-protective action. Heightened awareness and knowledge of health risks are important preconditions for self-directed change. Unfortunately, information alone does not necessarily exert much influence on refractory health-impairing habits.

To achieve self-directed change, people need to be given not only reasons to alter risky habits but also the means and resources to do so. Effective self-regulation of behavior is not achieved by an act of will. It requires certain skills in self-motivation and self-guidance (Bandura, 1986). Moreover, there is a difference between possessing coping skills and being able to use them effectively and consistently under difficult circumstances. Success, therefore, requires not only skills, but also strong self-belief in one's capabilities to exercise personal control.

Perceived self-efficacy is concerned with people's beliefs that they can exert control over their motivation and behavior and over their

Author's Note: This research was supported by Public Health Research Grant MH-5162–25 from the National Institute of Mental Health. This chapter is an abridged version of a chapter on this topic originally published in S. J. Blumenthal, A. Eichler, and G. Weissman (Eds.), *Women and AIDS*. Washington, DC: American Psychiatric Press, 1989. Correspondence concerning this chapter should be addressed to Albert Bandura, Department of Psychology, Jordan Hall, Building 420, Stanford University, Stanford, CA 94305, USA.

social environment. People's beliefs about their capabilities affect what they choose to do, how much effort they mobilize, how long they will persevere in the face of difficulties, whether they engage in self-debilitating or self-encouraging thought patterns, and the amount of stress and depression they experience in taxing situations. When people lack a sense of self-efficacy, they do not manage situations effectively even though they know what to do and possess the requisite skills. Self-inefficacious thinking creates discrepancies between knowledge and action.

Numerous studies have been conducted linking perceived self-efficacy to health-promoting and health-impairing behavior (Bandura, 1986, 1989; O'Leary, 1985). The results show that perceived efficacy can affect every phase of personal change—whether people even consider changing their health habits, how hard they try should they choose to do so, how much they change, and how well they maintain the changes they have achieved. In addition to influencing health habits, perceived coping inefficacy increases vulnerability to stress and depression and activates biochemical changes that can affect various facets of immune function (Bandura, 1989; Maier, Laudenslager, & Ryan, 1985).

Translating health knowledge into effective self-protection action against AIDS infection requires social skills and a sense of personal power to exercise control over sexual situations. As Gagnon and Simon (1973) have correctly observed, managing sexuality involves managing interpersonal relationships. Problems arise in following safer sex practices because self-protection often conflicts with interpersonal pressures and sentiments. In these interpersonal situations the sway of coercive power, allurements, desire for social acceptance, social pressures, situational constraints, and fear of rejection and personal embarrassment can override the influence of the best of informed judgment. The weaker the perceived self-efficacy, the more such social and affective factors can increase the likelihood of risky sexual behavior.

In managing sexuality, people have to exercise influence over themselves as well as over others. This requires self-regulatory skills in guiding and motivating one's actions. Self-regulation operates through internal standards, affective reactions to one's conduct, use of motivating self-incentives, and other forms of cognitive self-guidance. Self-regulatory skills thus form an integral part of risk-reduction capabilities. They partly determine the social situations into which people get themselves, how well they navigate through them, and how effectively they can resist social inducements to potentially risky behavior. It is easier to wield control over preliminary choice behavior that may lead to troublesome social situations than to try to extricate oneself from such situations. This is because the antecedent phase involves mainly anticipatory motivators that are amenable to cognitive control; the entanglement phase includes stronger social inducements to engage in high-risk behavior that are less easily manageable.

The route of heterosexual transmission of AIDS is mainly via bisexuals and intravenous drug users infected by sharing contaminated needles. Control of the spread of the AIDS virus by intravenous drug users requires risk-reduction strategies aimed at both drug and sexual practices.

Components of Effective Self-Directed Change

An effective program of widespread change in detrimental lifestyle practices includes four major components. The first is informational, designed to increase people's awareness and knowledge of health risks. The second component is concerned with development of the social and self-regulatory skills needed to translate informed concerns into effective preventive action. The third component is aimed at skill enhancement and building resilient self-efficacy by providing opportunities for guided practice and corrective feedback in applying the skills in high-risk situations. The final component involves enlisting social supports for desired personal changes. Let us consider how each of these four components would apply to self-directed change of behaviors that pose high risk of AIDS infection.

Informational Component

The preconditions for change are created by increasing people's awareness and knowledge of the profound threat of AIDS. They need to be provided with a great deal of factual information about the nature of AIDS, its modes of transmission, what constitute high-risk sexual and drug practices, and how to achieve protection from infection. This is easier said than done. Our society does not provide much in the way of treatment for drug addiction, nor is it about to provide refractory drug users with easy access to sterile needles and other drug paraphernalia.

Society has little experience in how to reach and educate drug users on how to disinfect needles to reduce the risk of AIDS infection. In the sexual domain, our society has always had difficulty talking frankly about sex and imparting sexual information to the public at large. Since parents generally do a poor job of it as well, most young-sters pick up their sex education from other, often less trustworthy and reputable, sources outside the home or from the consequences of uninformed sexual experimentation. To complicate matters further, some sectors of the society lobby actively for maintaining a veil of silence regarding protective sexual practices, in the belief that such information will promote indiscriminate sexuality. In their view, the remedy for the spreading AIDS epidemic is a national celibacy cam-paign for unweds and gays and faithful monogamy among the wed-ded. They oppose educational programs in the schools that talk about sex methods that provide protection against AIDS infection. The net result is that many of our public education campaigns regarding AIDS are couched in desexualized generalities that leave some igno-rance in their wake. To those most at risk, such sanitized expressions as "exchange of bodily fluids" not only are uninformative but may invest safe bodily substances with perceived infective properties. Even those more skilled in deciphering medical locutions do not always know what the preventive messages are talking about. For example, an intensive campaign spanning a full week was conducted on the Stanford University campus, including public lectures, numerous panel discussions, presentations in dormitories, and condom distribu-tion, all of which were widely reported in the campus newspaper. A systematic assessment of students' beliefs and sexual practices con-ducted several weeks later revealed that more than a quarter of the students did not know what constitutes "safer sex," and some of them had misconceptions of safer sex practices that, in fact, would present high risk of infection. Other findings of this study, which will be reviewed below, underscore the severe limitations of efforts to change sexual practices through information alone.

The informational component of the model of self-directed change includes two main factors—the informational content of the health communications and the mechanisms of social diffusion. Detailed fac-tual information about AIDS must be socially imparted in an under-standable, credible, and persuasive manner. Social cognitive theories provide a number of guidelines on how this might best be accom-plished (Bandura, 1986; McGuire, 1984; Zimbardo, Ebbesen, & Maslach, 1977). However, developing effective AIDS prevention pro-grams is only the first step; they must also be disseminated. Unlike other health risk-reduction campaigns that involve relatively prosaic habits, the risky habits associated with AIDS infection are laden with matters of illegalities and judged immoralities.

Informative health messages, however well designed, cannot have much social impact without effective means of dissemination. Because of their wide reach and influence, the mass media, especially television, can serve as a major vehicle of social diffusion of information regarding health guidelines. However, a variety of diffusion vehicles must be enlisted in a public health campaign for several reasons. High costs and restricted access to television limit its availability. Moreover, television networks typically adopt a conservative stance on controversial matters. They have resisted getting into the act for fear that talk of protective sex practices will jeopardize advertising revenue by arousing the wrath of some sectors of their viewing audience. This resistance may eventually weaken as the AIDS virus is increasingly transmitted heterosexually, thus making it a more general societal problem rather than one confined to gays and drug users. However, it is unlikely that the television industry will offer much help if AIDS becomes mainly a disease of poor minorities. Existing social, religious, recreational, occupational, and educational organizations can serve as highly effective disseminators of preventive health guidelines. Wide cultural diversity requires that the messages of risk-reduction campaigns for AIDS be tailored to socioeconomic, racial, and ethnic differences in value orientations and disseminated through multiple sources to ensure adequate exposure (Mantell, Schinke, & Akabas, 1989). Nontraditional social networks must be enlisted for high-risk groups who are beyond the reach of the usual community organizations. For example, in an educational program in San Francisco, "street-wise" counselors have been highly successful in reaching drug populations (Watters, 1987). After they become known in the social circles of drug users, the counselors help them with referrals to drug treatment programs. They offer explicit instruction in safer sex practices. They teach intravenous drug users how to reduce the risk of AIDS by disinfecting needles with ordinary household bleach, which kills HIV. The disinfection procedure, which rarely had been used before, was widely adopted and consistently applied. Although this outreach program also increased the use of condoms, the drug users were much more conscientious in disinfecting needles than in protecting their sexual partners against sexually transmitted infection. Such findings underscore the need for sexual partners to exercise personal control in protecting their own health.

A comprehensive national program regarding the growing AIDS threat must address broader social issues as well as risky health practices. This is because the AIDS epidemic has far-reaching social repercussions. One of these issues concerns the widespread public fear of AIDS infection. Many people continue to believe that the AIDS virus can be transmitted by casual contact or by insect transmission and food handling, despite evidence to the contrary. Efforts by health professionals to dispel misapprehensions are discounted by many of those who are alarmed on the grounds that what is proclaimed safe currently may be discovered to be risky later. Fear gets translated into advocacy of laws requiring sweeping mandatory blood testing and identification and social restriction of those with antibodies to HIV.

As AIDS imposes mounting financial burdens on society and strains medical and social service systems, members of high-risk groups may become targets of growing public hostility. Once entire groups become stigmatized because some of their members behave in high-risk ways, those who do not also become the objects of fear and hostility. The way in which they are treated socially may be dictated more by group identity than by their personal characteristics. Public alarm, fueled by many misbeliefs, enhances such stigmatization. Policy debates on how to control the spread of AIDS have become highly politicized. Prohibitionists argue that public health campaigns promote indiscriminate sex. Their critics argue that knowledge does not foster sexuality and that prohibitionists are intent on curtailing sex practices they find morally objectionable rather than concerned with increasing the safety of sex. Uninformed public reactions to the AIDS threat require serious attention, as do the risky health practices themselves, because they help to shape public policies and impose constraints on health education programs.

Development of Self-Protective Skills and Controlling Self-Efficacy

It is not enough to convince people that they should alter risky habits. Most of them also need guidance on how to translate their concerns into efficacious actions. In the Stanford survey mentioned above, after exposure to an intensive educational campaign, less than half of the students who were sexually active used safer sex methods designed to prevent infection with sexually transmitted diseases. Most of them even avoided talking about the matter with their sexual partners. Studies conducted on other campuses similarly reveal that most sexually active students who are knowledgeable about AIDS do not adopt safer sex practices (Edgar, Freimuth, & Hammond, 1988). McKusick, Horstman, and Coates (1986) found that gay men were uniformly well-informed about safer sex methods for protecting against AIDS infection, but those who had a low sense of efficacy that they could manage their behavior and sexual relationships were unable to act on their knowledge.

The ability to learn through social modeling provides a highly effective method for increasing human knowledge and skills. A special power of modeling is that it can simultaneously transmit knowledge and valuable skills to large numbers of people through the medium of videotape. Knowledge of modeling processes identifies a number of factors that can be used to enhance the instructive power of modeling. Applications of modeling principles to AIDS prevention would focus on how to manage interpersonal situations and one's own behavior in ways that afford protection against infection with the AIDS virus. Both self-regulatory and risk-reduction strategies for dealing with a variety of situations would be modeled to convey general guides that can be applied and adjusted to fit changing circumstances.

As mentioned earlier, human competency requires not only skills but also self-belief in one's capability to use those skills well. Indeed, results of numerous studies of diverse health habits and physical dysfunctions reveal that the impact of different methods of influence on health behavior is partly mediated through their effects on perceived self-efficacy (Bandura, 1989). The stronger the self-efficacy beliefs instilled, the more likely people are to enlist and sustain the effort needed to change habits detrimental to health. Modeling influences should, therefore, be designed to build self-assurance as well as to convey rules for how to deal effectively with troublesome situations. The influence of modeling on beliefs about one's capabilities relies on comparison with others. People judge their own capabilities, in part, by how well those whom they regard as similar to themselves exercise control over situations. People develop stronger belief in their capabilities and more readily adopt modeled ways if they see models similar to themselves solve problems successfully with the modeled strategies than if they see the models as very different from themselves (Bandura, 1986). To increase the impact of modeling, the characteristics of models—such as their age, sex, and status, the type of problems with which they cope, and the situations in which they apply their skills—should be made to appear similar to those of the group one is trying to reach.

Enhancement of Social Proficiency and Resilience of Self-Efficacy

Proficiency requires extensive practice, and this is no less true of managing the interpersonal aspects of sexuality. After people gain knowledge of new skills and social strategies, they need guidance and opportunities to perfect those skills. Initially, people practice in simulated situations, where they need not fear making mistakes or appearing inadequate. This is best achieved by role playing in which they practice handling the types of situations they have to manage in their social environments. They then receive informative feedback on how they are doing and the corrective changes that need to be made. The simulated practice is continued until the skills are performed proficiently and spontaneously. Not all the benefits of guided practice are due to skill improvement. Some of the gains result from raising people's beliefs in their capabilities. Experiences in exercising control over social situations serve as self-efficacy builders. This is an important aspect of self-directed change, because if people are not fully convinced of their personal efficacy they undermine their efforts in situations that tax capabilities and readily abandon the skills they have been taught when they fail to get quick results or when they suffer reverses. The important matter is not that difficulties rouse self-doubts, which is a natural immediate reaction, but rather the degree and speed of recovery from setbacks. It is resilience in perceived self-efficacy that counts in maintenance of changes in health habits. The higher the perceived self-efficacy, the greater the success in maintenance of health-promoting behavior (Bandura, 1989).

The influential role played by perceived self-efficacy in the management of sexual activities is documented in studies of contraceptive use by teenage women at high risk because they often engage in unprotected intercourse (Levinson, 1982). Such research shows that perceived self-efficacy in managing sexual relationships is associated with more effective use of contraceptives. The relationship remains when controls are applied for demographic factors, knowledge, and sexual experience.

Gilchrist and Schinke (1983) applied the main features of the multicomponent model of personal change to teach teenagers how to exercise self-protective control over sexual situations. The subjects received essential factual information about high-risk sexual behavior and self-protective measures. Through modeling, they were taught how to communicate frankly about sexual matters and contraceptives, how to deal with conflicts regarding sexual activities, and how to resist unwanted sexual advances. They practiced applying these social skills by role playing in simulated situations, and received instructive feedback. The program significantly enhanced perceived self-efficacy and skill in managing sexuality.

Research by Kelly, St. Lawrence, Hood, and Brasfield (1989) attests to the substantial value of self-regulatory programs for AIDS risk reduction. Gay men were taught—through modeling, role playing, and corrective feedback—how to exercise self-protective control in sexual relationships and to resist coercions for high-risk sex. Multifaceted assessments showed that they became more skillful in handling sexual relationships and coercions, markedly reduced risky sexual practices, and used condoms on a regular basis. These self-protective practices were fully maintained in follow-up assessments. In contrast, matched control subjects continued to engage in unprotected high-risk sexual practices.

Combining factual information about health risks with development of risk-reduction efficacy produces good results. Because people learn and perfect effective ways of behaving under lifelike conditions, problems of transferring the new skills to everyday life are reduced. The mastery-modeling approach is readily adaptable in audio- or videocassette format to self-protective behavior with regard to AIDS. Large-scale applications of self-instructional programs sacrifice the guided role-playing component. However, instruction in imaginal rehearsal, in which people mentally practice dealing with prototypic troublesome situations, boosts perceived self-efficacy and improves actual performance (Bandura, 1986; Kazdin, 1978). The self-instructional approach, designed in a format suitable for mass distribution, has been shown to achieve some success in changing other refractory health-impairing behaviors (Sallis et al., 1986).

Because of the high level of unprotected sexual activity and experimentation with drugs by teenagers, they are vulnerable to becoming the new high-risk group as transmitters of the AIDS virus (Mantell & Schinke, 1989). Training materials need to be developed to assist parents and teachers in educating youngsters about AIDS. The mastery-modeling program developed by Gilchrist and Schinke (1983) provides a good prototype for application in schools. However, other channels of dissemination must be created to reach teenagers because of factional opposition to educational efforts in the schools that address self-protective behavior in an explicitly informative manner. A major segment of the teenage population can be reached by making informative audiotapes and videocassettes readily available in the settings they frequent, such as record and video stores.

Social Supports for Personal Change

People effect self-directed change when they understand how personal habits threaten their well-being, are taught how to modify them, and believe in their capabilities to marshal the effort and resources needed to exercise control. However, personal change occurs within a network of social influences. Depending on their nature, social factors can aid, retard, or undermine efforts at personal change. This is especially true in the case of sexual and drug practices.

People who are fully informed on the modes of HIV transmission and effective self-protective methods acquire the virus only if they allow it to happen. They often allow it to happen because interpersonal, sociocultural, religious, and economic factors operate as constraints on self-protective behavior. Some of those most at risk must contend with sociocultural obstacles to the use of prophylactic methods that afford protection against HIV infection. The major burden for self-protection against sexually transmitted diseases usually falls on women. Unlike protection against pregnancy, where women can exercise independent control, use of condoms requires them to exercise control over the behavior of men. Those men who possess coercive power over their partners resist the use of condoms if, in their view, it reduces their sexual pleasure, threatens their sense of manliness and authority, casts aspersions on their faithfulness, or carries the frightening implication that they may be carriers of disease. It is difficult for women to press the issue in the face of emotional and economic dependence, coercive threat, and subcultural prescription of compliant roles for them. Women who are enmeshed in relationships of imbalanced power need to be taught how to negotiate protected sex nonconfrontationally. At the broader societal level, attitudes and social norms must be altered to increase men's sense of responsibility for the consequences of their sexuality.

Risk reduction through alteration of subcommunity norms is an especially important vehicle for curbing the spread of AIDS among intravenous drug users. This is because drug use is often a socially shared activity. Restricted access to drug injection equipment and the legal problems of being caught with it promote risky common use of drug paraphernalia. "Shooting galleries" involving widespread sharing of contaminated needles provide the most fertile ground for spreading the virus. Preventive efforts aimed at drug subcultures show that drug users are reachable and instructable in safer practices. Thus provision of protective information by outreach workers about AIDS transmission, needle-exchange programs, and instruction on how to sterilize needles can substantially reduce risky injection practices, thus lowering infection rates among those who continue the drug habit (Des Jarlais, 1988; Watters, 1987). Needle-exchange programs do not propagate drug use, as some people have feared it might (Buning, van Brussel, & van Santen, 1988). As Des Jarlais notes, most drug users now know about the modes of AIDS transmission, but many are inadequately informed or misinformed about risk-reduction techniques. For example, some dutifully wash needles in solutions that do not kill the virus. Although the subcommunity approach also serves as an excellent vehicle for enlisting drug users in treatment programs, there is not much that outreach workers can offer them because of the scarcity of treatment services.

Social influences rooted in indigenous sources generally have greater impact and sustaining power than those applied by outsiders for a limited time. A major benefit of community-mediated programs is that they can mobilize the power of formal and informal networks of influence for transmitting knowledge and cultivating beneficial patterns of behavior. A community-mediated approach is a potentially powerful vehicle for promoting both personal and social change in several ways. It provides an effective means for creating the motivational preconditions of change, for modeling requisite skills, for enlisting natural social incentives for adopting and maintaining beneficial habits, and for establishing protective practices as the normative standards of conduct. Generic principles of effective programs are readily adaptable at the subcommunity level to sociocultural differences in the populations being served. In the social diffusion of new behavior patterns, indigenous adopters usually serve as more influential exemplars and persuaders than do outsiders. Moreover, behavioral practices that create widespread health problems require group solutions that are best achieved through community-mediated efforts.

In their pioneering health-promoting programs, Farquhar and Maccoby have drawn heavily on existing community networks for transmitting knowledge and cultivating beneficial patterns of health behavior (see, e.g., Farquhar, Maccoby, & Solomon, 1984). This work provides a model of how to mobilize community resources to disseminate health information and to convey explicit guides on how to change refractory health habits. A program of self-directed change should be applied in ways designed to create self-sustaining structures within the community for promoting behavioral practices conducive to health. Persons in the community, who serve as local organizers, are taught how to design, coordinate, and implement the programs. Teaching communities how to take charge of their own changes fosters self-directedness at the community level as well as at the personal level.

The substantial reduction of high-risk sexual practices by gay subgroups was achieved largely through effective self-empowering organization. They educated themselves, made safer sex practices the social norm, devised their own instructional programs to prevent HIV transmission, established mechanisms for diffusing this knowledge, issued regular updates on new research findings and available treatments, created social support systems to counteract despair and encourage meaningful life pursuits, and actively fostered life-style changes that might enhance immune function in those infected with the virus but not yet experiencing any symptoms. There have been some attempts at self-mobilization by drug-user subgroups for self-protective change, but these have been less successful (Friedman, de Jong, & Des Jarlais, 1988). Lack of educational and financial resources, illegalities surrounding drug activities, mistrust, and the large amount of time devoted to supporting the drug habit impede efforts at self-organization. These conditions create a greater need for external aid in subgroup organization for risk reduction.

Attitudinal Impediments to Development of Psychosocial Models

Several attitudes exist that downgrade the priority for the development of psychosocial approaches to this deadly epidemic. One such view trivializes psychosocial approaches by regarding them as merely stopgap measures to be used until a vaccine is discovered. The AIDS virus appears in many forms; it mutates rapidly, invades immune cells, and not only evades destruction by the body's defense system but turns infected cells into producers of more viruses and destroys the very cells that provide protective immunity. It remains latent for long periods, and it may become more virulent over time. Considering these baffling biological properties, the quest for a vaccine that will provide protective immunity against the changing forms of this virus is likely to be a lengthy and frustrating one. Because viruses merge genetically into the host cells, the task of developing antiviral treatments that can kill the AIDS virus without destroying the host immune cells is a formidable one.

Even the more limited goal of keeping the condition in check with antiviral drugs that do not produce serious toxicogenic side effects presents an immense challenge. Sexually transmitted diseases such as gonorrhea and syphilis, which have been with us for ages, have thwarted vaccine development. Whether our advanced biotechnology will triumph over the AIDS virus or the mutable virus will foil our biotechnology remains to be seen. In any event, AIDS will remain with us for a long time to come.

Another downgrading view rests on the belief that psychosocial influences cannot effect much change in the transmissive risky behaviors because they serve potent drives. Amenability of behavior to change differs considerably depending on whether one seeks to eliminate certain kinds of gratifications or to alter the means of gaining those gratifications. It is much more difficult to get people to relinquish behavior that is powerfully reinforced than it is to get them to adopt safer forms of the behavior that serve the same function. In the case of AIDS prevention, people who are not about to give up drugs or their preferred forms of sexuality can achieve substantial protection against HIV infection by substituting safer behaviors for risky ones. Multifaceted psychosocial programs that equip people with protective knowledge, with the means and self-beliefs to exercise effective personal control, and provide social supports for their efforts at personal change can achieve highly beneficial results. Indeed, prevention programs that incorporate many of these elements have produced substantial reductions in risky sexual and drug-injection behaviors. Neglect or downgrading of psychosocial models for AIDS prevention will exact heavy personal tolls and impose mounting financial and social burdens on society.

References

Bandura, A. (1986). *Social foundations of thought and action: A social cognitive theory*. Englewood Cliffs, NJ: Prentice-Hall.

Bandura, A. (1989). Self-efficacy mechanism in physiological activation and health-promoting behavior. In J. Madden IV, S. Matthysse, & J. Barchas (Eds.), *Adaptation, learning and affect*. New York: Raven.

Buning, E. C., van Brussel, G.H.A., & van Santen, G. (1988). Amsterdam's drug policy and its implications for controlling needle sharing. In R. Battjes & R. Pickens (Eds.), *Needle sharing among intravenous drug abusers: National and international perspectives* (Research Monograph Series No. 80, pp. 59–74). Bethesda, MD: National Institute on Drug Abuse.

Des Jarlais, D. C. (1988). *Effectiveness of AIDS educational programs for intravenous drug users*. Unpublished manuscript, State of New York, Division of Substance Abuse Services.

Edgar, T., Freimuth, V. S., & Hammond, S. L. (1988). Communicating the AIDS risk to college students: The problem of motivating change. *Health Education Research, 3*, 59–65.

Farquhar, J. W., Maccoby, N., & Solomon, D. S. (1984). Community applications of behavioral medicine. In W. D. Gentry (Ed.), *Handbook of behavioral medicine* (pp. 437–478). New York: Guilford.

Friedman, S. R., de Jong, W. M., & Des Jarlais, D. C. (1988). Problems and dynamics of organizing intravenous drug users for AIDS prevention. *Health Education Research, 3*, 49–57.

Gagnon, J., & Simon, W. (1973). *Sexual conduct: The social sources of human sexuality.* Chicago: Aldine.

Gilchrist, L. D., & Schinke, S. P. (1983). Coping with contraception: Cognitive and behavioral methods with adolescents. *Cognitive Therapy and Research, 7*, 379–388.

Kazdin, A. E. (1978). Covert modeling: Therapeutic application of imagined rehearsal. In J. L. Singer & K. S. Pope (Eds.), *The power of human imagination: New methods in psychotherapy. Emotions, personality, and psychotherapy* (pp. 255–278). New York: Plenum.

Kelly, J. A., St. Lawrence, J. S., Hood, H. V., & Brasfield, T. L. (1989, in press). Behavioral intervention to reduce AIDS risk activities. *Journal of Consulting and Clinical Psychology.*

Levinson, R. A. (1982). Teenage women and contraceptive behavior: Focus on self-efficacy in sexual and contraceptive situations (Doctoral dissertation, Stanford University, 1982). *Dissertation Abstracts International, 42*, 4769A.

Maier, S. F., Laudenslager, M. L., & Ryan, S. M. (1985). Stressor controllability, immune function, and endogenous opiates. In F. R. Brush & J. B. Overmier (Eds.), *Affect, conditioning, and cognition: Essays on the determinants of behavior* (pp. 183–201). Hillsdale, NJ: Lawrence Erlbaum.

Mantell, J. E., & Schinke, S. P. (1989). The crisis of AIDS for adolescents: The need for preventive risk-reduction interventions. In A. R. Roberts (Ed.), *Contemporary perspectives on crisis intervention and prevention.* Englewood Cliffs, NJ: Prentice-Hall.

Mantell, J. E., Schinke, S. P., & Akabas, S. H. (1988). Women and AIDS prevention. *Journal of Primary Prevention, 9*, 18–40.

McGuire, W. J. (1984). Public communication as a strategy for inducing health-promoting behavioral change. *Preventive Medicine, 13*, 299–319.

McKusick, L., Horstman, W., & Coates, T. J. (1986). *AIDS and sexual behavior of gay men in San Francisco.* Unpublished manuscript, University of California, San Francisco.

O'Leary, A. (1985). Self-efficacy and health. *Behavior Research Therapy, 23*, 437–451.

Sallis, J. F., Hill, R. D., Killen, J. D., Telch, M. J., Flora, J. A., Girard, J., & Taylor, C. B. (1986). Efficacy of self-help behavior modification materials in smoking cessation. *American Journal of Preventive Medicine, 2*, 342–344.

Watters, J. K. (1987). *Preventing human immunodeficiency virus contagion among intravenous drug users: The impact of street-based education on risk-behavior.* Unpublished manuscript, San Francisco.

Zimbardo, P. G., Ebbesen, E. B., & Maslach, C. (1977). *Influencing attitudes and changing behavior.* Reading, MA: Addison-Wesley.

10

Perceptions of Personal Susceptibility to Harm

Neil D. Weinstein

As researchers investigate illnesses, natural disasters, and environmental and occupational hazards, they often identify precautions that can reduce individuals' susceptibility to harm. Yet people often fail to take these precautions. They suffer disease and injury that could have been avoided.

If the benefits of a preventive measure are uncertain and the burden of change substantial, it is not surprising that few people respond. But there are also situations, such as with acquired immunodeficiency syndrome, in which the chance of death for those continuing high-risk actions is considerable, the argument for self-protective action appears unequivocal, and yet prevention action is still limited. It sometimes seems that people think they are invulnerable.

The failure to acknowledge personal vulnerability has long been thought to be a barrier to the adoption of precautions. In fact, recent investigations do show that people tend to be unrealistically optimistic about their own susceptibility to harm (Kamler & Stone, 1988; Kulik & Mahler, 1987; Larwood, 1978; Perloff & Fetzer, 1986; Svenson, Fischhoff, & MacGregor, 1985; Weinstein, 1980, 1982, 1984, 1987). They may not claim that they are invulnerable, but they do claim that their chances of suffering negative events are smaller than the chances of their peers.

The goal of this chapter is to examine some of the factors that shape beliefs about risk susceptibility, to describe errors and optimistic biases in these beliefs, and to discuss the relationship between perceived susceptibility and precautionary behavior.[1] Many of the find-

---

Author's Note: The suggestions made by Peter Guernaccia, Karolynn Siegel, and Ann O'Leary during the preparation of this chapter are gratefully acknowledged.

142

ings will be drawn from my own research. This chapter is not specifically about perceptions of susceptibility to AIDS, but it does attempt to provide background that will help researchers understand how people react to all types of hazards and to suggest possible applications to AIDS prevention efforts.

Before beginning these topics, however, two other issues will be addressed briefly. The first is a warning about the many motivations for self-protective behavior that are not considered here. The second concerns the relationship between two key concepts, an individual's overall feeling of threat and his or her specific belief about the likelihood of personal harm.

Motivations Governing Risk-Relevant Behaviors

When professionals concerned with public health and safety study a hazard or promote a particular preventive measure, the goal of risk reduction is uppermost in their minds. It is natural for them to assume that the public is also concerned with the matter of risk, that if people change their behavior it is to lower their risk, and that if people do not follow recommendations it is because they underestimate the risk. But there are many motives that determine behavior, and the motives that shape particular risk-relevant behaviors may have nothing to do with risk reduction. Condoms, for example, may reduce the risk of AIDS transmission, but their use is also tied up with the desire to maximize sexual satisfaction, to demonstrate trust in one's partner, and to appear intelligent and sophisticated.

Theoretical models that are capable of fully explaining risk behaviors and of guiding us to effective behavior change strategies must reflect all the motives involved in a particular situation (Cleary, 1987). To discourage smoking among adolescents, for example, it may be more important to increase the ability to withstand peer pressure than to provide additional information about the dangers of cigarettes (for references, see Hansen, Malotte, & Fielding, 1988). Because drug use or sexual contact is involved in nearly all AIDS transmission, it should be obvious that hazard reduction is only one motive to be considered. In fact, motivations associated with drugs and sexuality (including the interpersonal pressures associated with these behaviors) may be more powerful than the desire to avoid risk.

Risk issues will probably be most important to the early adopters of new preventive measures. It is their desire for threat reduction that leads these individuals to engage in behaviors that are not normative.

When precautions become more widely accepted, however, social influence is likely to take precedence as the determinant of precautionary behavior. This chapter, however, will deal only with risk issues, that is, risk perceptions and their relationship to self-protective behavior.

The Threat of Harm

Most current models of individual preventive action see behavior change as the consequence of a decision about the costs and benefits of different options (Becker & Maiman, 1983; Cleary, 1987; Maddux & Rogers, 1983; Pagel & Davidson, 1984; Rogers, 1983; Wallston & Wallston, 1984; Weinstein, 1988). In these theories, the principal benefit sought from taking a precaution is a reduction in the magnitude of the threat. Thus the perception of threat and the expectation of threat reduction are the stimuli for self-protective behavior. Models in which fear, rather than cognitive expectations of threat reduction, drives protective action (see Janis, 1967; Leventhal, Safer, & Panygris, 1983) are employed much less frequently in research, perhaps because they do not provide predictions about the amount of fear produced by different hazards. Fear and fear reduction are not considered by the decision-oriented models.[2]

The cost-benefit theories usually describe the perceived magnitude of a threat in terms of two variables: *Perceived susceptibility* refers to the likelihood of experiencing personal harm if no action is taken; *perceived severity* denotes the amount of harm that will be experienced if the illness or event does occur. The importance of these two components appears self-evident. In probability theory, too, they form the optimum measure of threat, since the average outcome over many risky events is given by the product of event likelihood and magnitude (severity). If one were programming a computer to gamble, likelihood times magnitude would be the measure of threat that would yield the greatest winnings. Two forms of cost-benefit models, expectancy-value theories (such as the theory of reasoned action: Ajzen & Fishbein, 1980; Fishbein, 1980; Fishbein & Ajzen, 1975) and subjective expected-utility theories (e.g., Beach, Campbell, & Townes, 1979; Edwards, 1954; Sutton, 1982), assume that people use this multiplicative rule to calculate the size of the threat. It has also been suggested (Leventhal et al., 1983; Wallston & Wallston, 1984) that the multiplication of perceived severity by perceived likelihood is implicit in the health belief model (Becker, 1974; Janz & Becker, 1984; Maiman & Becker, 1974; Rosenstock, 1974).

Though these theories have had considerable success in predicting preventive behavior, questions about the way they treat the threat of harm remain. Two questions that will be explored in the following paragraphs concern the way in which likelihood and severity are combined and roles of other hazard attributes in shaping perceptions of threat.

Combining Risk Likelihood and Risk Severity

Do people combine severity and likelihood to create a composite measure of threat magnitude as described in these models? Although the multiplication of these two variables leads to "optimal" decisions, decision analysts no longer believe that people always combine likelihood and severity in this way (Fischhoff, Goitein, & Shapira, 1982; Schoemaker, 1982). For examples, terms such as "satisficing" and "elimination by aspects" have been coined to denote processes in which hazard attributes are considered one at a time (Beach & Mitchell, 1978; Kuhl, 1982; Svenson, 1979).

When hazard attributes enter into a decision in some sort of sequential fashion, it no longer makes sense to speak of the magnitude of the threat as if it were a single quantity. The profile of these different qualities, not just their sum, product, or other combination, determines the decision. For example, Kruglanski and Klar (1985) suggest that severity is considered first. Below some minimum level of severity, hazards get little attention. Once severity passes this threshold, this variable is no longer important and behavior is governed only by the perceived probability of harm. Because the severity of AIDS is widely recognized, this rule would suggest that differences in perceptions of threat are shaped only by differences in beliefs about personal susceptibility to AIDS. Kruglanski and Klar's idea is consistent with the finding that perceived severity is not a good predictor of preventive behavior in studies of serious health problems (Janz & Becker, 1984).

Although investigators have identified a variety of multiattribute strategies that people use to handle complex decision problems, the relevance of these strategies to everyday precautionary behavior is uncertain. Understandably, decision researchers tend to study choices (usually laboratory-posed dilemmas) in which the competing options are well described; the risk probabilities, risk severities, and precaution payoffs are all fully explained to subjects. Real-world situations, in contrast, are often messy. The alternatives and their consequences are usually poorly described, probabilities are uncertain, and detailed information is difficult or impossible to obtain. For most health and safety problems, people may be forced to use simpler decision rules and a vaguer overall notion of threat magnitude. The fact that we commonly speak of problems as "serious," "dangerous," or "threatening" suggests that global appraisals of hazards are natural to us.

Determinants of Threat Perceptions

In addition to questioning how people combine perceptions of severity and likelihood, there is also the issue of other threat characteristics to which people may respond. It seems likely that hazard appraisal reflects many factors, not just the two variables prescribed by probability theory. In real life, people often appear to acquire their notion of a threat's seriousness directly from acquaintances or from the mass media rather than deriving it from separate beliefs about likelihood and severity. For instance, many people believe that refined sugar is unhealthy (and act in accordance with this belief) without having the slightest idea of the diseases that might be caused, the likelihoods of these diseases, or their severities. Community groups often object to mental health centers, chemical plants, and AIDS treatment facilities without appearing to have thought about the likelihood that negative consequences will occur. Risk is not just an individual judgment, but also a social and cultural construct reflecting values, symbols, history, and ideology (Johnson & Covello, 1987).

Among the additional variables that might heighten perceptions of threat are any that increase salience (such as vivid images and frequent reminders). Thus people who have clear mental images of the ways in which asbestos fibers lodge in lung tissue and eventually cause disease may see this hazard as more threatening than people who have the same abstract information about probability and severity but lack an image of the disease-inducing process. AIDS may be perceived as especially threatening because schemas of infectious disease transmission are familiar, making the possibility of infection seem concrete and plausible.

Since salience influences many social processes (Nisbett & Ross, 1980), it would be surprising if it did not influence hazard response as well. Hazards that receive a lot of press attention tend to be rated as more risky (Lichtenstein, Slovic, Fischhoff, Layman, & Combs, 1978). Furthermore, decisions about hazards are influenced by the ways in which the problems are "framed" or presented (Slovic, Fischhoff, &

Lichtenstein, 1982; Tversky & Kahneman, 1981). Stating the probability of death, for example, makes a hazard seem more serious than stating the probability of survival, though the actual information is identical. Informing people that there is a 10% chance of acquiring AIDS from a particular behavior makes this behavior seem more risky than speaking of the 90% chance that they will not be infected. A study by Larson, Olsen, Cole, and Shortell (1979) bearing upon the issue of salience showed that reminders could increase self-protective behavior even when they did not affect beliefs about likelihood and severity.

A distinct "risk perception" literature (Cole & Withey, 1981; Schwartz, White, & Hughes, 1985; Slovic, Fischhoff, & Lichtenstein, 1985; Vaughan, 1986; Von Winterfeldt, John, & Borcherding, 1981) has grown up around the study of the disagreements between the judgments of experts and ordinary citizens (especially disagreements over the safety of nuclear power). This research has been concerned with policy and public opinion rather than with self-protective behavior. Investigators working in this tradition have identified many different hazard characteristics that influence estimates of the risk presented by diverse technologies, chemicals, occupations, and recreational activities.

Participants in these investigations are typically asked "to consider the risk of dying (across all U.S. society as a whole) as a consequence of this activity or technology" (Slovic et al., 1985, p. 93). Experts tend to respond to this question in terms of the actual fatality rate; their answers correlate highly with fatality statistics, reflecting risk probabilities. The public's answers indicate a broader conception of risk, varying not only with the fatality rate, but also with other hazard attributes, especially those that form a "dread risk" dimension. Dread risks are those rated high on the following scales: dread, certain to be fatal, risk is increasing, affects me personally, threat to future generations, globally catastrophic, risks and benefits inequitably distributed, and involuntary. AIDS seems to be an example of a dread risk, since it would rate high on several of these scales. The dread risk dimension may help to explain why people at very low risk often show extreme reactions when they think others are exposing them to AIDS. They protest treatment centers for infants with AIDS and refuse to work near someone who has AIDS.

Some hazard attributes that do not affect ratings of risk include whether or not effects are delayed, the newness of the risk, and whether or not the risk is understood by science (Slovic et al., 1985).

Other researchers have studied additional hazard characteristics that may affect risk perceptions (reviewed in Vaughan, 1986).

It seems likely that some of these attributes also influence perceptions of personal risk. However, people can distinguish between the social problems that they think are important and the problems that affect them personally. In surveys, for example, individuals who report being very concerned about crime tend to mean that they believe crime is a serious social problem, not that they are frightened by the threat of criminal victimization in their own lives (Furstenberg, 1971; see also Tyler & Cook, 1984). Just because people rate a technology, chemical, or activity as risky for society, and suggest that society should take measures to reduce the risk, does not automatically mean that they would be motivated to take self-protective measures. Consequently, the risk perception literature should be viewed as a source of hypotheses rather than as a set of proven relationships about the factors that govern perceptions of personal threats and influence personal preventive behavior.

Perceptions of Personal Vulnerability

For the purpose of explaining protective behavior, it is not yet clear whether the threat of AIDS and other real-life hazards should be viewed as a single, composite quantity or as a complex entity with several irreducible attributes. Neither is it clear how many different attributes affect threat perceptions. Nevertheless, one attribute, personal susceptibility, is included in almost all major theories of preventive action (Cummings, Becker, & Maile, 1980) and there are abundant data showing that perceptions of susceptibility are often closely related to precautionary behavior (Becker, 1974; Drabek, 1986; Janz & Becker, 1984; Kunreuther, 1978; Skogan, 1981). Unless other motivations intrude, people seldom take precautions when they believe that they are not at risk.[3]

If beliefs about personal vulnerability were accurate reflections of objective reality, this section of the chapter could be quite short. But subjective and objective risk are quite separate matters. In everyday life, it is often impossible to determine our own objective risk of harm. Aggregate statistics about automobile fatalities, for example, are readily available. But do these numbers apply to me? What is my own risk considering the type of car I drive, the distance I travel, the traffic I experience, my driving style and reflexes, and the extent to which I use alcohol? For AIDS, the difficulties of estimating personal susceptibility are even more severe. Most information about hazards comes from the mass media or from acquaintances. It refers to people in general or to major subgroups of the population, not to us as individuals, and it contains only crude hints about the effects of various risk factors on the probability of harm.

Given this ambiguity, it would not be surprising if perceptions of personal susceptibility were frequently in error. The errors, however, do not seem to be random. People tend to show a consistent optimistic bias; they think that their own vulnerability to harm is less than that of their peers.

Assessing Personal Susceptibility and Optimistic Bias

Although researchers have measured the perceived magnitude of many probability terms, deriving numerical equivalents for "unlikely," "probable," "seldom," and so forth (Wallsten & Budescu, 1983; Wallsten, Budescu, Rapoport, Zwick, & Forsyth, 1986), their findings do not provide clear guidance about the response scales that are best for eliciting beliefs about event likelihood. Laboratory experiments in decision making use quantitative scales that are essentially continuous. In community controversies, however, people often act as though risk is a dichotomy—either negligible or serious—and show little interest in information about degrees of risk. The scales used in research investigations demonstrate this full range, from two categories to an infinite number of gradations.

Like many researchers, I am skeptical of the public's ability to understand risk probabilities and prefer to use ordinal scales with a limited number of labeled categories. In my own studies respondents typically have the following options: no chance, very unlikely, unlikely, moderate chance, likely, very likely, and certain to happen.

Because accurate risk probabilities for individuals are usually unobtainable, it is difficult to determine whether someone's risk estimates are in error. However, if comparative, rather than absolute, risk judgments are gathered, it is easy—on a group basis—to demonstrate the existence of an optimistic or pessimistic bias. If a randomly selected group of people report their beliefs on a scale that ranges from −3 (much below average) to +3 (much above average), with zero (average for men or women my age) as the midpoint, the mean of the responses should lie at zero if there is no systematic bias. Those who claim below-average risk should be balanced by those who admit above-average risk. If the mean is significantly less than zero, it indicates an optimistic bias, a consistent tendency to view one's own risk as less than the risk faced by others. Means significantly greater than zero indicate a pessimistic bias.

Another way to demonstrate optimistic tendencies is to compute comparative risk estimates from two absolute risk scales, one asking about the individual's own risk, the second referring to a broader category of people to which the individual belongs. The difference between the two responses can be analyzed for optimistic or pessimistic tendencies according to the procedure described in the preceding paragraph.

To compare these two approaches for assessing optimistic biases, I asked the members of a college class in health psychology (n = 82) to give comparative risk judgments for 16 different health and safety problems. The students in the health psychology class the following semester (n = 60) used two absolute risk scales for each problem (the same problems used the semester before). One scale indicated their own risk and the other scale referred to the chances for an average college student.[4] Within each class, the mean score (mean difference score for the second class) was calculated for each hazard. The correlation across the 16 problems for these two different indicators of bias was .84, demonstrating that the amount of bias associated with a given problem is insensitive to the measurement method used. (AIDS elicited one of the largest optimistic biases among the hazards considered, with group means of −1.6 and −1.8 from the comparative risk scales and from the separate absolute risk scales, respectively.)

Extent of Optimistic Bias

Data collected in a growing number of investigations of a wide range of health and safety hazards and other negative life events show that unrealistic optimism is the norm (Kamler & Stone, 1988; Kulik & Mahler, 1987; Larwood, 1978; Perloff & Fetzer, 1986; Svenson et al., 1985; Weinstein, 1980, 1982, 1984, 1987). Optimism in comparative risk judgments is insensitive to age, sex, education, or occupational status (Weinstein, 1987). Table 10.1 shows the optimistic bias present in the comparative risk ratings of a diverse community sample (Weinstein, 1987). Clearly, whatever impression people receive from the media, friends, and public health messages about the likelihood of harm from negative life events, they tend to believe that their own risk is smaller. There is evidence that perception of the risk of AIDS follows this pattern. Several groups of researchers have reported that gay men tend to regard themselves as less likely to develop AIDS than

TABLE 10.1

Comparative Risk Judgments for Health Problems
and Other Hazards

Hazard	Mean	Standard Deviation
Drug addiction	-2.17	1.63
Drinking (alcohol) problem	-2.02	1.47
Attempting suicide	-1.94	1.69
Asthma	-1.36	1.38
Food poisoning	-1.25	1.43
Poison ivy rash	-1.19	1.73
Sunstroke	-1.17	1.53
Nervous breakdown	-1.15	1.56
Homicide victim	-1.14	1.50
Gallstone	-0.84	1.23
Deaf	-0.82	1.49
Pneumonia	-0.80	1.29
Lung cancer	-0.77	1.77
Skin cancer	-0.77	1.44
Cold sores	-0.77	1.53
Senile	-0.76	1.23
Laryngitis	-0.71	1.40
Gum disease	-0.69	1.49
Tooth decay	-0.58	1.38
Insomnia	-0.57	1.65
Ulcer	-0.55	1.40
Mugging victim	-0.54	1.45
Diabetes	-0.53	1.77
Overweight 30 or more pounds	-0.40	2.09
Influenza (flu)	-0.31	1.07
Stroke	-0.29	1.40
Serious auto injury	-0.27	1.24
Heart attack	-0.24	1.55
Arthritis	-0.24	1.52
Falling and breaking a bone	-0.10	1.27
High blood pressure	-0.02	1.57
Cancer	0.08	1.33

SOURCE: Weinstein (1987).
NOTE: Comparative risk judgments could range from -3 ("much below average") to +3 ("much above average"). A mean less than zero indicates an optimistic tendency to claim that one's risk is less than average. Significance levels refer to t-tests of the hypothesis that the mean is different from zero. N = 87–104.

are other gay men (Bauman & Siegel, 1987; Joseph et al., 1987; McKusick, Horstman, & Coates, 1985).

Although optimism is prevalent, the amount of bias varies greatly from hazard to hazard. The causes of this variation will be examined in a later section.

Downward Comparisons

There are two basic processes that could lead people to claim below-average susceptibility: They could underestimate their own risk (exaggerating the efficacy of their own preventive actions and denying the significance of personal risk-increasing factors), or they could exaggerate the risk of "average" individuals, comparing themselves with people unusually high in risk. The two processes might occur simultaneously. Without accurate individual-level data about risk, it is very difficult to distinguish errors in personal risk estimates from the choice of an inappropriate, high-risk reference point, a "downward comparison."

There is evidence, however, that people do engage in downward comparisons for risk judgments, choosing as reference points people who are particularly high in risk (Hakmiller, 1966; Perloff & Fetzer, 1986; Wills, 1981; Wood, Taylor, & Lichtman, 1985). Wood et al. (1985), for example, report that women with breast cancer tend to compare themselves to others whose disease (or associated problems) is more serious. Perloff and Fetzer (1986) found that when they asked students to pick "one of your friends" for a health risk comparison, their subjects tended to select individuals who were especially vulnerable to that risk. They also reported that college students' personal risk ratings were optimistically biased when compared to their ratings of an "average student" or "average person," but were no different from their perceptions of the risks faced by their closest friends, a sibling, or a parent.

Mull's (1988) subjects seemed to choose comparison groups that were literally downhill. She asked people who live on or near a floodplain to compare their own risk of a future flood with the risk of people who live "nearby." Her data are shown in Table 10.2. People who had never been flooded appeared to construe houses "nearby" to be ones at greatest risk, that is, downhill, close to the river. Only those who had been flooded several times (who could find no reference group that was worse off) finally began to concede that their risk may be as large as that of their neighbors.

Other data on comparison groups come from a study by Kamler and Stone (1988), who report that adolescent boys with hemophilia show optimistic biases when comparing themselves to other boys with hemophilia. Comparing themselves to boys without hemophilia, they

TABLE 10.2

Risk of Future Flooding Compared to Risk of Nearby Houses

Comparative Risk Judgment	Past Flooding Experience		
	Never Flooded (n = 22)	Flooded Once (n = 24)	Flooded Two or More Times (n = 26)
Much lower	14	8	4
Slightly lower	2	6	5
Same as nearby homes	6	9	12
Slightly higher	0	1	2
Much higher	0	0	3

SOURCE: Mull (1988).
NOTE: Entries indicate numbers of subjects. Effects of flooding experience on perceptions of future risk are statistically significant, $F(2,69) = 8.00$, $p < .001$.

show optimism with regard to risks unrelated to hemophilia but appropriate pessimism for several risks related to hemophilia.

Together, the limited data suggest that people tend to choose salient, high-risk individuals to represent "average" when making a comparative risk judgment. Health promotion programs sometimes deliberately attempt to create vivid images of individuals with multiple risk factors (for example, a potential heart attack victim who chain smokes, is greatly overweight, never exercises, and eats high-cholesterol foods). By making this caricature serve as a reference point, the program may unintentionally increase optimistic biases. People will compare themselves with this caricature and conclude that their risk is much below average instead of concluding correctly that while they are not in the very highest risk category, they are at considerable risk. The fact that intravenous drug users and gay men have been identified as high-risk groups for AIDS will magnify the perceived invulnerability of any individuals who can convince themselves that they do not belong to these groups.

Of course, high salience and high risk need not coincide. Programs can try to create vivid images of people with no risk factors, people who do all the right things. One atypical finding may represent the operation of a positive image as a reference point. College students tend to claim that they engage in fewer risk-increasing behaviors and more risk-decreasing behaviors than their peers. Yet, they do not claim to exercise more (Weinstein, 1984). Perhaps this is because a few hardworking joggers (not necessarily the same ones) are almost always visible on campus paths. Though these joggers make up only a small fraction of the student body, they serve as a concrete and readily available reference group. Compared to the people "always" out jogging, students cannot justify claiming that they exercise more than average. Research comparing the relative merits of stressing positive or negative images in prevention programs is much needed.

Relationships Between Risk Judgments and Objective Risk Factors

Comparative risk judgments are overly optimistic, but are they at least accurate in a relative sense, so that people who are higher in objective risk are less optimistic than those who are lower in risk? In other words, do personal risk judgments covary with objective risk factors? In several studies, I have asked individuals for risk judgments and for information about their standing on well-known risk factors (Weinstein, 1984, 1987; see also Svenson et al., 1985). Typical results are shown in Table 10.3. To summarize the findings it is useful to distinguish among different types of risk factors, ones referring to (a) family history, (b) physical and social environment, (c) psychological attributes, (d) constitution (i.e., physical and physiological characteristics), and (e) behaviors.

Significant correlations between risk judgments (either absolute or comparative judgments) and risk factors are often seen for categories a through d (especially a). However, correlations between risk judgments and self-reported behaviors are seldom significant. There is no association between seat belt use and perceived auto injury risk, between sugar consumption and expected tooth decay, or between walking alone at night and the perceived probability of being mugged. Overall, people seem willing and able to incorporate knowledge about their family history, personality, environment, and constitution into their views of their vulnerability to harm, at least to a limited extent, but they are much poorer at recognizing the relationships between their own actions and their vulnerability. They acknowledge that certain behaviors are relevant risk factors, but do not apply this knowledge to themselves.

Most of the risk factors for AIDS are matters of behavior. It seems likely that the correlations between these AIDS risk factors and individuals' views of their own susceptibility to AIDS are quite weak. Put another way, though AIDS researchers believe they know who is at high risk, many of these people will not acknowledge their increased vulnerability. People may think their risk is below average because they sometimes use condoms or believe they have relatively few sex partners, without admitting that intermittent condom use and changing sexual partners are major risk-increasing behaviors. To some extent, their

TABLE 10.3

Correlations Between Self-Rated Susceptibility and
Self-Ratings on Relevant Risk Factors

Risk and Risk Factors	Correlation with Absolute Risk Judgment	Correlation with Comparative Risk Judgment
Diabetes		
number of family members with diabetes	.48***	.36***
number of cigarettes smoked	.06	.20+
pounds overweight	.01	.02
Tooth decay		
*average number of cavities in dentist visits	.43***	.32**
*sweet baked goods consumed	.22+	.18
*candy consumed	.03	.17
*frequency of brushing	−.14	−.04
Automobile accident injury		
*frequency of driving and drinking	.12	.06
average highway driving speed	.12	.07
hours in car per week	−.02	.17
frequency of using seat belt	−.01	−.07
Lung cancer		
number of family members with cancer	.21+	.16
number of cigarettes smoked	.58***	.64***
Heart attack		
*number of family members with heart attacks	.34**	.42***
number of cigarettes smoked	.33**	.39***
*hard-driving (versus easygoing) personality	.20+	.27*
hours of exercise per week	.14	.08
*red meat consumed	−.03	.00
*eggs consumed	−.14	−.15
Mugging victim (females only)		
height	−.14	−.43**
frequency of walking alone at night	.20	−.07
*frequency of being out past midnight	−.07	.15
*avoids unlit and secluded areas at night	−.10	.05

NOTE: An asterisk in front of a risk factor indicates that subjects rated other students higher in risk than they rated themselves ($p < .05$).
$+p < .1$; $*p < .05$; $**p < .01$; $***p < .001$.

claims are understandable; what constitutes typical condom use or typical numbers of sexual partners is not at all clear. However, it seems that the consequences of risk factor ambiguity tend to be unidirectional. People use ambiguity in a one-sided fashion to bolster claims for relative invulnerability (see Siegel & Gibson, 1988; Weinstein, Sandman, & Klotz, 1987). Thus Bauman and Siegel (1987) report that gay men underestimate the seriousness of risk-increasing behaviors and overestimate the value of what they perceive to be risk-decreasing behaviors.

Because of this biased use of risk information, prevention-oriented brochures containing lists of risk factors but lacking norms, specific recommendations, and any way to combine risk factor information to arrive at an overall sense of risk may have unintended negative effects. Because few people will score high on all risk factors, such brochures may decrease the sense of risk for most individuals and may actually increase optimistic biases. In one study, giving subjects lists of risk factors magnified optimism, but adding information about the status of peers on these same factors eliminated optimistic biases (Weinstein, 1983).

The fact that some risk factors for AIDS—needle sharing and anal sex—are relatively unambiguous should help in convincing people who engage in these behaviors that they are increasing their risk. Yet, even if people acknowledge that their drug use or sexual behavior increases their susceptibility, they may be so reluctant to admit above-average risk that they may invent or exaggerate risk-decreasing factors. In spite of participation in needle sharing or anal sex, these individuals may assert that their overall risk is average or only slightly above average. Furthermore, members of high-risk groups—drug users, gay men who engage in anal sex, heterosexuals with many partners—are likely to compare themselves with similar others—with other drug users, other gay men, other heterosexuals. If they do engage in some risk-increasing practices, they will still tend to conclude that their peers perform even more risky behaviors, that they are not particularly susceptible (compared to their peers), and that they do not need to attend to prevention messages.

Pointing out risky behaviors is not sufficient. It appears necessary, in addition, to emphasize the link between behavior and risk status. People who engage in high-risk behaviors for AIDS should be encouraged to see themselves as the ones most likely to become victims, because they will tend to resist this conclusion. People who do not engage in these behaviors can give themselves credit for a low-risk life-style. Public health campaigns against smoking have succeeded in getting smokers to admit that they are in a high-risk group for cancer (Hansen & Malotte, 1986; Weinstein, 1984, 1987), and this seems to increase the motivation to quit.

Origins and Correlates of Optimistic Biases

At least three different processes have been suggested as underlying unrealistic optimism. One proposal is that these biases represent defensive denial (Kirscht, Haefner, Kegeles, & Rosenstock, 1966), an attempt to avoid the anxiety one would feel from admitting vulnerability to harm. If this hypothesis were correct, hazards that are more serious or life threatening would produce greater optimism than minor problems. Comparing different hazards, we would expect a positive correlation between optimistic bias (determined from the mean comparative risk rating for the hazard) and seriousness. For a specific hazard, we would expect a negative between-subject correlation between comparative risk judgments and perceived seriousness. Surprisingly, neither of these predictions is supported by the data (Weinstein, 1980, 1982, 1987). Optimism is no greater for life-threatening risks than for minor problems.

Since some life-threatening risks may seem too improbable to be threatening (too weak to elicit a defensive response), a second measure of threat, the extent to which others are thought to worry about the problem, might give a better test of the defensive denial hypothesis. However, worry tends to be negatively, not positively, correlated with optimistic biases (Weinstein, 1982, 1987). Available data do not support the position that denial is responsible for unrealistic optimism.

A second notion is that people claim that they are less at risk than their peers in order to enhance or preserve their self-esteem. Downward comparisons have often been described as instances of self-esteem enhancement (Wills, 1981; Wood et al., 1985). However, high-risk status does not necessarily threaten our self-esteem. Self-esteem seems to be most involved if hazards are preventable by personal action. High vulnerability to preventable problems suggests that we are ignorant, lack self-control, or are incapable of coping effectively. Thus the more preventable the hazard, the greater the threat to self-esteem and the stronger should be the tendency to claim below-average risk. This predicted association between perceived preventability and optimistic bias has indeed received strong confirmation (Weinstein, 1980, 1982, 1987).

Other hazards that can threaten self-esteem are those associated with social stigma or disapproval. Gonorrhea, alcoholism, and mental illness are examples. In one test of this idea, ratings of hazard embarrassment were positively correlated with optimistic bias ($r = .48$, $p < .01$) (Weinstein, 1987). AIDS would seem to rate high on both preventability and social stigma, implying the existence of a particularly strong optimistic bias.

A third line of reasoning suggests that optimistic biases may result from simple cognitive errors rather than from motivated distortions.

One such error is egocentrism. Any factor that makes us think our own risk is low could lead us to claim that we are below average in risk if we fail to recognize that the same factor may apply to others as well. And information about the self is generally more salient than information about others. Consequently, problems that seldom occur could lead to optimistic biases in comparative risk judgments simply because we forget that the probability is small for others, too.

Probability judgments are also affected by "availability," the ease with which relevant examples or plausible scenarios come to mind (Tversky & Kahneman, 1974). Thus lack of experience with a problem may make it seem unlikely, and, because we do not consider that few others have experienced it either, we may conclude that our own risk is below average. The predictions that low frequency and lack of experience would be associated with greater optimistic biases have received repeated empirical support (Hoch, 1985; Weinstein, 1980, 1982, 1987).

The details of the effects of experience are interesting. If, for a particular problem, one compares people with different degrees of experience, it appears that indirect experience is much less potent in overcoming unrealistic optimism than personal experience (Weinstein, 1989). This finding (averaged over many health problems) is shown in Figure 10.1. Close involvement with AIDS, as in caring for someone who is ill, or having several friends who have died from AIDS, as is common in the gay community, may be able to substitute for this personal experience. But secondhand knowledge of AIDS victims is unlikely to reduce optimistic biases or stimulate protective behavior.

People show a general overreliance on past experience to predict their future (Osberg & Shrauger, 1986). In the absence of past victimization experience, they may mistakenly conclude that they are exempt from future risk (absent/exempt). People may think the problem has a hereditary basis and will appear early in life if it is going to appear at all (e.g., juvenile diabetes and asthma). For other problems, such as tooth decay, they may believe that vulnerability is a constitutional matter, so if the problem has not appeared, their bodies must be resistant. Still, people realize that past experience is a better predictor in some cases than in others. In the case of cancer, for example, people recognize that not suffering harm in the past provides no guarantee about the future. In three studies, the correlations between subjects' ratings of the extent to which absence implies exemption for different hazards and the amount of optimism evoked by these haz-

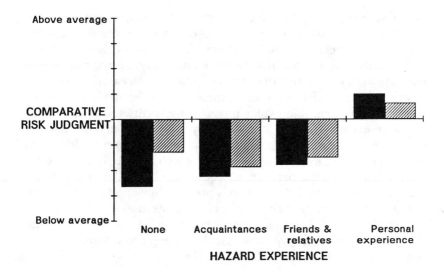

Figure 10.1 Comparative Risk Judgments at Different Levels of Hazard Experience
SOURCE: Weinstein (1989).
NOTE: Solid and striped bars represent data from a community sample and from college students, respectively. Data represent averages over many different hazards.

ards were .57, .67, and .81, $ps < .001$ (Weinstein, 1987), showing that the absent/exempt attribute is a very powerful predictor.

People who have engaged in risk-increasing behaviors for AIDS but have not become infected are likely to use this fact to conclude that they are not susceptible. They may infer that their bodies are resistant to this infection, that the protective measures they take are sufficient, or that the people from whom they could acquire the disease (such as sexual partners or individuals with whom they share needles) are not infected. All these beliefs lead to the conclusion that no change in behavior is needed. Education can probably help to prevent such faulty inferences, but in the absence of effective education, people who violate recommendations but are free of AIDS will tend to conclude that they are not susceptible.

The factors reviewed in this section provide predictions about the types of hazards that provoke the greatest unrealistic optimism. In multiple regression analyses, these variables explain over half the between-hazard variation in the magnitude of optimistic biases that is evident in Table 10.1 (Weinstein, 1987). It should be emphasized that although these hazard attributes modify the amount of optimism,

optimism is the norm. Perceived susceptibility is seldom unbiased, and hardly any hazards have been associated with a pessimistic bias (an exception has been reported by Dolinski, Gromski, & Zawisza, 1987).

The hazard attributes that have been discussed do not yield a simple explanation for the underlying cause of unrealistic optimism. There is no empirical support in these studies for defensive denial, but two other plausible explanations, self-esteem enhancement and cognitive errors, are both supported by available data, and they are very difficult to disentangle. For example, preventability could lead to optimism simply because the precautions we take are so much better known to us than the precautions taken by others. This would be an argument for a correlation between preventability and optimism due to cognitive error rather than self-esteem protection.

What is quite clear is that optimistic biases are widespread and that AIDS has several of the qualities that lead people to believe that their risk is much lower than that faced by others.

Relationship Between Perceived Susceptibility and Self-Protective Behavior

Although studies have found associations between perceptions of vulnerability and protective action, our understanding of the relationship between these two variables is still quite limited. One problem concerns the types of data that are available. Most findings come from cross-sectional surveys. Ratings of susceptibility and action are positively correlated, but the direction of causation is unclear. It is possible that actions shape risk perceptions rather than the other way around. People who choose not to take a precaution may justify their inaction (to themselves and to others) by claiming that their risk is low. Prospective studies, however, also find that perceptions of vulnerability predict the adoption of preventive measures (Janz & Becker, 1984). Yet, only a few investigations have used controlled, experimental designs (e.g., Rogers & Mewborn, 1976) and have attempted to manipulate perceptions of susceptibility. These are typically laboratory studies. Field experiments in health promotion are certainly common, but they usually involve multifaceted interventions in which the roles of individual variables are unclear. Additional field experiments are badly needed to clarify the mechanisms that lead to precautionary behavior.

One recent field experiment found a strong correlation between individuals' beliefs about the likelihood of radon problems in their homes and their intentions to test for radon, r = .50, p < .0001 (Weinstein, Roberts, & Sandman, 1988). There was also a moderate association between perceived likelihood and actual test orders, r = .24, p < .0001. Yet, information brochures stressing that radon problems are quite likely did not change testing intentions or behavior when compared to brochures that did not emphasize the probability of radon contamination, even though the increase in perceived likelihood produced was highly significant, p < .0001.

Additional calculations used the within-condition correlation between perceptions and behavior to predict the amount of behavior change that would be expected from the between-conditions difference in risk perceptions. These analyses showed that the effects of the different brochures on beliefs about susceptibility were too small to produce a detectable change in action. Perceptions of relative invulnerability to AIDS and other hazards are likely to be difficult to change. Researchers need to be cautious because, as in this radon study, an intervention may change perceptions, fail to change preventive behavior, and yet not provide an adequate test of the effect of these perceptions on behavior.

A second issue concerns the precise nature of the relationship between perceptions of susceptibility and protective behavior. When a positive correlation is reported, is it because people who believe that they have no risk behave differently from those who believe they face some risk, or does the degree of perceived risk make a difference? Officials of government environmental agencies, after failing to convince community groups that the risk from a proposed new facility is negligible, often feel that the public does not differentiate among different levels of risk. Zero risk is the only outcome that appears acceptable to local residents in such cases. As mentioned earlier, in the discussion of measurement issues, we know very little concerning how people think about risk likelihood and what categories they use to store their perceptions. It would be helpful if large-scale studies gave more detailed information about the association between beliefs and behavior.

A third question concerns the roles of comparative risk judgments and absolute risk judgments. From a purely rational perspective, the value of taking a precaution depends on the actual size of the risk and the degree to which preventive measures would reduce that risk. It would seem that our own risk of AIDS is what counts, and that comparisons to others' risks are irrelevant. Protective behavior, from this point of view, is solely a function of the individual's estimate of his or her absolute risk. The identification of optimistic biases in comparative risk judgments would then be informative only for what those biases tell us about absolute risk judgments. They warn us that whatever impression about the likelihood of harm is produced by the media, social interactions, and organized programs, people will tend to believe that their own risk is lower.

Yet, interpersonal risk comparisons may be quite important. Even when risk likelihood information is available, it is not easy to determine the appropriate response. We cannot eliminate our risk of heart disease or cancer, but must live with probabilities that are still substantial. We may ask ourselves whether all the measures recommended for avoiding AIDS are warranted. At what level of risk and after how many precautions should we feel satisfied? When situations are ambiguous or complex, and most hazard situations are, people use social comparisons to help them make decisions. They use the actions of others to decide whether they should be doing more than they are already doing. If people believe that their own risk is already lower than the risk faced by their peers, they may decide that additional precautions are unnecessary. From this point of view, comparative risk judgments may directly shape behavior.

Absolute and comparative risk judgments will usually be positively correlated (median $r = .64$ in Weinstein, 1984), but they are not interchangeable. It is worth investigating whether precautions are influenced solely by absolute risk judgments, as suggested in current theories of self-protective behavior, or whether comparative risk judgments provide predictive power distinct from that yielded by absolute risk judgments.

A final issue concerns some apparent inconsistencies in reactions to the same hazard. For example, community residents appear to be vigilant and vigorous in opposing anything, such as treatment centers, that they think will expose them or their children to AIDS. Classes in cardiopulmonary resuscitation (CPR) have even been canceled when the students, company employees, said they would not perform CPR on a co-worker for fear of contracting AIDS. In contrast, many well-informed people continue to perform truly high-risk behaviors. Similar over- and underreactions to radon risks have also been observed (Weinstein et al., 1987).

Can we explain these reactions? One idea is that these differing responses simply reflect the variation in risk sensitivity among different citizens. The protests against perceived AIDS threats may come from people who are especially risk averse, whereas risk taking may occur among those who are unusually risk tolerant. Another possibility is that differences in behavior may be related to subtle differences among the hazard situations. People may be strongly motivated to avoid incurring new risks (especially when the risks will be imposed by government authorities), but are less concerned about reducing current risks to which they may have become accustomed. A third hypothesis is that people will demand action from others, but are reluctant to expend any effort of their own to reduce hazard exposure. All three explanations are plausible, but why we see both overreactions and underreactions to the risk of AIDS is not at all clear.

Much is known about personal risk judgments, optimistic biases, and the conditions under which these biases appear. However, the issues raised in this concluding section show that there is much we do not know about the relationship between beliefs about personal susceptibility and the adoption of precautions. Often such beliefs appear to be important, but, as noted earlier, motives other than risk reduction may be still more powerful, especially when we seek to alter the drug use and sexual behaviors that increase the risk of AIDS. This chapter has pointed out barriers to the acknowledgment of personal vulnerability and strategies that should help to reduce unrealistic optimism. Whether interventions that follow the suggestions offered here will actually increase self-protective behavior remains to be tested.

Notes

1. The terms *susceptibility, risk likelihood,* and *vulnerability* are used interchangeably in this chapter.

2. For a thoughtful discussion of the relative roles of emotion and cognition in preventive action, see Averill (1987).

3. Joseph et al. (1987) report that gay men's perceptions of susceptibility to AIDS were associated with reductions in the number of anonymous partners and in the number of receptive anal exposures from an initial measurement to a follow-up six months later. (Several other risk behaviors showed no change.) However, when covariance analysis rather than a change score was used, the relationships were not significant. It may be that well-informed gay men who continue high-risk behaviors have other factors, such as uncooperative partners, keeping them from reducing their risk. Perceiving oneself to be susceptible is certainly not sufficient for behavior change.

4. The hazards used were heart attack, stroke, lung cancer, sunstroke, insomnia, being mugged, pneumonia, deafness, attempting suicide, being a murder victim, addiction to drugs, gallstones, nervous breakdown, AIDS, being 30 pounds overweight, and senility. The comparative risk scales had the following choices: much below average, below average, a little below average, average for men/women my age, a little above average, above average, and much above average. The absolute risk scales offered these options: no chance, almost no chance, very unlikely, unlikely, moderate chance, likely, very likely, almost certain, and certain.

References

Ajzen, I., & Fishbein, I. (1980). *Understanding attitudes and predicting behavior.* Englewood Cliffs, NJ: Prentice-Hall.

Averill, J. R. (1987). The role of emotion and psychological defense in self-protective behavior (pp. 54–78). In N. D. Weinstein (Ed.), *Taking care: Understanding and encouraging self-protective behavior.* New York: Cambridge University Press.

Bauman, L. J., & Siegel, K. (1987). Misperceptions among gay men of the risk for AIDS associated with their sexual behavior. *Journal of Applied Social Psychology, 17*(3), 329–350.

Beach, L. R., Campbell, F. L., & Townes, B. D. (1979). Subjected expected utility and the prediction of birth planning decision. *Organizational Behavior and Human Performance, 24*, 18–28.

Beach, L. R., & Mitchell, T. R. (1978). A contingency model for the selection of decision strategies. *Academy of Management Review, 3*, 439–449.

Becker, M. H. (Ed.). (1974). The health belief model and personal health behavior [Special issue]. *Health Education Monographs, 2*(4).

Becker, M. H., & Maiman, L. A. (1983). Models of health-related behavior. In D. Mechanic (Ed.), *Handbook of health, health care, and the health professions* (pp. 539–568). New York: Free Press.

Cleary, P. (1987). Why people take precautions against health risks. In N. D. Weinstein (Ed.), *Taking care: Understanding and encouraging self-protective behavior* (pp. 119–149). New York: Cambridge University Press.

Cole, G. A., & Withey, S. B. (1981). Perspectives on risk perceptions. *Risk Analysis, 1*(2), 143–163.

Cummings, K. M., Becker, M. H., & Maile, M. C. (1980). Bringing the models together: An empirical approach to combining variables used to explain health actions. *Journal of Behavioral Medicine, 3*, 123–145.

Dolinski, D., Gromski, W., & Zawisza, E. (1987). Unrealistic pessimism. *Journal of Social Psychology, 127*(5), 511–516.

Drabek, T. E. (1986). *Human system responses to disaster.* New York: Springer-Verlag.

Edwards, W. (1954). The theory of decision making. *Psychological Bulletin, 51*, 380–417.

Fischhoff, B., Goitein, B., & Shapira, Z. (1982). The experienced utility of expected utility approaches. In N. Feather (Ed.), *Expectations and actions: Expectancy value models in psychology* (pp. 315–339). Hillsdale, NJ: Lawrence Erlbaum.

Fishbein, M. (1980). A theory of reasoned action: Some applications and implications. In H. E. Howse, Jr. (Ed.), *Nebraska Symposium on Motivation* (Vol. 27, pp. 65–110). Lincoln: University of Nebraska Press.

Fishbein, M., & Ajzen, I. (1975). *Belief, attitude, intention and behavior: An introduction to theory and research.* Reading, MA: Addison-Wesley.

Furstenberg, F. F., Jr. (1971). Public reactions to crime in the streets. *American Scholar, 40*(4), 601–610.

Hakmiller, K. L. (1966). Threat as a determinant of downward comparison. *Journal of Experimental Social Psychology, 1*, 32–39.

Hansen, W. B., & Malotte, C. K. (1986). Perceived personal immunity: The development of beliefs about susceptibility to the consequences of smoking. *Preventive Medicine, 15*, 363–372.

Hansen, W. B., Malotte, C. K., & Fielding, J. E. (1988). Evaluation of a tobacco and alcohol abuse prevention curriculum for adolescents. *Health Education Quarterly, 15*(1), 93–114.

Hoch, S. J. (1985). Counterfactual reasoning and accuracy in predicting personal events. *Journal of Experimental Psychology: Learning, Memory, & Cognition, 11*, 719–731.

Janis, I. L. (1967). Effects of fear arousal on attitude change: Recent developments in theory and experimental research. In L. Berkowitz (Ed.), *Advances in experimental social psychology* (Vol. 19, pp. 41–79). New York: Academic Press.

Janz, N. K., & Becker, M. H. (1984). The health belief model: A decade later. *Health Education Quarterly, 11*(1), 1–47.

Johnson, B. B., & Covello, V. T. (Eds.). (1987). *The social and cultural construction of risk.* Dordrecht, Netherlands: D. Reidel.

Joseph, J. G., Montgomery, S. B., Emmons, C. A., Kirscht, J. P., Kessler, R. C., Ostrow, D. G., Wortman, C. B., O'Brien, K., Eller, M., & Eshleman, S. (1987). Perceived risk of AIDS: Assessing the behavioral and psychological consequences in a cohort of gay men. *Journal of Applied Social Psychology, 17*(3), 231–250.

Kahneman, D., & Tversky, A. (1979). Prospect theory: An analysis of decision under risk. *Econometrica, 47*(2), 263–291.

Kamler, J. A., & Stone, G. C. (1988). *Optimistic bias in adolescents with hemophilia.* Unpublished manuscript, University of California, San Francisco, Health Psychology Program.

Kirscht, J. P., Haefner, D. P., Kegeles, F. S., & Rosenstock, I. M. (1966). A national study of health beliefs. *Journal of Health and Human Behavior, 7*, 248–254.

Kruglanski, A. W., & Klar, Y. (1985). Knowing what to do: On the epistemology of actions. In J. Kuhl & J. Beckmann (Eds.), *Action control: From cognition to behavior* (pp. 41–60). Berlin: Springer-Verlag.

Kuhl, J. (1982). The expectancy-value approach within the theory of social motivation: Elaborations, extensions, critique. In N. T. Feather (Ed.), *Expectations and actions: Expectancy-value models in psychology.* Hillsdale, NJ: Lawrence Erlbaum.

Kulik, J. A., & Mahler, H. I. M. (1987). Health status, perceptions of risk and prevention interest for health and nonhealth problems. *Health Psychology, 6*, 15–27.

Kunreuther, H. (1978). *Disaster insurance protection.* New York: John Wiley.

Larson, E. B., Olsen, E., Cole, W., & Shortell, S. (1979). The relationship of health beliefs and a postcard reminder to influenza vaccination. *Journal of Family Practice, 8*(6), 1207–1211.

Larwood, L. (1978). Swine flu: A field study of self-serving biases. *Journal of Applied Social Psychology, 8*(3), 283–289.

Leventhal, H., Safer, M., Panygris, F. D. (1983). The impact of communications on the self-regulation of health beliefs, decisions, and behavior. *Health Education Quarterly, 10*(1), 3–29.

Lichtenstein, S., Slovic, P., Fischhoff, B., Layman, M., & Combs, B. (1978). Judged frequency of lethal events. *Journal of Experimental Psychology: Human Learning and Memory, 4*, 551–578.

Maddux, J. E., & Rogers, R. W. (1983). Protection motivation and self-efficacy: A revised theory of fear appeals and attitude change. *Journal of Experimental Social Psychology, 19*, 469–479.

Maiman, L. A., & Becker, M. H. (1974). The health belief model: Origins and correlates in psychological theory. *Health Education Monographs, 2*(4), 336–353.

McKusick, L., Horstman, W., & Coates, T. J. (1985). AIDS and sexual behavior reported by gay men in San Francisco. *American Journal of Public Health, 75*(5), 493–496.

Mull, J. (1988). *Helplessness effects of repeated flooding experiences.* Unpublished master's thesis, Rutgers University, Department of Psychology.

Nisbett, R., & Ross, L. (1980). *Human inference: Strategies and shortcomings of social judgment.* Englewood Cliffs, NJ: Prentice-Hall.

Osberg, T. M., & Shrauger, J. S. (1986). Self-prediction: Exploring the parameters of accuracy. *Journal of Personality and Social Psychology, 51*, 1044–1057.

Pagel, M. D., & Davidson, A. R. (1984). A comparison of three social-psychological models of attitudes and behavioral plans: Prediction of contraceptive behavior. *Journal of Personality and Social Psychology, 47*(3), 517–533.

Perloff, L. S., & Fetzer, B. K. (1986). Self-other judgments and perceived vulnerability to victimization. *Journal of Personality and Social Psychology, 50*(3), 502–511.

Rogers, R. W. (1983). Cognitive and physiological processes in fear appeals and attitude change: A revised theory of protection motivation. In J. T. Cacioppo & R. E. Petty (Eds.), *Social psychophysiology* (pp. 153–176). New York: Guilford.

Rogers, R. W., & Mewborn, C. R. (1976). Fear appeals and attitude change: Effects of a threat's noxiousness, probability of occurrence, and the efficacy of coping responses. *Journal of Personality and Social Psychology, 34*, 54–61.

Rosenstock, I. M. (1974). Historical origins of the health belief model. *Health Education Monographs, 2*(4), 328–335.

Schoemaker, P.J.H. (1982). The expected utility model: Its variants, purposes, evidence and limitations. *Journal of Economic Literature, 20*, 529–563.

Schwartz, S. P., White, P. E., & Hughes, R. G. (1985). Environmental threats, communities, and hysteria. *Journal of Public Health Policy, 6*, 58–77.

Siegel, K., & Gibson, W. C. (1988). Barriers to the modification of sexual behavior among heterosexuals at risk for acquired immuno-deficiency syndrome. *New York State Journal of Medicine, 88*, 66–70.

Skogan, W. G. (1981). On attitudes and behaviors. In D. A. Lewis (Ed.), *Reactions to crime* (pp. 19–46). Beverly Hills, CA: Sage.

Slovic, P., Fischhoff, B., & Lichtenstein, S. (1982). Response mode, framing, and information-processing effects in risk assessment. In R. Hogarth (Ed.), *New directions for methodology of social and behavioral science: Question framing and response consistency* (pp. 21–36). San Francisco: Jossey-Bass.

Slovic, P., Fischhoff, B., & Lichtenstein, S. (1985). Characterizing perceived risk. In R. Kates, C. Hohenemser, & J. Kasperson (Eds.), *Perilous progress: Managing the hazards of technology* (pp. 91–125). Boulder, CO: Westview.

Sutton, S. R. (1982). Fear arousing communications: A critical examination of theory and research. In J. R. Eiser (Ed.), *Social psychology and behavioral medicine* (pp. 303–338). New York: John Wiley.

Svenson, O. (1979). Process descriptions of decision making. *Organizational Behavior and Human Performance, 23*, 86–112.

Svenson, O., Fischhoff, B., & MacGregor, D. (1985). Perceived driving safety and seatbelt usage. *Accident Analysis and Prevention, 17*(2), 119–133.

Tversky, A., & Kahneman, D. (1974). Judgment under uncertainty: Heuristics and biases. *Science, 185*, 1124–1131.

Tversky, A., & Kahneman, D. (1981). The framing of decisions and the psychology of choice. *Science, 211*, 1453–1458.

Tyler, T. R., & Cook, F. L. (1984). The mass media and judgments of risk: Distinguishing impact on personal and societal risk judgments. *Journal of Personality and Social Psychology, 47*(4), 693–708.

Vaughan, E. (1986, March). *Some factors influencing the nonexpert's perception and evalua-*

tion of environmental risk. Unpublished doctoral dissertation, Stanford University, Department of Psychology.

Von Winterfeldt, D., John, R. S., & Borcherding, K. (1981). Cognitive components of risk ratings. *Risk Analysis, 1*(4), 277–287.

Wallsten, T. S., & Budescu, D. V. (1983). Encoding subjective probabilities: A psychological and psychometric review. *Management Science, 29*(2), 151–173.

Wallsten, T. S., Budescu, D. V., Rapoport, A., Zwick, R., & Forsyth, B. (1986). Measuring the vaguer meanings of probability terms. *Journal of Experimental Psychology: General, 115*(4), 348–365.

Wallston, B. S., & Wallston, K. A. (1984). Social psychological models of health behavior: An examination and integration. In A. Baum, S. E. Taylor, & J. E. Singer (Eds.), *Handbook of psychology and health* (Vol. 4, pp. 23–54). Hillsdale, NJ: Lawrence Erlbaum.

Weinstein, N. D. (1980). Unrealistic optimism about future life events. *Journal of Personality and Social Psychology, 39*, 806–820.

Weinstein, N. D. (1982). Unrealistic optimism about susceptibility to health problems. *Journal of Behavioral Medicine, 5*, 441–460.

Weinstein, N. D. (1983). Reducing unrealistic optimism about illness susceptibility. *Health Psychology, 2*, 11–20.

Weinstein, N. D. (1984). Why it won't happen to me: Perceptions of risk factors and illness susceptibility. *Health Psychology, 3*, 431–457.

Weinstein, N. D. (1987). Unrealistic optimism about illness susceptibility: Conclusions from a community-wide sample. *Journal of Behavioral Medicine, 10*(5), 481–500.

Weinstein, N. D. (1988). The precaution adoption process. *Health Psychology, 7*(4), 355–396.

Weinstein, N. D. (1989). Effects of personal experience on self-protective behavior. *Psychological Bulletin, 105*, 31–50.

Weinstein, N. D., Roberts, N., & Sandman, P. M. (1988). *Determinants of home radon testing.* Unpublished manuscript, Rutgers University, Department of Human Ecology.

Weinstein, N. D., Sandman, P. M., & Klotz, M. L. (1987, August 28). *Underestimation and overestimation in radon risk perception.* Paper presented at the annual meetings of the American Psychological Association, New York.

Weinstein, N. D., Sandman, P. M., & Klotz, M. L. (1988). Optimistic biases in public perceptions of the risk from radon. *American Journal of Public Health, 78*, 796–800.

Wills, T. A. (1981). Downward comparison principles in social psychology. *Psychological Bulletin, 90*, 245–271.

Wood, J. V., Taylor, S. E., & Lichtman, R. R. (1985). Social comparison processes in adjustment to cancer. *Journal of Personality and Social Psychology, 49*(5), 1169–1183.

11

Making Decisions About AIDS

Baruch Fischhoff

What Are AIDS Decisions?

Decisions

Decisions are choices among alternative courses of actions (including, perhaps, inaction). Decisions can be characterized qualitatively by the following:

- a set of actions (or options), describing what one can do
- a set of possible consequences of those actions, describing what might happen (in terms of desirable and undesirable effects)
- a set of sources of uncertainty, describing the obstacles to predicting the connection between actions and consequences

Decisions can be characterized quantitatively by the following:

- trade-offs among consequences, describing their relative importance
- probabilities of consequences, describing the chances that they will actually be obtained

This basic conceptual scheme has been used by investigators to describe a very wide variety of decisions, from decisions to go to war (Jervis, 1976; Lebow & Stein, 1987), to decisions to have children

Author's Note: Preparation of this chapter was supported by a grant from the Carnegie Corporation of New York, "Adolescent Decision Making." The unpublished research reported here was partially supported by the National Science Foundation, Grant SES-8715564, "Understanding and Improving Risk Perception and Communication." Their support is gratefully acknowledged. I thank Robyn Dawes, Greg Fischer, Lita Furby, Marilyn Jacobs, Patty Linville, Harriet Shaklee, and the members of the CMU Risk Communication Group for their contributions. The views expressed are those of the author.

(Beach, Campbell, & Townes, 1979), to decisions to operate on the basis of X-rays (Eddy, 1982), to decisions regarding which of two simultaneously presented lights is brighter (Coombs, Dawes, & Tversky, 1970). In some cases, the usage has been descriptive, attempting to show how people actually make decisions in these situations. In other cases, the usage has been normative, attempting to show how decisions ought to be made, if decision makers are to choose the action in their own best interests. In some cases, both approaches are used, in order to show the difference between how well people make decisions and how well they might. In some of these cases, there is an additional, prescriptive purpose, attempting to tell people how to go about making decisions in a way that will bring them closer to the normative ideal than if they were left to their own devices (von Winterfeldt & Edwards, 1986; Watson & Buede, 1987).

This chapter extends this behavioral decision theory perspective to decisions about AIDS. The remainder of this section discusses how AIDS decisions can be characterized in these general terms. It is followed by a section raising some of the hard questions about the appropriateness of this perspective for AIDS decisions. The next section addresses the normative question of how to identify the right decision options. It is followed by an analysis of how decisions can go wrong, illustrated, in part, by previously unpublished results regarding AIDS decisions. Methodological issues associated with determining how people make decisions are then addressed. The chapter concludes with a discussion of how the methods and results of the behavioral approach might be used to help people make better decisions.

AIDS Decisions

The left-hand column of Table 11.1 lists four representative decisions concerning AIDS: deciding whether to be tested for (antibodies to) the virus; deciding whether to read the U.S. Surgeon General's (1988) brochure, *Understanding AIDS*; deciding whether to ask a sexual partner to use condoms; and deciding whether to support legislation ensuring the confidentiality of the results of AIDS tests. Obviously, these are very different decisions, in terms of the actions considered, the magnitude of their personal consequences, their potential impact on others, and the sort of factual considerations that could inform them. The remainder of the table details some of these differences.

Testing. For the testing decision, the options are (obviously) taking the test and not taking the test. The most salient possible consequences

TABLE 11.1

The Structure of Some AIDS Decisions

Decision	Options	Consequences	Uncertainties
Get tested	Take test Don't take test	Physical health Mental health Social costs Economic costs	Test result Ability to forget
Read *Understanding AIDS*	Read Don't read	All of above Competence	Informativeness
Ask partner to use condoms	Ask Don't ask or Ask_1, Ask_2, . . . , Ask_n Don't ask	All of above Sexual pleasure	Partner's response Nature of experience Effectiveness (protection)
Support confidentiality	Support Oppose Remain neutral Ignore issue	Hedonic Political balance Social values	Public opinion Effects of policy Personal vulnerability

of this decision are changes in the state of one's physical health, of one's mental health, of one's social relations, and of one's economic situation. Just how these states will be affected depends (obviously) on the results of the test and (perhaps less obviously) on how well one can forget unpleasant considerations (e.g., the possibility of having AIDS if one does not get tested or the result of the test if it is positive).

For example, testing positive might lead to an improvement in one's physical health if it prompted one to take better care of oneself, in the hopes of postponing (or even avoiding) progression to AIDS-related complex or to the disease itself. On the other hand, it might have no effect at all if one put the thought out of one's mind. A negative result might improve physical health for people who respond, "If I've made it this far, I should protect what I've still got." It might reduce physical health if it discouraged taking precautions in the future (e.g., "If I haven't gotten it, after all I have done, then I must be immune. I guess I can do whatever I want."). Being able to predict the outcome of these events would help one to anticipate the full consequences of the testing decision (and to identify the best course of action).

One's mental health ought to be improved greatly by a negative result; how bad an effect a positive result would have depends both on one's ability to deal with the result and on one's ability to put it out of mind. Conceivably, a mature individual who received proper counseling and community support might be better off psychologically after receiving a positive result than worrying about what the result might be and coping with the side effects of such a blatant attempt at denial as refusing to be tested. The impacts of the testing decision (and test result) on one's social relations follow similar (complicated) lines.

The most direct economic impact of the decision, the cost of the test, ought to be relatively unimportant in the overall scheme of things—compared, say, with the impact of a clear result on employment, housing, or insurance. However, it may loom large for low-income people who need to come up with the cash.[1]

Reading. Analogous considerations can be sketched for the other decisions in the table. The consequences of deciding to read the official AIDS brochure are like those of the testing decision, if only because it can affect testing. Reading may affect one's feeling of competence for dealing with the crisis. Those effects might be subsumed under mental health consequences (e.g., if perceived competence affected feelings of control, anxiety, or self-esteem) or even under social relations (e.g., to the extent that it affected one's ability to act knowledgeably and confidently with others).

How the reading decision affects perceived competence and the other consequences will depend on how much the brochure has to offer. Does it contain anything new? Does it at least confirm beliefs that one held already, but shakily? Is it written comprehensibly? Is it logically structured? Or does it take a shotgun approach, scattering facts without pattern? Does it help readers to "organize their work" for the purpose of reaching personally relevant decisions? Or does it just give uncompromising directives, telling readers what some official thinks they should do—rather than trusting them to make their own decisions? Being able to predict the brochure's informativeness should help one decide whether or not to read it. In this case, there is a simple, familiar, and effective way to reduce this uncertainty: Give the brochure a quick look-over. Moreover, its cost is so low that it does not pay to think about whether or not to do it—just give it a look.

Asking. Deciding whether to ask a partner to use condoms can affect all of the above consequences. For example, the decision can change physical health by facilitating or impeding transmission of the virus. Deciding to ask can weaken a specific social relationship (e.g., by implicitly impugning the past of one's partner) or strengthen it (e.g., by showing concern for one another's health, by showing that the relationship is already strong enough to handle a difficult topic), and so on. It has the added possible consequence of affecting sexual pleasure, perhaps reducing it (e.g., if condoms are uncomfortable), perhaps enhancing it (e.g., if condom use eliminates a gnawing worry).

What happens depends, of course, on how one's partner responds. It may be hard to reduce this source of uncertainty as much as one would like. Hearing about others' experiences may provide some (base-rate) information; however, it cannot reflect all the chemistry of a specific relationship. What happens also depends on just how much protection condom use affords. Reading about condom effectiveness may reduce this uncertainty enough to justify the transaction costs of acquiring that information.

What happens depends also on how the initiating partner brings up the subject. That is, there are different ways of asking, varying in their degree of coerciveness and in the concerns that apparently motivate them (among other things). Each way of asking may have its own "profile" of effects on the different consequence dimensions. As a result, each distinct way could be conceptualized as a separate action option (Ask 1, Ask 2, . . . Ask n). The price paid for such refinement is an increasingly large set of option-consequence-uncertainty combinations to consider.[2]

Supporting. Social policy is determined, in part, by the cumulative effect of such individual decisions as testing, reading, and asking. It is also determined more directly by individuals' responses to policy issues, like the current national debate over the confidentiality of AIDS test results. In deciding what position, if any, to take on such issues, individuals may consider personal, hedonic consequences, such as how confidentiality will affect their physical health (as a result of its effect on the spread of the disease). Anticipating these effects means estimating how one's own actions affect the political process, how that process will resolve itself, how that resolution will affect the disease, and how vulnerable one is to the fate of those who take (or avoid) tests.

Analogous uncertainties affect two consequences that are particular to political action: the impact of those actions on the balance of political power in a society and on its ensemble of social values. These are complicated assessments. Indeed, the transaction costs of figuring out what difference political action will make may be one reason people often seem to choose inaction.

AIDS Decisions as Decisions

Two generic criticisms might be leveled at casting AIDS-related behavior in a decision-making perspective. One is that it does too little, merely invoking a different nomenclature (that of decision making) for the familiar phenomena of AIDS. The second is that it does too much, imposing a framework that obscures what people really are doing.

Does Too Little

Given the diversity of the settings in which it can be invoked, the language of decision theory might seem a bit like Esperanto. Anything can be translated into it, with a modest loss in meaning but little addition to understanding. Like any universal language, decision theory's usefulness can be defended on either semantic or syntactic grounds: Translating diverse situations into common terms can help one understand related elements in them; having those elements be related by a central grammar can clarify the logical relations among them. The test of decision theory is the ability to identify such relations whether or not characterizations like those in Table 11.1 reveal similarities that would not otherwise be apparent to those making or studying decisions.

The usefulness of identifying semantic similarities depends on the answers to questions such as, Does it help to see which consequences repeat themselves across decisions? Or to see how the importance of a particular consequence (e.g., physical health) varies from decision to decision? Or to see that each option might have an effect on all consequences, not just those it is intended to influence? Or to realize that inaction is an option in most decisions? Does it help individuals to examine the consistency of their values and beliefs across decisions? Does it help the investigators who study them?

The usefulness of identifying syntactic similarities depends on issues such as, Does it help to see such structural properties as the interdependence of actions, consequences, and uncertainties? Does recognizing the complexity of these interrelations help to clarify (and overcome) the obstacles to systematic, comprehensive decision making? Without the framework, would it have been as easy to characterize concepts such as transaction costs, base-rate information, or the optimal degree of refinement for options?

In both respects, the language of decision theory is essential for analyzing actual behavior as a deviation from optimal behavior. From a practical standpoint, such discrepancies identify opportunities for intervention. Indeed, the quantitative mechanics of decision theory allow one to say something not only about where decision making could stand improvement, but also about where improvements could have the greatest effect. From a theoretical standpoint, such discrepancies prompt a search for the reasons people are not performing better. That is, what aspects of their experience limit people's ability to acquire the needed skills?

The remainder of this chapter should be read with an eye to whether the decision-making perspective provides enough added value to be worth the effort of applying it when studying AIDS-related behavior. The chapter offers both AIDS-specific data and speculations produced by generalizing data from studies of decisions about quite different topics.

Does Too Much

A theoretical perspective can do too much both descriptively and prescriptively. Descriptively, it can make erroneous claims about people's behavior. The decision-making perspective could be faulted, for example, if it assumed that people always implement it perfectly. Although such claims have been made, they need not be. Indeed, a focus of behavioral decision theory is identifying how and why people perform suboptimally (e.g., emotion, fatigue, laziness, confusion, deliberate misinformation).

The key empirical claim that is made by the behavioral decision-making approach is that it is able to capture the significant aspects of people's decision making. One aspect that it might seem to miss is the social context of that behavior. Table 11.1 describes mental states of a single individual, but it is clearly the case that people influence one another's behavior. One way that the decision-making perspective can represent such influences is by including social impacts of a decision among its consequences, showing how much the decision maker cares about what others think. A second expression of social influences is through decision makers' perceptions, which summarize information and impressions from a variety of sources, including other people. One basic reason for maintaining an individual focus is that, in the end, individuals decide what they will do, even if it is only to do as they are told.

Another aspect of behavior that the decision-making perspective might seem to exclude is stable individual differences (e.g., risk-taking propensity), since each decision is analyzed in its own right. In principle, however, individuals with stable characteristics will just interpret decisions in similar ways. One might still ask (a) whether this case-by-case analysis is an efficient research strategy and (b) how well it represents the way individuals approach their decision problems. That is, do they examine each on its merit and then reach consistent conclusions, rather than having global preferences, determined by their personality characteristics? Perhaps surprisingly, investigators have had relatively little success in detecting consistent differences in risk-taking propensity (e.g., Davidshofer, 1976; Slovic, 1962).[3] This result may reflect either the absence of such propensities or the difficulty of developing personality measures. The fact that this seems surprising may reflect the tendency to see in others more stable personalities than we see in ourselves (Nisbett & Ross, 1980).

Normatively, this theoretical scheme could be faulted if it made controversial assumptions about how decisions should be made. One implicit assumption of Table 11.1 that might raise some eyebrows is that of individual sovereignty in decision making, that is, the idea that individual decision makers ought to be the final arbiters of what decisions they choose to make. They are the ones to choose, for example, which consequences to consider and how to weigh their importance— rather than there being an official "right" way to think about decisions.[4]

A second potentially controversial normative assumption of this approach is that it does not characterize risky options in terms of whether or not they have acceptable levels of risk. In fact, it does not even recognize the concept (Fischhoff, Lichtenstein, Slovic, Derby, & Keeney, 1981). Rather, it views a decision as a choice among options, each of which has a set of consequences, including perhaps some risk. The option chosen need not be the least risky, if it has compensating benefits. Nor need its risks be "acceptable" in any absolute sense. The decision maker may be quite unhappy with that level of risk, but may have no safer option (at least at reasonable cost).

Making Risky Decisions

In these lights, there is an essential difference between thinking of what people do as risk taking or as decision making. Taking risks is but a by-product of making decisions involving risky outcomes. Moreover, risks are defined in the eye of the beholder. One person may stick with a job rather than risk the outside world; another may leave the same job rather than risk stagnating personally or being stuck in a declining firm or industry. Knowing people's perceptions is a precondition for interpreting their decisions. It is all too easy to assume that people who make apparently riskier choices than we imagine we would make in their stead are "risk takers" (if we give them credit for identifying the course of action in their own best interests) or as fools (if we do not). Such assumptions can hamper our ability to understand, aid, and respect other people's decision making.

How Should AIDS Decisions Be Made?

Volumes of decision theory detail the intricacies of how to choose the best course of action in a wide variety of situations. These techniques convert the raw materials of Table 11.1 (options, consequences, uncertainties) into defensible recommendations. Although these procedures can be quite elaborate, their underlying principles are relatively straightforward (Behn & Vaupel, 1983; Raiffa, 1968; von Winterfeldt & Edwards, 1986; Watson & Buede, 1987). Decision makers face two fundamental challenges in integrating the pieces of their decisions: (a) balancing conflicting objectives and (b) incorporating the uncertainty regarding which of those objectives will be obtained. Decision theory offers some help in each respect.

Evaluation

Decision making can be difficult, even when we know what we are going to get, whenever we cannot get all that we want. As a result, we are forced to make trade-offs among objectives. Thus deciding whether or not to ask a partner to use condoms would be easy if asking were certain to strengthen the relationship, protect physical and mental health, increase sexual pleasure, and be cheaper than the alternative. In decision theory terms, it would dominate other alternatives by being at least as good in all respects. However, the world of consequences is seldom that benign, forcing us to determine which consequence matters most.

There is no mechanical way to make trade-offs. Unless one is comfortable reducing all consequences to a single "objective measure" (e.g., their market price), then there is no substitute for personally determining what is really important.[5] Where decision theory hopes to help is in organizing those deliberations. One form of help is in decomposing the complex outcomes of decisions into a set of essential consequence dimensions (as depicted in Table 11.1). Doing so facilitates thinking about what is important and comparing the consequences of different actions.

A second form of help is in offering orderly procedures for evaluating consequences. For example, decision makers might be directed to assign values of 0 and 100, respectively, to the worst and best possible outcomes on each consequence dimension, with appropriate values going to intermediate states. Then, the relative importance of each pair of dimensions is determined by considering the relative impact of going from the best to worst state on each. This procedure initially focuses attention on what ought to be the simpler task of comparing similar consequences (Tversky, 1969; Tversky, Sattath, & Slovic, 1988). Regarding comparisons across consequences, the procedure makes it clear that importance depends on the range of possible outcomes rather than on some intrinsic importance of each dimension. Thus, for example, although "economic costs" are important in some general sense, there may not be many at stake in a particular decision (e.g., going with or without a condom).[6]

Considering each consequence dimension for every option helps to ensure that proper attention is paid to opportunity costs (i.e., the benefits forgone by selecting one option rather than another). For example, in deciding whether or not to read the Surgeon General's brochure, one should consider how that time could otherwise be used. This procedure also deliberately ignores any sunk costs associated with previous actions, focusing on what will happen as the result of subsequent actions. In deciding whether or not to invest effort in supporting confidentiality, it should not matter how much effort one has already put in, only what fruit future investment would bring (Dawes, 1988; Thaler, 1980, 1985).[7]

Expectations

Decision theory does offer a mechanical way of accommodating the uncertainty surrounding the consequences of actions. It is the expectation rule, whereby the overall attractiveness of an option is calculated by multiplying the value of each possible consequence by the probability that it will actually be obtained if that option is chosen. This is a compensatory rule, in the sense that making a consequence more positive can compensate for lowering the probability that it will be obtained. Conversely, no negative consequence is unacceptably bad, insofar as it could always be tolerated if its probability were sufficiently low. It is also a compensatory rule in the sense that attractive expectations regarding one consequence can compensate for unattractive expectations regarding another.

Explications

Calculating expectations is a familiar rule that formalizes a familiar intuition. One could use it without endorsing decision theory per se, as is done in a variety of less formal approaches to decision making

178   Baruch Fischhoff

(Feather, 1982; Janis, 1982). Perhaps a unique contribution of decision theory is in helping to clarify the relationships between a decision's outcomes and uncertainties. Figure 11.1 shows one common
device, the decision tree. In it, decision points (or nodes) are represented by squares, from which options emanate. The fate of undertaking these options depends on various uncertain events, represented
by their own circular nodes. Each action-event sequence leads to some
profile of consequences. The probability that it will occur is determined by the probability associated with that event. If the values of
the consequences have been quantified, then the expected values of
the sequences can be computed.

Figure 11.1 shows these relations with a testing decision regarding
another risk, radon concentrations in people's homes.[8] The consequences here parallel those with the HIV testing decision. This decision differs in offering the option of moving and leaving the problem
behind. Analysis of these options suggests that testing is generally
beneficial, except perhaps in cases where one is unprepared to take
any action in response to high radon levels. In that case, testing could
result in significant unrequited worry.[9]

Figure 11.2 offers an analogous tree for the HIV testing decision.
Whether to test is the focal decision, the outcome of which depends
both on the test results and on one's ability to put unpleasant thoughts
out of mind. The decision to test does not, of course, influence the
probability of having the virus; it may, however, affect the probability
of forgetting (by affecting what there is to forget). Applying the expectation rule is now straightforward, once quantitative values are assigned to the relative importance of these consequences. If there is
uncertainty about any of these numbers (the probabilities and values),
then sensitivity analyses can be conducted, recalculating the expectation with different possible numbers.

How Can AIDS Decisions Go Wrong?

Subjective Optimization

As mentioned, the behavioral decision-making approach does not
claim that people intuitively make optimal decisions. It should also be
mentioned that this is a controversial nonclaim. Standard economic
theory holds that people are able to identify the courses of action in
their own best interest, based on an accurate understanding of risks
and benefits, subject to the transaction costs of acquiring information
(Bentkover, Covello, & Mumpower, 1985). These assumptions are mir-

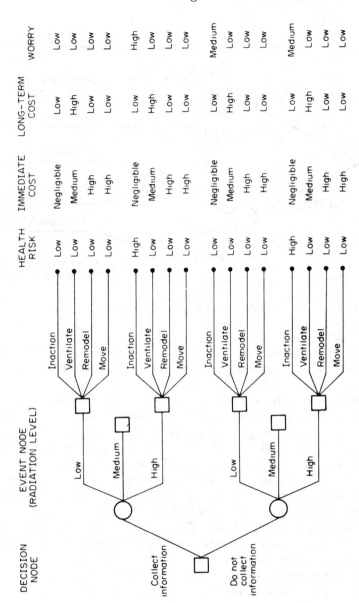

Figure 11.1 Decision Tree for Testing for Radon

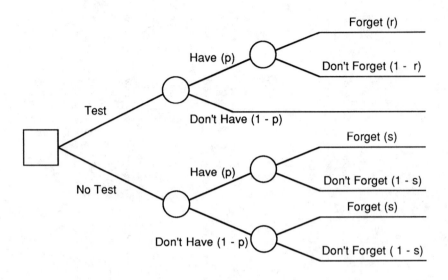

Figure 11.2 Decision Tree for Testing for HIV

rored, with less theoretical superstructure, by behavioral models with an underlying expectation rule. These include the health belief model and the expectancy-value family of models (Feather, 1982).

Applied sensitively, optimizing models typically show some, albeit imperfect, ability to predict people's behavior. Unfortunately, these successes have ambiguous implications for the descriptive validity of the models. If one has a rough idea of what consequences concern people, then many compensatory rules for aggregating the attractiveness of options will produce similar rankings (Dawes, 1979). As a result, it is relatively easy to predict the results of people's intuitive aggregation procedures. However, it is also relatively difficult to know just what those procedures are. Thus good predictions can affirm hypotheses about what goes into people's decisions more than they can affirm hypotheses about how those decisions are made.

From an applied perspective, these models provide general encouragement to those hoping to influence people's behavior. One can expect people to like a risky option less if one can make its unattractive options seem worse or more likely (and, conversely, with its attractive options). On the other hand, the models' lack of insight regarding the psychological processes involved gives them little leverage for affecting those perceptions.

The following subsections describe ways in which decision-making processes can go awry. Compared with the single, tidy, coherent theoretical scheme allowed by the assumption of optimization, they may seem like a hodgepodge of locally relevant effects. Three basic kinds of suboptimality might be distinguished: having the right structure for a decision, but misestimating some of its components; having the wrong structure, with or without appropriate component estimates; and having no structure.

Quantitative suboptimality. Decisions require two kinds of quantitative estimate: probabilities and values. From a measurement perspective, their estimation is obviously subject to some random error (Wallsten & Budescu, 1983), as people summarize their feelings and beliefs for the specific purposes of a decision. The importance of this measurement error would be revealed by sensitivity analyses examining the choices indicated by alternative possible estimates. Von Winterfeldt and Edwards (1982) have shown that, for many decisions involving continuous options (e.g., invest $X), modest errors in single estimates have little effect on the expected outcome of the decision-making process where everything else is done right (e.g., the expectation rule is applied accurately to the inaccurate estimates). Studies of the reliability of probability assessments suggest that the random error of a single estimate would typically be within these limits (Wallsten & Budescu, 1983). Less is known about how the effects of errors accumulate when a decision depends on multiple fallible estimates, or how such errors affect decisions with discrete alternatives (e.g., test/don't test; ask/don't ask).

Even more troublesome are studies suggesting systematic errors in subjective estimation processes. They also reveal some consistent strengths. Together, these provide an empirical foundation for helping people with AIDS decisions.[10]

Frequency estimates. How frequent are AIDS cases in this area? How often do condoms fail? How many people use them? How often are government brochures useful? How likely are physicians to help me make my own decisions (rather than preach to me)? One obvious resource for making such estimates is the individual's personal experiences: How many AIDS cases have I heard about? How often have condoms failed me? How often have friends mentioned failures?

Numerous laboratory studies have shown moderate to high correlations between observed and estimated frequencies. Indeed, it has even been suggested that the encoding of frequency is an automatic process, as though people had counters in their minds (Hasher & Zacks, 1984; Hintzman, 1969). In generalizing these results to the real world, it is essential to examine the conditions under which they were ob-

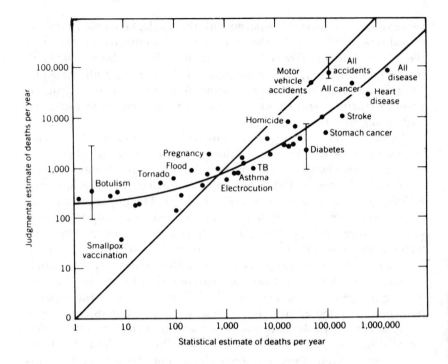

Figure 11.3 Estimates of the Frequency of Causes of Death in the United States

tained. Typically, experimental events have been clearly presented, unambiguously defined, concentrated in time, and relatively equal in relative frequency (i.e., differing by a factor of ten, rather than hundreds, thousands, or millions, like many real-life events). Life often provides less favorable conditions.

Complicating conditions can be found in the voluminous research into how the memorability of events can be enhanced by factors such as recency, meaningfulness, and salience (Fiske & Taylor, 1984). These factors are problematic precisely because it has taken voluminous research to establish their existence and estimate their magnitude. Were they matters of common knowledge, people might know enough about them to undo their effects on memory. As it is, any factor that makes events more memorable also makes them seem more frequent (Tversky & Kahneman, 1973).

Figure 11.3 shows one example of the difficulty of adjusting for systematic biases in memorability. It is drawn from a study of laypeople's estimates of the frequency of different causes of death in the United States (Lichtenstein, Slovic, Fischhoff, Layman, & Combs, 1978). Overall, there is a positive correlation between judged frequencies and statistical estimates. However, the curve shows some compression, with judgments ranging over three or four orders of magnitude, while statistics range over six. This could reflect problems with using such numbers, inability to discriminate such large frequency differences on the basis of life experiences, unrecognized overreporting (and, hence, overestimation) of infrequent events (the novelty of which provides newsworthiness), and corresponding underreporting of common causes of death. Deviations from the best-fit line might be thought of as specific biases, above and beyond this overall tendency. These deviations could be predicted both from subjects' reports of their personal experiences with each event (as a cause of death or suffering for people they know) and from counts of newspaper reports (Combs & Slovic, 1979). Unfortunately, subjects told about such potential sources of bias were not able to adjust their frequency estimates to more appropriate values.

An apparently related bias is the tendency for people to see themselves as being less at risk than other people. For example, most people view themselves as safer than average drivers (Svenson, 1979; Weinstein, 1980). A motivational account of these results is possible: People distort reality in defense of their own egos. However, an information-processing account is also possible (Langer, 1975). It may be much easier to see other drivers' mistakes (and one's own defensive responses) than it is to see the risks that one creates for others. One may not realize that serious accidents with clear culprits are so rare that even poor drivers can go a long time without incontrovertible evidence of their deficiencies.

One might ask about comparable biases in estimating the frequency of AIDS. How do people assess their own vulnerability, given the AIDS stories depicted in the news media? Do they have any idea what common reporting biases might be? Do they think to apply these ideas to their own experiences? What do they conclude regarding the relative risks to men and women from the disproportionate representation of women in the pictures of victims in the Surgeon General's brochure? Did that lead to exaggerating the risks to women, or did it counter prior underestimates of women's vulnerability? Do people who test negative believe that they are immune to the virus? Do people who believe that they are immune see any need to confirm this belief with a test?

Recently, Patty Linville, Greg Fischer, and I asked several hundred college students to estimate the chances that they personally would get the AIDS virus during the next three years. Median answers were around 5% for both sexual and nonsexual transmission, for both men and women, from an educated population that overwhelmingly reported heterosexual orientation. When asked about the probability of male-to-female transmission in a single case of sexual intercourse, their median estimates were about 5% with condom use and 50% without. All of these seem to be great overestimates, considering current scientific estimates (e.g., Fineberg, 1987; Padian, 1987). At this point, one can only speculate about their source.[11]

Numerical estimates. A hidden strength in these results is the ordinal consistency of the estimates produced using different response modes. For example, the ordering of the events in Figure 11.3 matches that derived from a parallel study in which subjects judged paired causes of death, deciding which was more frequent and by how much. Given how unusual it must be to answer such specific quantitative questions, these results suggest that people have a stable feeling for the relative frequency of these events that emerges no matter how the question is worded.

Nonetheless, people's absolute estimates can vary greatly depending on how the question is put. For example, the subjects depicted in Figure 11.3 were told that 50,000 people die annually in the United States from motor vehicle accidents, as a way of stabilizing their responses. (Without such an anchor, subjects had only a vague idea of how many annual deaths there are overall.) A second group received the identical task, except that they were told that 1,000 people die from electrocution. The latters' estimates were lower for almost all causes of death, typically by a factor of 2 to 5 (for low and high estimates, respectively).

Such difficulties with quantitative estimates, especially when using somewhat unfamiliar units, are well known in experimental psychology (Poulton, 1968, 1977). From a methodological point of view, they complicate the task of determining what subjects currently believe. For example, depending on which question was asked, one might conclude that people overestimated or underestimated the risks. From a theoretical perspective, these results suggest that people have difficulty understanding and using such quantitative information. For example, we must wonder what estimates of AIDS risk we would have obtained had we used a different response mode in the study just cited (Linville, Fischhoff, & Fischer, 1988). We made a special effort to make very small probabilities a viable response mode, showing subjects' response options ranging down to .01%. They did not hesitate to

TABLE 11.2
Median Judged Probability (× 100) of AIDS Virus
Transmission

| | Male to Female | | Female to Male | |
| | Condoms | | Condoms | |
Exposures	Yes	No	Yes	No
1	4	50	3	40
10	10	80	6	60
100	20	98	20	90

use such probabilities, so we believe that their apparent overestimates were actually smaller than they would have been had we simply asked, "Please estimate the probability that . . . ."[12]

Cumulative risk. As with many other hazards, the risks of contracting the AIDS virus add up over time. For example, Fineberg (1987) calculates that there is a 99% chance of contracting AIDS from 20 cases of unprotected sex with each of 50 partners having a 50% chance of having the virus—even if one assumes that the single-exposure transmission probability is just 1%. One must wonder to what extent this cumulative risk perspective occurs to people spontaneously. To the extent that it does, how well are they able to assess the cumulative probabilities?

Various studies have found that people underestimate the rate at which the probability of failure adds up (e.g., see Bar Hillel, 1973). Slovic, Fischhoff, and Lichtenstein (1978) found that drivers reported finding seat belts considerably less attractive when told that the risk of death on an average trip was about 1 in 4 million, compared to drivers told that the lifelong risk was closer to 1 in 100. Shaklee, Fischhoff, and Furby (1988) found that estimates of the cumulative risk of contraceptive failure were very insensitive to the estimated failure rate for a single year. For methods described as having single-year failure rates of 1% to 13%, respondents estimated the chances of getting through 15 years of use without a failure as 78% to 57%, respectively, whereas the actual chances ranged from 87% to 12%.

Table 11.2 shows median estimates of AIDS transmission for 1, 10, and 100 exposures, as given by Linville et al.'s (1988) subjects. For someone who believes that the single-exposure chance of transmission without condoms is 50%, the 100-exposure risk should be a virtual certainty. The same is true for someone who believes that the single-exposure risk is 10% with a condom. These subjects seem to have a very poor idea of how these risks mount up. Compared with the statistical estimates, subjects' responses greatly overestimate the single-exposure risks of transmission, but are roughly accurate for multiple exposures. In this case, providing accurate information about single-exposure risks would likely lead them to underestimate the cumulative risk greatly, whereas providing accurate cumulative risk figures would lead to overestimated single-exposure risks. A striking feature of our results was that 15% of the time subjects' risk estimates did not increase monotonically with the number of exposures, violating a fundamental rule of probability theory. This was twice as likely to happen when the question involved condom use as when it did not (a result we are currently trying to clarify).

Combining information. Estimating cumulative risk means integrating several pieces of similar information. Other risk estimates require integrating diverse pieces of information. One common task is to integrate case-specific information with background information describing the base rate of a particular event (Fischhoff & Beyth-Marom, 1983). For example, radiologists must consider the frequency of various problems when analyzing individual mammograms; social workers must consider the rate of welfare cheaters when interviewing individual candidates; auto buyers must consider the cumulative repair records appearing in *Consumer Reports* along with their impressions of a particular used car; bank managers must consider the typical fate of start-up restaurants when analyzing business plans. Case-specific judgments should be very strong if one is to ignore solid statistical estimates. Voluminous research has found people to be overly reliant on their impressions, neglecting base rates in favor of impressions that even they admit to be of limited validity (Bar Hillel, 1980; Eddy, 1982; Kahneman & Tversky, 1973; Nisbett & Ross, 1980).

On the basis of these results, one would expect people to exaggerate how well they can tell whether someone else has AIDS. If so, then they might believe that the base rate of AIDS is high enough to mandate a change in sexual practices, but do nothing because they believe that they can reduce their personal risk by diagnosing the status of potential sexual partners. One relevant piece of data can be found in a National Center for Health Statistics (1987) study titled "Knowledge and Attitudes About AIDS." In response to the statement "You can tell if people have the AIDS virus just by looking at them," 65% of respondents said "definitely false," while an additional 18% said "probably false." Although these results seem encouraging, the specific wording of the question makes a very strong claim. Respondents who exaggerate their ability to discern others' health status might feel, "Of course, you can't tell just by looking at them. However, I can ask people a few well-chosen questions, or just see how they act, and get a pretty good idea." Clarifying these beliefs requires more specific questions.

Another context in which people must combine base-rate and case-specific information is in estimating the effectiveness of risk-control strategies. Consider, for example, a request that effectively convinces one kind of sexual partner to use condoms, but has no effect on others. If it is always used, then its overall effectiveness will depend on the prevalence of that kind of partner. Furby, Fischhoff, and Morgan (1989) asked people to estimate the effectiveness of various strategies for reducing the threat of sexual assault. They found that even when a strategy was applicable in only a small pro-portion of assault situations, judgments of its overall effectiveness seemed insensitive to these limits. For example, on average, "always look in the backseat of your car before getting in" was estimated to eliminate 65% of all assaults.

Framing. The laws of probability theory and the statistics of govern-ment agencies provide a ready standard against which to evaluate judgments of fact. It is more difficult to evaluate judgments of worth. As a result, the typical standard of quality has been internal consis-tency. There is an elaborate literature in psychometrics for evaluating the quality of evaluative responses and for adapting elicitation meth-ods to the kind of information that people have to offer (e.g., Coombs, 1964; Coombs et al., 1970; Dawes, 1972). This literature typically assumes that people have a value for any consequence; what varies is how precisely they know it. Where expressed values are unreliable, they can add noise to people's decision-making processes analogous to that added by uncertainty about the facts.

More troubling is the discovery of systematic biases in value esti-mates. One well-documented bias is the "range-frequency effect," whereby people's expressed satisfaction with a consequence depends on the range of consequences being considered and the frequency with which different portions of the range are sampled (Johnson, 1972; Parducci, 1974; Poulton, 1977, 1982).

Several interpretations of such effects are possible, each with some-what different implications for the quality of people's intuitive decision-making processes. One is that subjects are uncertain about how to use the response scale (so that the alternatives define what "very satisfied" and "very unsatisfied" mean for present purposes); in that case, the result is just an experimental artifact. A second possibil-ity is that subjects are uncertain about what they are expected to say (so that the alternatives provide clues to investigator expectations); in that case, the result reflects people's normal sensitivity to what other people think—although the investigator may be an otherwise irrelevant "other." A third possibility is that people do not really know what they want in advance, but assemble an evaluation on the basis of whatever thoughts come to mind at the time of the experiment; in that case, the result reflects a "deep" susceptibility of expressed values to transient influences.

Indeed, there is extensive, if somewhat scattered, literature showing how expressed values can be influenced by seemingly irrelevant features of how questions are asked (Fischhoff & Furby, 1988; Fischhoff, Slovic, & Lichtenstein, 1980; National Research Council, 1982; Turner & Martin, 1985; Tversky & Kahneman, 1981; Tversky et al., 1988). For example: (a) When asked to choose between a gamble with a 0.25 chance of losing $200 (and a 0.75 chance of losing nothing) and a sure loss of $50, most people prefer the gamble; however, when the sure loss is called an "insurance premium," most people will forgo the $50 (Hershey & Schoemaker, 1980). (b) Turner and Krauss (1978) observed that, in two contemporaneous national surveys, people who had first answered six questions relating to political alienation were less favorable in their evaluations of national institutions than people who had not received the alienation questions. (c) Fischhoff, Slovic, Lichtenstein, Read, and Combs (1978) found that people found the risks of various technologies to be more acceptable following a judgment task that involved estimating the benefits of those technologies than after estimating their risks.

If people are as sensitive to such influences in their lives as they are in experiments, then the decisions that they make may not reflect their own deeply held values. If people cannot access their basic feelings and integrate them into articulated values, then they are handicapped in making decisions in their own best interests (Rokeach, 1973). Such risks are greatest in situations where people are least sure of their values, where neither habit nor tradition dictates their response. Unfortunately, modern life creates many decisions with novel trade-offs, with many AIDS decisions falling squarely into this category. Just how much social awkwardness is it worth to achieve an X% reduction in the probability of virus transmission? Exploring one aspect of the instability of evaluative standards, Linville et al. (1988) asked people whether the government should allow a condom to be advertised and sold as an "effective method for preventing the spread of AIDS" if it were 95% effective. Some 88% answered affirmatively. A second group was asked the same question about a condom having a 5% failure rate. Although these two questions are formally equivalent, only 42% answered the second question affirmatively. The change in wording also produced a drop from 95% to 81% in the percentage of subjects who answered yes to the question, "Would you use it or encourage your partner to use it?" One can only guess how adequately the perspectives that life spontaneously makes available capture the richness of such decisions. For example, do condom manufacturers publicize both effectiveness and failure rates?

Qualitative Suboptimality

Missing parts. The difficulty of making trade-offs is, in part, an estimation problem. People cannot tell what they want precisely enough to guide their own decision making. However, it can also be a structural problem, if the trade-offs are based on an incomplete definition of the decision problem. First, consequences, such as those listed in Table 11.1, must be coded at a somewhat arbitrary level of abstraction. We care about physical health because we care about its constituents, such as absence of pain and unrestricted mobility. We run the risk of misestimating the value of physical health if we fail to recognize these factors. Second, even at a given level of abstraction, the label used (by investigators or by ourselves) to characterize a consequence may capture only a portion of its significance. Thus part of what one cares about with condoms is how well they work. However, their effectiveness rate apparently does not immediately invoke or capture the associated failure rate, which is formally, but not psychologically, complementary.

A decision maker who recognizes the possibility of omissions might try to take them into account. One might allow for random error (e.g., "I haven't thought very hard about this. It's not impossible that I've left something out. I shouldn't be too surprised if I don't really like what I think I'm going to like."). One might even allow for systematic error (e.g., "I know myself well enough to realize that I tend to give too much weight to what I am afraid of doing wrong and overlook positive reasons for taking action.").

Whether or not people undertake such strategies depends on whether or not they recognize the possibility of incompleteness. A few studies suggest, however, that people are insensitive to even large omissions in problem representations, whether these are produced by themselves or by others (Fischhoff, Slovic, & Lichtenstein, 1978; Gettys, Pliske, Manning, & Casey, 1987). How well people might undertake such strategies (when they do) depends on how much insight they have into their own thought processes. For thought processes at this level of inferential complexity, there would be reason to doubt the validity of people's introspections (Ericsson & Simon, 1980; Nisbett & Wilson, 1977).

In the terms of Table 11.1, the definition of a decision problem can be deficient in three basic respects: options, uncertainties, or consequences. The same concerns about awareness and introspection apply to neglected options and uncertainties as were just discussed for neglected consequences. What may differ are the specific reasons for omissions. For example, people might tend to miss consequences with more distant effects, with less visible effects, with effects on other people, or with unpleasant effects. On the other hand, people tend to omit options involving collective action, inaction, complex actions, or contingent actions (actions dependent on how events develop). People might tend to ignore uncertainties concerning background (i.e., base-rate) information, the quality of their knowledge, or the subtleties of other people's behavior.

There are some generic strategies for partially completing a problem definition, such as "think through the implications of doing nothing" or "think about collecting information." However, getting many of the pieces requires a substantive understanding of the specific decision problem. As a result, the greatest difficulties should be expected with the most unfamiliar problems. AIDS decisions offer a mixture of the old and the new. People know something about reading brochures, about getting medical tests, about discussing sex, and about undertaking political action. So they have some background to draw on. The helpfulness of this background will depend on both how well people can analyze the unique features of new situations and how well they have done in the past (e.g., a long history of difficulty in talking about sex is unlikely to help with talking about AIDS). Thus people are likely to define AIDS decisions in the same way and with the same success as they have defined other decisions that seem relevant to them.

Extra parts. A problem definition can frustrate decision making by containing too much, as well as too little. For example, it can contain irrelevant options, consequences, and uncertainties, thereby diverting attention from more important considerations. Options are irrelevant when they are dominated by other ones or when they have very similar consequence profiles. Consequences and uncertainties are irrelevant when they fail to discriminate among options (e.g., costs are irrelevant when everything costs the same).

These excesses mainly threaten the efficiency of the decision-making process, by wasting valuable time and thought. Other extra parts distort the problem definition, by introducing considerations that people ought to ignore. For example, people frequently pay attention to sunk costs by attending to past investments, rather than just to the return on future investments (Dawes, 1988; Thaler, 1985). One example in AIDS decisions might be reluctance to abandon a long-term sexual relationship even though it is likely to have more risks than benefits in the future. Another might be wanting to use up a supply of condoms even after learning that they are less effective than a competing brand.

Other extra features involve distinctions missing from decision theory. For example, laypeople may assign money to distinct categories, each with its own spending rules (e.g., clothing money, leisure money, food money, mad money) (Thaler, 1985). By contrast, economists consider all money to be fungible, or interchangeable, in principle. One should not forgo the freedom of being able to move money around among accounts.

Economics also holds that the consequences of a decision should be evaluated in terms of how they leave one overall. By contrast, laypeople seem to evaluate outcomes relative to some reference point (e.g., where they are now, where they expect to be when the consequences are experienced, where other people are) (Kahneman & Tversky, 1979; Tversky & Kahneman, 1981). The result is instability in preferences, which comes with shifts in those points.

AIDS decisions seem to be particularly vulnerable to such difficulties. They are insufficiently familiar to be formulated efficiently. Popular reports are full of irrelevant factors that people might be tempted to worry about. Witness the concern over such apparently negligible worries as transmission by mosquitoes and blood donations. The result can be searching for useless information and analyzing ineffective options. Unfamiliarity also increases exposure to manipulations of perspective, such as the shift in evaluations that we found when describing condoms in terms of their effectiveness or their failure rate (with the implicit shift in reference point between how much they do and how much they do not do).

Nonoptimality

Even individuals unschooled in decision theory must have some feeling for how difficult it is even to identify all the pieces of a decision, much less to analyze their logical interrelations and estimate quantitative parameters (like probabilities and trade-offs). That awareness may make them reluctant to try to think through decisions. The obvious alternative to analysis is experience. For individuals, experience is summarized in habits; for societies, in traditions. These summaries may be explicit, in the form of rules of thumb, or implicit, in the form of learned behaviors. In either case, their usefulness depends on how good they were in the first place and how well they fit new circumstances. Good, applicable rules are most likely to be found in stable, repeated situations providing prompt, unambiguous feedback.

AIDS decisions seem unlikely to enjoy these circumstances. The most similar prior experiences are often ones in which people are unhappy with their decision making. Patients often ask physicians whether it was appropriate to request medical tests (or are told that they came in too late). Even long-time sexual partners are often uncertain about how to approach each other with requests. Moreover, even the most similar prior decisions may be sufficiently different from AIDS decisions that they are not applicable.

The obvious alternative to having experience is creating it, arriving at a preferred course of action through trial and error. Unfortunately, AIDS decisions often lack the conditions needed for such learning. Often, they are not repeatable, in the fundamental sense that errors are so costly that decision makers and their worlds are changed by them. Contracting AIDS is one such irreversible "learning experience"; losing a partner is another; having an unforgettable test result is a third. A second threat to learning is that the feedback must be integrated over several consequence dimensions that reveal themselves at very different rates. The impacts on health are particularly slow in coming (compared, say, to the impacts on sexual satisfaction). It may never be clear what the chances of transmission were in a particular encounter, or even where a transmission came from.

These obstacles are unfortunate because people are often quite good at learning—when they have the chance. Indeed, they may be so good at trial and error that they fail to develop the skills needed for analytical decision making—creating problems when they need to get it right the first time.

Finally, it is hard to make decisions optimally when decisions are not obviously being made. At times, big decisions emerge from a series of small decisions, none of which received (or even seemed to merit) systematic analysis. People may look back on such creeping decisions and wonder, "How did I get into this situation?" Other "decisions" emerge from a series of nondecisions, the result of whatever options are chosen de facto when people refuse to decide. Still other "choices" are the result of shaping by social forces.

The language of decision theory can be used to illuminate even these situations (Corbin, 1980). Any choice involves some rudimentary set of options, consequences, and uncertainties. Descriptively, one can ask how it has been selected from the set of possibilities that might have been considered in a more deliberative process. For example, what fragments of a decision flit through people's minds when they put off thinking seriously about getting tested for AIDS, or broaching the topic of condom use, or resisting social pressure to deny civil rights to people living with AIDS? Prescriptively, these omissions show where to begin helping them to make better decisions, or to make decisions at all. However, some account is also needed for the sheer magnitude of these discrepancies between possible and actual decision-making richness. Lack of time is a possible contributing factor, but not one that would account for the apparent shallowness of decision making in many situations where plenty of time is available. Emotional involvement is another possible barrier to thoughtfulness. However, it may be an effect as well as a cause. That is, not knowing how to make decisions thoughtfully can be frustrating. In this light, a significant contribution to people's decision making about AIDS may be giving them the feeling that they can make sense out of these decisions—in cases where they cannot rely on their skill at trial-and-error decision making.

How Can We Tell How AIDS Decisions Are Being Made?

Actions and Words

Two complementary strategies can be used to describe a decision-making process: the revealed preference and the expressed preference approaches. The former focuses on actual choices and attempts to infer the considerations that motivated them. The latter asks people how they perceive problems and attempts to infer their links with the ensuing decisions (Bentkover et al., 1985). Revealed preference approaches have the strength of observing actual choices, but the weakness of allowing many possible accounts of any given choice. In addition, these approaches typically make strong assumptions regarding the accuracy of people's perceptions and the sophistication of their information-integration strategies. By contrast, the expressed preference approach must rely on the candor of people's reports and the accuracy of their introspections. Given the rudimentary state of our understanding of AIDS decisions and the potentially incoherent state of people's thinking about those decisions, this more open-ended approach seems called for initially. It could, in time, bound the set of models used for revealed preference studies.

Holistic Approaches

Among expressed preference approaches, one might distinguish between holistic and decomposition approaches. In the former, one observes what people say and do as they solve decision problems. The result could be a unique description for each subject, with the researcher hoping that some recurrent patterns emerge (Blackshaw & Fischhoff, in press; Ericsson & Simon, 1984; Montgomery & Svenson, in press). Or each subject's behavior could be mapped onto a common conception of the problem. For example, subjects could be asked to think through whether and how they would ask a sexual partner about using condoms. The considerations that they mention could then be compared with those listed in Table 11.1. Which options did they note? Which consequences concerned them? What uncertainties were they aware of? Such a mapping makes minimal assumptions regarding the structure of people's thinking. All it assumes is that the contents mentioned during the experiment resemble those that would emerge were subjects to face the decision on their own. An even more assertive mapping procedure would map what people say onto a proper decision model. Doing so would assume that people intuitively structure these pieces in that way. If subjects said enough to suggest their quantitative estimates for the model's parameters, then one could even compute the option that should follow.

These procedures, like those described below, can be applied to different populations, to understand the differences in their perceptions, or to a given population at different points in time, to understand the effects of AIDS-related events on their perceptions. For example, can a few media reports get the risk of mosquito-borne AIDS onto people's agenda? Did the Surgeon General's report remove it? Do hard-to-educate populations have deficient mental models of their decision problems, or do they just have difficulty putting the pieces together? One could even perform such mappings at several times during an extended decision-making session (or repeated sessions devoted to the same problem), in order to see how perceptions evolve through reflection.

Decomposition Approaches

Listing. Rather than have people consider everything at once, and taking what occurs to them, investigators can have subjects focus on particular components of decision-making problems. A qualitative strategy, applicable to any of the three components, is to have people list all the examples that they have considered. For example, we asked groups of women, men, and sexual assault experts to list options for reducing the threat of such assaults, consequences that could be affected by their choice of option, and uncertainties obscuring the impact of options on consequences (Fischhoff, Furby, & Morgan, 1987; Furby et al., 1989).

In the study of options, we derived a list of some 1,100 different strategies. Although individuals seldom produced more than a couple of dozen, the sheer number of possibilities represents a significant obstacle for women or investigators attempting to analyze alternatives systematically. To overcome this problem, we developed a theoretically based categorization scheme. When applied in a secondary analysis of studies of the effectiveness of self-defense strategies, it revealed a consistent pattern of results that was blurred when each strategy was treated distinctively (Furby & Fischhoff, in press). Analogous studies could reveal the structure of the option, consequence, and uncertainty spaces for AIDS decisions.

Such intensive studies are necessarily reactive, in the sense that they may change subjects through the process of asking them questions. People seldom spontaneously attempt to list explicitly exhaustive lists of options. Doing so may make them organize their thoughts as they never have before, and even to generate options that are novel for them. The results of such studies are better thought of as representing how people can think, rather than what they do. They may also show how well people can think, and how that limit to behavior changes with experience. Although these studies seem to create very favorable conditions for people to analyze decisions, studies have found that the lists produced frequently have substantial omissions (Fischhoff, Slovic, Lichtenstein, Read, & Combs, 1978; Gettys et al., 1987; Hoch, 1985).

Estimating

As mentioned, two kinds of estimates are needed to derive a recommendation from a decision-making model (except in the case of a dominating option): judgments of fact and judgments of value. In addition to the methodological problems of making unfamiliar tasks and response modes clear, two additional topics bear attention.

Task definition. For twenty years or so, the U.S. National Weather Service has been providing probability of precipitation forecasts (Murphy & Winkler, 1984). Periodically, there are reports that these fore-casts confuse listeners. Murphy and Winkler (1984) examined this issue and found that the confusion came not from the probability, but from the event. People were uncertain whether a 70% forecast meant rain 70% of the time, rain over 70% of the area, or 70% chance of at least some rain.

An analogous ambiguity can be seen in a recent survey asking, "How likely do you think it is that a person will get AIDS or the AIDS virus infection from having sex with a person who has AIDS?" (National Center for Health Statistics, 1987). Linville et al. (1988) posed this question to a group of students and then asked how they inter-preted the event in question, offering a fixed set of options: having vaginal intercourse without a condom (chosen by 72.5%), having vagi-nal intercourse with a condom (4.3%), and having other kinds of sex (6.5%). Another 8.7% reported being uncertain what the event was (even though all of them provided a likelihood estimate), while 8.0% endorsed more than one alternative. A second question asked whether they interpreted this sex as occurring on a single occasion (61.6%), occurring on several occasions (22.5%), or occurring on many occasions (7.2%). The rest were uncertain (5.1%) or chose more than one alternative (3.6%). For responses to be usable, all respon-dents must interpret each question in the same way and investigators must know what that way is.

A second complication with this study (and others) is the use of an ambiguous response mode. The alternatives were very likely, some-what likely, somewhat unlikely, very unlikely, not possible, and don't know. However, individuals vary in how they interpret such verbal quantifiers; interpretations vary even for the same individual across contexts (Beyth-Marom, 1982). Using an unbalanced response scale, without a "certain" option to parallel "not possible," creates the possi-bility of systematic bias in addition to the random error.

Similar difficulties may arise whenever terms lack a consensual societal definition (e.g., effectiveness, reliability, exposure, risk, work-ing near someone with AIDS). Developing unambiguous definitions is straightforward, if cumbersome (Turner & Martin, 1985). Failing to do so risks producing uninterpretable judgments of facts. Analogous problems arise in defining judgments of value (Fischhoff & Furby, 1988).

Nonquantitative mental models. These studies asked for the probabil-ity that various statements of fact are true. Clearly, people can and do use probabilities in this explicit way. However, it seems very unlikely that they have their answers tidily stored in their minds in the form of propositions and associated their probabilities. Rather, people must have some general-purpose representation on a topic, from which they derive specific probability estimates. For AIDS, these might include mental models of what the virus is like and how it behaves, of how social institutions divide up responsibility for its control, and of how other people think about it. Indeed, so many different probability estimates might be needed for different decisions that people could not have all of them precalculated.

Because this substantive knowledge forms the basis for the summary judgments needed in decisions, it merits study in its own right. Some rationale is needed, however, for determining what facts are relevant. For example, the Institute of Medicine's (1986) fine report, *Confronting AIDS*, mentions discouragingly the results of a study finding that only 41% of respondents knew that AIDS was caused by a virus. This would be troubling only if there were decisions that depended on this knowledge or if people knew enough about the behavior of viruses that such knowledge could help them make other inferences. Neither seems likely.

Such a rationale could direct the composition of tests regarding risk-related knowledge. It could also serve as a template against which to compare the knowledge produced in response to more open-ended tasks—just as decision-related considerations could be mapped into Table 11.1 or an associated decision tree.

How Might We Help in AIDS Decisions?

Analyzing the Need for Help

The point of departure for most of the descriptive research proposed here is an analysis of how AIDS decisions ought to be viewed. Performing such analyses is a critical first step for professionals planning to present facts or recommendations. It forces explicit consideration of what needs to be said and how much latitude is possible in people's responses (e.g., Need they follow the professionals' recommendations in order to be considered rational? How precise must their technical knowledge be?). Unfairly chastising the public for failing to be like experts is poisonous for public—expert relations. It makes the public seem stupid to the experts, and it makes experts look haughty to the public (National Research Council, 1988).

The analytical perspective also provides guidance for what to do when people's current perceptions diverge from how they ought to view AIDS decisions. With it, one can analyze how critical various pieces of information are to people's understanding. Focusing communications on that information serves the cognitive goal of using people's limited attention span wisely and the affective goal of showing that the communicator understands them well enough to address their most pressing concerns.

Addressing Psychological Difficulties

Having decided what to communicate, one can begin to worry about how to communicate. The research literatures cited here describe various systematic biases in people's information processing that need to be considered by communicators. For example, if people have difficulty seeing how small risks accumulate, then those implications need to be made clear. If people are misled by systematic biases in media reports on AIDS (or their own direct experiences), then those biases must be addressed. If people are subject to framing effects, then alternative ways of looking at problems need to be brought to their attention. If they have difficulty "organizing their work" regarding AIDS decisions, then they need help in assembling the pieces of those decisions.

In some cases, the literature offers tested techniques. In others, methods need to be developed. In still others, the methods are there, but the means of delivery are lacking. For example, when different decisions are defensible, people need help to determine personally relevant conclusions. Decision analysis offers such techniques, but primarily for corporate clients able to pay for personal attention. It is a challenge to make such contingent advice available to the masses. One partial possibility is to solve the decision problems facing archetypal individuals, then allow individual readers to figure out where they fit into the space defined by the archetypes. Addressing and respecting the uniqueness of individuals' AIDS decisions may be both difficult and critical to effective communication.

Ensuring Comprehensiveness

The methodological issues described here provide several messages regarding the best ways to help people with their AIDS decisions. One is obvious: Avoid bad research. Misreading how much people know or why they fail to behave as experts would can have serious implications. There seem to be nuances to studying AIDS decisions that are not immediately obvious either to experts in AIDS or to experts in decision making.

A second message is that what we tell people should be driven by what they need to know. For example, there should be protocols for reporting AIDS-related information so that it can be readily incorporated into people's thinking (Fischhoff, 1985). One component would be some indication of the quality of scientific studies regarding AIDS. Reports should describe the scientific (and practical) significance of results, not just their statistical significance. Reports should link new knowledge to existing knowledge, so that a coherent picture can be built. There is no guarantee that even the best formulated message will be relayed accurately (by the news media or by word of mouth). However, poor messages will only get worse in the retelling.

Finally, when it is hard to get information out of people, it is probably difficult to get information into them. For example, the ambiguities noted in the survey questions about the likelihood of AIDS risks need to be resolved in communications about those risks. That is, both the event and the associated probability need to be defined unambiguously. The same conclusion holds for the communication of any technical information. I recently saw a television report to the effect that some brands of condoms are only 22% reliable. How many viewers assumed that this means that users have a 78% chance of AIDS transmission (or pregnancy) if they use those condoms? How many interpreted it as meaning that 22% of shipments have fewer than 3 defective condoms per 1,000 (or whatever the actual definition is)? Similarly, if it is hard to get people to talk about their multifaceted decisions in an orderly way, then it will be hard to describe those decisions in an orderly way. If the choice of unit affects people's expressed estimates of risk, then it can also affect understanding of quantitative risk messages.

These are generic suggestions, applicable to helping people with any decisions. Working out the implications of the existing research for AIDS decisions will require detailed analysis. Testing those implications will require empirical research. There seem to be methods (and suggestive hypotheses) in place for undertaking those efforts.

Conclusion

Describing people's current perceptions is the first step toward understanding, predicting, and assisting their decisions. Describing these perceptions in the language of decision theory provides a common methodology for achieving these three aims: (a) It allows the description of many decisions in a single framework with clear logical relations among its terms. (b) That framework provides predictions of the decisions that might follow from people's more or less perfect perceptions of their decisions. (c) It allows identification of imperfections in decision making and the assessment of their importance. The associated behavioral research suggests a variety of possible biases that might be expected with AIDS decisions. It also provides some methods for improving these deficiencies and measuring the impact of such measures.

Decision making will seldom be perfect. People lack the time, concentration, and training for perfection. Some decisions are so complex that a very satisfactory resolution is unlikely. What an intervention can hope to do is help people get a little further into decisions before throwing up their hands and going with their intuitions.

Notes

1. Whether they used whatever subsidized testing was available might depend on what assurances of confidentiality were made—just one way in which AIDS decisions are interdependent.

2. In a series of studies regarding women's decision making about the threat of sexual assault, we identified 1,100 different action options sufficiently distinct that one could readily see how they might have different impacts on the consequence dimensions most salient to women (Fischhoff et al., 1987). Combined with multiple significant consequences and sources of uncertainty (mentioned by most participants in our studies), the result is an almost unfathomable matrix of possibilities facing the woman hoping to choose strategies with complete thoroughness.

3. This result should be distinguished from Zuckerman's (in press) finding of stable individual differences in sensation seeking. That refers to the amount of stimulus that people derive and want from the outcomes of their actions. Such stimulation is, however, thought of as another consequence of decision making. The actions chosen by people who desire more sensation might also have higher levels of risk. However, such apparent risk seeking is an effect rather than a cause of their sensation seeking.

4. One salient contrast to this perspective might be the current "Just Say 'No'" campaign, designed to discourage drug use among youth. In decision-making terms, it disallows consideration of consequences that might support drug use (e.g., social acceptability, new experiences). Another contrast can be found in the advice literature telling women how to defend themselves against the threat of sexual assault. It, too, offers categorical advice on what all women should do, ignoring any differences in their personal situations or values. Unlike the drug advice, however, this literature is internally inconsistent, with different experts offering different universal advice (Morgan, 1986).

5. Economic procedures go the furthest toward reducing all consequences to a common denominator (in this case, money). These procedures prove controversial even for many consequences that are in commerce; they are almost hopeless for ones that are not (e.g., Bentkover et al., 1985; Cummings, Brookshire, & Schulze, 1986).

6. The nuances of such procedures have been worked out in great detail for a wide

variety of different situations, with much more complex interdependencies than can be considered here (Keeney & Raiffa, 1976).

7. One might, however, consider previous investments as a source of information (showing the effects of such effort) or as creating a public commitment that it is hard to abandon (so that "saving face" becomes a consequence).

8. Svenson and Fischhoff (1985) contrast the focal radon decision facing laypeople (shown in Figure 11.1) with the decision most occupying radon officials—what level of radon concentration to designate as requiring remedial action. Used in that way, decision trees can help clarify the differences in perspectives between experts and laypeople, potential barriers to communication and understanding.

9. Radon is a radioactive gas, the short-lived decay products of which can lodge in the lungs. Released from the ground, it can reach sufficiently dangerous concentrations that some 20,000 annual lung cancer deaths have been attributed to it (U.S. Environmental Protection Agency, 1987).

10. The alternative to relying on one's own subjective estimates is relying on the estimates produced by others. The susceptibility of expert estimates to judgmental biases is a topic in its own right (e.g., Dawes, 1988; Einhorn & Hogarth, 1978; Fischhoff, in press; Henrion & Fischhoff, 1986; Kahneman, Slovic, & Tversky, 1982; Murphy & Brown, 1984). One summary is that the judgmental processes of experts resemble those of other people when they are forced to go beyond hard data and rely on intuition, unless they have had the conditions needed to learn particular judgments as learned skills.

11. Further details can be found in Linville et al. (1988).

12. As elsewhere, these estimates showed considerable internal consistency. For example, estimates of personal AIDS risk from sexual activity were highly correlated with estimates of personal herpes risk ($r = .90$), but not so highly correlated with AIDS risk from nonsexual sources ($r = .41$).

References

Bar Hillel, M. (1973). The subjective probability of compound events. *Organizational Behavior and Human Performance, 9*, 396–406.

Bar Hillel, M. (1980). The base-rate fallacy in probability judgments. *Acta Psychologica, 44*, 211–233.

Beach, L. R., Campbell, F. L., & Townes, B. D. (1979). Subjective expected utility and the prediction of birth-planning decisions. *Organizational Behavior & Human Performance, 24*, 18–28.

Behn, R. D., & Vaupel, J. W. (1983). *Quick analysis for busy decision makers.* New York: Basic Books.

Bentkover, J., Covello, V. T., & Mumpower, J. (Eds.). (1985). *Benefits assessment: The state of the art.* Amsterdam: Reidel.

Beyth-Marom, R. (1982). How probable is probable? *Journal of Forecasting, 1*, 257–269.

Blackshaw, L., & Fischhoff, B. (in press). Decision making in online search. *Journal of American Society for Information Sciences.*

Combs, B., & Slovic, P. (1979). Newspaper coverage of causes of death. *Journalism Quarterly, 56*(4), 837–843, 849.

Coombs, C. (1964). *A theory of data.* New York: John Wiley.

Coombs, C., Dawes, R. M., & Tversky, A. (1970). *Mathematical psychology: An elementary introduction.* Englewood Cliffs, NJ: Prentice-Hall.

Corbin, R. M. (1980). Decisions that might not get made. In T. Wallsten (Ed.), *Cognitive processes in choice and decision behavior.* Hillsdale, NJ: Lawrence Erlbaum.

Cummings, R. G., Brookshire, D. S., & Schulze, W. D. (1986). *Valuing environmental goods: An assessment of the contingent valuation method.* Totowa, NJ: Rowman & Allenheld.

Davidshofer, I. O. (1976). Risk taking and vocational choice: Reevaluation. *Journal of Counseling Psychology, 23,* 151–154.

Dawes, R. M. (1972). *Fundamentals of attitude measurement.* New York: John Wiley.

Dawes, R. M. (1979). The robust beauty of improper linear models in decision making. *American Psychologist, 34,* 571–582.

Dawes, R. M. (1988). *Rational choice in an uncertain world.* San Diego: Harcourt Brace Jovanovich.

Eddy, D. M. (1982). Probabilistic reasoning in clinical medicine: Problems and opportunities. In D. Kahneman, P. Slovic, & A. Tversky (Eds.), *Judgment under uncertainty: Heuristics and biases.* New York: Cambridge University Press.

Einhorn, H., & Hogarth, R. (1978). Confidence in judgment: Persistence in the illusion of validity. *Psychological Review, 85,* 395–416.

Ericsson, K. A., & Simon, H. A. (1980). Verbal reports as data. *Psychological Review, 87,* 215–251.

Ericsson, K. A., & Simon, H. A. (1984). *Verbal reports as data.* Cambridge: MIT Press.

Feather, N. T. (1982). *Expectancy, incentive and action.* Hillsdale, NJ: Lawrence Erlbaum.

Fineberg, H. V. (1987). Education to prevent AIDS: Prospects and obstacles. *Science, 239,* 592–596.

Fischhoff, B. (in press). Eliciting expert judgment. *IEEE Transactions on Systems, Man, and Cybernetics.*

Fischhoff, B. (1985, Winter). Environmental reporting: What to ask the experts. *Journalist,* pp. 11–15.

Fischhoff, B., & Beyth-Marom, R. (1983). Hypothesis evaluation from a Baysian perspective. *Psychological Review, 90,* 239–260.

Fischhoff, B., & Furby, L. (1988). Measuring values: A conceptual framework for interpreting transactions with special reference to contingent valuation of visibility. *Journal of Risk and Uncertainty, 1,* 147–184.

Fischhoff, B., Furby, L., & Morgan, M. (1987). Rape prevention: A typology and list of strategies. *Journal of Interpersonal Violence, 2*(3), 292–308.

Fischhoff, B., Lichtenstein, S., Slovic, P., Derby, S. L., & Keeney, R. L. (1981). *Acceptable risk.* New York: Cambridge University Press.

Fischhoff, B., Slovic, P., & Lichtenstein, S. (1978). Fault trees: Sensitivity of estimated failure probabilities to problem representation. *Journal of Experimental Psychology: Human Perception and Performance, 4,* 330–344.

Fischhoff, B., Slovic, P., & Lichtenstein, S. (1980). Knowing what you want: Measuring labile values. In T. Wallsten (Ed.), *Cognitive processes in choice and decision behavior.* Hillsdale, NJ: Lawrence Erlbaum.

Fischhoff, B., Slovic, P., Lichtenstein, S., Read, S., & Combs, B. (1978). How safe is safe enough? A psychometric study of attitudes towards technological risks and benefits. *Policy Sciences, 8,* 127–152.

Fiske, S. T., & Taylor, S. (1984). *Social cognition.* Reading, MA: Addison-Wesley.

Furby, L., & Fischhoff, B. (in press). Rape self-defense strategies: A review of their effectiveness. *Victimology.*

Furby, L., Fischhoff, B., & Morgan, M. (1989). Judged effectiveness of common rape prevention and self-defense strategies. *Journal of Interpersonal Violence, 4*, 44–64.

Gettys, C. F., Pliske, R. M., Manning, C. A., & Casey, J. T. (1987). An evaluation of human act generation performance. *Organizational Behavior and Human Decision Processes, 39*, 23–51.

Hasher, L., & Zacks, R. T. (1984). Automatic and effortful processes in memory. *Journal of Experimental Psychology: General, 108*, 356–388.

Henrion, M., & Fischhoff, B. (1986). Assessing uncertainty in physical constants. *American Journal of Physics, 54*(9), 791–798.

Hershey, J. C., & Schoemaker, P.J.H. (1980). Risk taking and problem solving in the domain of losses. *Journal of Risk and Insurance, 47*, 111–132.

Hintzman, D. (1969). Apparent frequency as a function of frequency and spacing. *Journal of Experimental Psychology, 80*, 139–145.

Hoch, S. J. (1985). Counterfactual reasoning and accuracy in predicting personal events. *Journal of Experimental Psychology: Learning, Memory, & Cognition, 11*, 719–731.

Institute of Medicine, National Academy of Sciences. (1986). *Confronting AIDS: Directions for public health, health care and research.* Washington, DC: National Academy Press.

Janis, I. L. (Ed.). (1982). *Victims of groupthink.* Boston: Houghton Mifflin.

Jervis R. (1976). *Perception and misperception in international relations.* Princeton, NJ: Princeton University Press.

Johnson, D. (1972). *A systematic introduction to the psychology of thinking and judgment.* New York: Harper & Row.

Kahneman, D., Slovic, P., & Tversky, A. (Eds.). (1982). *Judgment under uncertainty: Heuristics and biases.* New York: Cambridge University Press.

Kahneman, D., & Tversky, A. (1973). On the psychology of prediction. *Psychological Review, 80*, 237–251.

Kahneman, D., & Tversky, A. (1979). Prospect theory: An analysis of decision under risk. *Econometrica, 47*, 263–281.

Keeney, R., & Raiffa, H. (1976). *Decisions with multiple objectives: Preferences and value trade-offs.* New York: John Wiley.

Langer, J. (1975). The illusion of control. *Journal of Personality and Social Psychology, 32*, 311–328.

Lebow, R. N., & Stein, J. (1987). Beyond deterrence. *Journal of Social Issues, 43*, 5–72.

Lichtenstein, S., Slovic, P., Fischhoff, B., Layman, M., & Combs, B. (1978). Judged frequency of lethal events. *Journal of Experimental Psychology: Human Learning and Memory, 4*, 551–578.

Linville, P., Fischhoff, B., & Fischer, G. (1988). *Judgments of AIDS risks.* Unpublished manuscript, Carnegie Mellon University.

Montgomery, H., & Svenson, O. (Eds.). (in press). *Process and structure in decision making.* London: John Wiley.

Morgan, M. (1986). Conflict and confusion: What rape prevention experts are telling women. *Sexual Assault and Coercion, 1*(5), 160–168.

Murphy, A. H., & Brown, B. (1984). Comparable evaluation of subjective weather forecasts in the United States. *Journal of Forecasting, 3*, 369–393.

Murphy, A. H., & Winkler, R. (1984). Probability of precipitation forecasts: A review. *Journal of the American Statistical Association, 79*, 391–400.

National Center for Health Statistics. (1987). Knowledge and attitudes about AIDS: Data from the National Health Interview Survey, August 10–30, 1987. *Advance Data, 146.*

204   Baruch Fischhoff

National Research Council. (1982). *Survey measure of subjective phenomena*. Washington, DC: Author.
National Research Council. (1988). *Human factors issues in color displays*. Washington, DC: Author, Committee on Human Factors.
Nisbett, R., & Ross, L. (1980). *Human inference: Strategies and shortcomings of social judgment*. Englewood Cliffs, NJ: Prentice-Hall.
Nisbett, R. E., & Wilson, T. D. (1977). Telling more than we know: Verbal reports on mental processes. *Psychological Review, 84*(3), 231–259.
Padian, N. S. (1987). Heterosexual transmission of acquired immunodeficiency syndrome: International perspectives and national projections. *Review of Infectious Diseases, 9*, 947–960.
Parducci, A. (1974). Contextual effects: A range-frequency analysis. In E. C. Carterette & M. P. Friedman (Eds.), *Handbook of perceptions* (Vol. 2). New York: Academic Press.
Poulton, E. C. (1968). The new psychophysics: Six models for magnitude estimation. *Psychological Bulletin, 69*, 1–19.
Poulton, E. C. (1977). Quantitative subjective assessments are almost always biased, sometimes completely misleading. *British Journal of Psychology, 68*, 409–425.
Poulton, E. C. (1982). Biases in quantitative judgments. *Ergonomics, 13*, 31–42.
Raiffa, H. (1968). *Decision analysis*. Reading, MA: Addison-Wesley.
Rokeach, M. (1973). *The nature of human values*. New York: Free Press.
Shaklee, H., Fischhoff, B., & Furby, L. (1988). *The psychology of contraceptive surprises: Cumulative risk and contraceptive effectiveness*. Eugene, OR: Eugene Research Institute.
Slovic, P. (1962). Convergent validation of risk-taking measures. *Psychological Bulletin, 65*, 68–71.
Slovic, P., Fischhoff, B., & Lichtenstein, S. (1978). Accident probabilities and seat belt usage: A psychological perspective. *Accident Analysis and Prevention, 10*, 281–285.
Svenson, O. (1979). Process descriptions of decision making. *Organizational Behavior and Human Performance, 23*, 86–112.
Svenson, O., & Fischhoff, B. (1985). Levels of environmental decisions: A case study of radiation in Swedish homes. *Journal of Environmental Psychology, 5*, 55–68.
Thaler, R. (1980). Toward a positive theory of consumer choice. *Journal of Economic Behavior and Organization, 1*, 39–60.
Thaler, R. (1985). Mental accounting and consumer choice. *Marketing Science, 4*, 199–214.
Turner, C. F., & Krauss, E. (1978). Fallible indicators of the subjective state of the nation. *American Psychologist, 33*, 456–470.
Turner, C. F., & Martin, E. (Eds.). (1985). *Surveying subjective phenomena*. New York: Russell Sage.
Tversky, A. (1969). The intransitivity of preferences. *Psychological Review, 76*, 31–48.
Tversky, A., & Kahneman, D. (1973). Availability: A heuristic for judging frequency and probability. *Cognitive Psychology, 4*, 207–232.
Tversky, A., & Kahneman, D. (1981). The framing of decisions and the psychology of choice. *Science, 211*, 453–458.
Tversky, A., Sattath, S., & Slovic, P. (1988). Contingent weighting in judgment and choice. *Psychological Review, 95*, 371–384.
U.S. Environmental Protection Agency. (1987). *Citizen's guide to radon protection*. Washington, DC: Government Printing Office.
U.S. Surgeon General. (1988). *Understanding AIDS*. Washington, DC: Government Printing Office.

von Winterfeldt, D., & Edwards, W. (1982). Costs and payoffs in perceptual research. *Psychological Bulletin, 93*, 609–622.

von Winterfeldt, D., & Edwards, W. (1986). *Decision analysis and behavioral research.* New York: Cambridge University Press.

Wallsten, T., & Budescu, D. (1983). Encoding subjective possibilities: A psychological and psychometric review. *Management Science, 29*, 151–173.

Watson, S., & Buede, D. (1987). *Decision synthesis.* New York: Cambridge University Press.

Weinstein, N. D. (1980). Unrealistic optimism about future events. *Journal of Personality and Social Psychology, 39*, 806–820

Zuckerman, M. (in press). Sensation seeking. In L. Lipsitt & L. Mitnick (Eds.), *Self-regulation and risk-taking behavior.* New York: Ablex.

PART IV

Prevention in Targeted Populations

Although the first reported AIDS cases appeared in White gay men, this section clearly illustrates that it would be incorrect to view AIDS as a disease limited in its impact to one specific subpopulation. Instead, HIV, like all diseases to afflict human beings, has followed multiple infectious paths wherever the opportunity created through human behavior and geographic proximity has allowed transmission. In reality, AIDS has affected diverse segments of our society, recognizing only behavioral boundaries, not our artificial and socially constructed definitions of people, including differences in racial/ethnic status, creed, sexual orientation, age, and income.

HIV infects by very clear rules, as discussed in earlier chapters, so large numbers of cases have appeared in particular groups, such as gay and bisexual males, intravenous drug users, Blacks, and Latinos. But diagnosed AIDS cases have also appeared with less frequency in other groups—Native Americans, Asians, adolescents, women, and the elderly. While there are fewer total cases in these latter groups, it is important that we not forget or minimize our prevention efforts here. There is much that can be learned as to the importance of factors that may influence HIV transmission.

What the chapters in this section illustrate is how cultural norms related to sexual orientation, gender, ethnicity, economic status, or religion affect behaviors that may either facilitate or hinder HIV transmission. Each chapter, while focused on a particular population, provides the reader with basic information on the disease's epidemiology and the role of culture and community influences on HIV-related behaviors. The chapters also address the complex problems faced by those interested in working with individuals or communities who have been targeted as important in our prevention efforts. As an example, Aoki and his colleagues cogently remind us of the necessity to design interventions specific to subgroups within populations who themselves are never homogeneous when it comes to behavior, norms, or values. Among Asians, there is no single Asian community; rather, there are 32 distinct ethnic subgroups, each with different language, attitudes, traditions, and behaviors.

The importance of diversity should not be lost when the focus is on gay men, either. Joseph and her coauthors underscore that for some gay men the act of changing or not changing HIV-related behaviors may exact psychological costs. On the positive side, Morin points out in his commentary that distress associated with difficulties in behavior change may not be a negative event if it leads individuals to seek out sources of support and help. The utility of interventions tailored for gay men is illustrated in the chapter by Kelly and his colleagues. It is not enough merely to reach the population of gay men; it is important that we provide diverse prevention and intervention efforts effective in facilitating, not complicating, behavior change efforts. While factual HIV risk-reduction information is relevant for all gay men, it is that part of prevention focusing on expectancies, emotions, cognitions, and attitudes where differences may emerge as a function of individual differences within populations.

At the same time, this section highlights some of the similarities in issues across the distinct groups. In particular, on reading the chapters by Mata and Jorquez, Aoki and his colleagues, Cochran, Mays, and Tafoya, what emerges is the importance of acculturation, generational and immigration status, place of residence, class, and poverty to understanding risk for HIV infection across several different populations. There are common hurdles in the prevention of AIDS and HIV transmission, although it may be that the solutions differ as a function of each group's resources and norms. Catania and his colleagues explore the relationship of risk reduction to help-seeking behaviors among gay men, who may turn toward their community for support and help. In contrast, for others, families of origin may be a major part of a help-seeking solution. Ramos adeptly identifies the more difficult prevention efforts as those that are directed not at individuals, but at groups, families, and communities.

Finally, this section of the book includes commentaries to provide additional voices and guidance. Morin, who published one of the earliest articles on heterosexist bias in research on gay populations and continues to be an active AIDS researcher, again offers the reader an eloquently written view of the psychological context of gay men's behavior change. Ramos underscores the necessity of developing primary prevention strategies that incorporate the ideas outlined in the chapters on ethnic minorities and women. Morales, while focusing on the chapter by Mata and Jorquez, highlights many of the issues pertinent to all of the targeted populations. He offers readers a thoughtful commentary on the importance of subcultures within cultural and ethnic communities in the fight against AIDS.

12

Are There Psychological Costs Associated with Changes in Behavior to Reduce AIDS Risk?

Jill G. Joseph
Ronald C. Kessler
Camille B. Wortman
John P. Kirscht
Margalit Tal
Susan Caumartin
Suzann Eshleman
Michael Eller

Background

Following identification of the acquired immunodeficiency syndrome in 1981 (Friedman-Kier et al., 1981; Gottlieb et al., 1981), the importance of behavioral changes to reduce spread of the epidemic became apparent (Centers for Disease Control, 1983; Institute of Medicine, 1986). As the earliest identified and largest group of those contributing to the patient population, homosexual and bisexual men have been the focus of special intervention efforts. In particular, they have been urged to reduce their number of sexual partners, to avoid contact with anonymous partners, and to avoid, or modify through

Authors' Note: This work was supported by funding from the National Institute of Mental Health (2 RO1 MH39346–02A1) and the University of Michigan for the Coping and Change Study, and by the National Institute of Allergy and Infectious Diseases for the Chicago Multicenter AIDS Cohort Study (NO1-AI-32535), with partial funding by the National Cancer Institute. Special appreciation is expressed to participants in these concurrent studies, whose continuing assistance makes this research possible. Please refer questions, comments, and requests for reprints to Jill G. Joseph, Ph.D., Department of Epidemiology, School of Public Health, University of Michigan, 109 Observatory Street, Ann Arbor, MI 48109.

condom use, the practice of anal sex (Centers for Disease Control, 1988; Martin & Vance, 1984). Fortunately, a recent review suggests that in this population behavioral changes, although not uniform, are extensive (Becker & Joseph, 1988). Considerable recidivism has been observed, and there continue to be some men who maintain high-risk behaviors. Special concerns have also been expressed about the needs of minority gay men, those not living in urban centers, young men initiating homosexual activity, and "closeted" or bisexual men. In addition, active debate continues regarding the most appropriate methods for facilitating both the maintenance of established lower-risk behaviors and further behavioral risk reduction. For example, the special roles of "eroticized" educational materials, of peer support progress, and of HIV antibody testing remain controversial.

Permanent changes in sexual behavior are essential for preventing further transmission of the human immunodeficiency virus and thus extension of the AIDS epidemic. Those who are already infected will continue to carry the virus throughout their lifetimes, and those not yet infected will need to protect themselves for as long as they continue to be sexually active. In this context it becomes particularly important to specify carefully and respond to any unanticipated and negative consequences of behavioral risk reduction.

Qualitative investigations undertaken by our research group suggest that men who change their sexual behavior may do so at some psychological cost to themselves. Issues mentioned in focus group and individual discussions include accepting attributions of risk, dealing with potential personal implications of seeing friends or lovers diagnosed and ill with AIDS, and feelings of discouragement associated with unsuccessful attempts to change behavior. In addition, these men frequently described difficult alterations in both personal and community attitudes regarding sexuality. While recommendations for safer sex were endorsed as medically justified, they also were associated with similar historic and homophobic attempts to regulate or eliminate male homosexual behavior. For these men now to support and attempt to conform to such recommendations has often resulted in considerable dissonance. Similarly, the alteration of patterns of community socialization and sexual contact have been recognized as a source of distress. Some men referred, for example, to ways in which the bar scene was changing or to conflicts within gay organizations regarding appropriate responses to the AIDS epidemic. Finally, there was an ongoing and acute awareness of the political and policy environment within which they were attempting to restructure their lives. Proposals for mandatory testing and reporting of those who were seropositive, or even of quarantine, were frequent sources of distress (Ostrow, Eller, & Joseph, 1987). Even though many of these events and circumstances impinge on all gay men, those who are actively attempting to change their behavior may be more aware of or affected by these issues.

In addition to subjective impressions gained from focus groups and discussions with members of our cohort, there are multiple theoretical reasons for concern about the potentially negative sequelae of behavioral change. The life events literature suggests, for example, that both psychological and physical health may be influenced by alterations in life circumstances (Dohrenwend & Dohrenwend, 1974; Kasl, 1984). While voluntarily undertaken behavioral changes differ in many ways from imposed and often unanticipated events, it could be argued theoretically that such changes may also constitute potentially burdensome life events. Viewed in another way, the epidemic of AIDS might be seen as a social disaster; proximity to this disaster would be represented by variable awareness of the effects of AIDS, with those endeavoring to reduce their risk among the most aware. There is a provocative research literature that suggests that the experience of physical or natural disasters may negatively affect subsequent psychological functioning (Longue, Melick, & Hansen, 1981). Although it would be inappropriate to generalize the circumstances of gay men simplistically, this literature does suggest the value of exploring the question posed for this chapter.

Finally, there is a growing appreciation for the role of denial or illusion in the maintenance of psychological functioning (Lazarus & Delongis, 1983; Taylor & Brown, 1988). It seems possible that those men able to use denial in dealing with the AIDS epidemic might better be able to maintain psychological well-being, although at the cost of continued high-risk behavior. Put another way, those who understand and accept the enormity of the AIDS threat may be motivated to undertake behavioral changes, although such accurate perceptions might also be incompatible with a robust sense of psychological well-being.

In summary, both our own observations and theoretical considerations led us to ask if behavioral risk reduction is subsequently associated with adverse mental health effects. This investigation is in no way intended to diminish the importance of behavioral change; instead, it is meant to provide a more realistic understanding of the potentially complex relationship of behavior change to other aspects of the lives of gay men. As suggested above, we believe this is particularly important if safer sexual behaviors are to be maintained successfully. It is sobering

TABLE 12.1

Sociodemographic and Health Characteristics of the
Cohort

	Wave 1	Wave 4
Mean age (years)	34.4	
Mean income (1984 $)	24,000	
Mean education (years)	16.1	
Seropositive		36.0%
Symptomatic		39.0%

to note that emotional distress may precede and seemingly accounts for 30–70% of relapses from desired behavioral changes unrelated to AIDS (Shiffman, 1982). If this is also true for changes in sexual behavior, the question posed here is an especially important one.

Methods

Men participating in this study are enrolled in the Chicago Multicenter AIDS Cohort Study (MACS) (Kaslow et al., 1987) and visit the study center semiannually for physical examinations and laboratory studies. Standard methods are used to determine and confirm HIV serologic status at each of these visits. All MACS participants in Chicago were also invited to participate in the Coping and Change Study (CCS), a National Institute of Mental Health-funded study concerned with psychological and behavioral aspects of the AIDS epidemic. Thus both biomedical and psychosocial data are available describing participants. A summary of the sociodemographic, behavioral, and health characteristics of the cohort is provided in Table 12.1.

The results reported below are confined to those 525 men who participated in each of the first four biannual MACS and CCS assessments between spring 1984 and spring 1986. Recruited in a variety of ways from the Chicago gay male community, this cohort is not generally representative of all male homosexuals living in Chicago. Like cohorts being followed in other major metropolitan areas, it is a largely White, well-educated group of men whose mean age is in the mid-30s.

Serologic status was determined on the basis of standard ELISA and confirmatory Western Blot techniques on blood collected at each

MACS clinic visit. Beginning in the second year of the study (following the Wave 3 visit), participants were offered an opportunity to obtain their serologic test results. A careful protocol was established that required both pre- and postdisclosure counseling with appropriate referral, as necessary, to gay-sensitive psychological services. Special attention was paid to preventing release of personally identifiable test results to any study personnel, unless the participant chose to share this information himself. In Chicago during 1985 and 1986 there was considerable skepticism regarding the desirability of serologic testing and comparatively few men (N = 55) had obtained their test results by the Wave 4 visit, which concludes the observational period described here. Of these 55 men, 23 were seropositive. Health status was assessed by the MACS both on the basis of standardized physical examination and intercurrent medical history. Each participant was classified as symptomatic (including those with bilateral multisite lymphadenopathy only) or asymptomatic. Approximately one-third of the cohort was symptomatic at both Wave 1 and Wave 4.

Pilot studies had suggested that completion of psychosocial and behavioral questionnaires at the study center led to increased reporting of AIDS-relevant events and preoccupations. Therefore, participants were given the CCS questionnaire to complete at home approximately two weeks following their visit to the MACS study center. In this way psychological and social functioning data may be more representative of a participant's usual level of functioning.

Sexual behaviors associated in the epidemiologic literature with risk of HIV infection are assessed in some detail in the CCS questionnaire. Participants are asked to report the frequency and type of receptive male homosexual activity practiced with a variety of partners, ranging from the primary sexual partner to anonymous sexual partners. Behaviors are described for the preceding month, a period of time that was found to be sufficiently short to permit accurate recall yet long enough to provide representative data. A four-level summary behavioral Risk Index (RI) was constructed based on the number and type of sexual partners, the practice of receptive anal intercourse, and condom usage. The RI was validated by examining seroconversion data among those originally seronegative (not further reported). For the purposes of longitudinal analysis, the RI was dichotomized so that lower-risk (no-risk and low-risk categories combined) and higher-risk (modified high- and high-risk categories combined) participants are compared. Analyses reported below use the dichotomized risk index (lower risk versus higher risk) to describe intraindividual patterns of

TABLE 12.2

Behavioral Patterns During Two Years of Observation (N = 525)

Behavioral Pattern	Number	Percentage
Consistently low risk behavior LLLL	154	29.3
Improving risk behavior HHHL HHLL HLLL	139	26.5
Inconsistent risk behavior all other e.g. HLLH LHLL	141	26.9
Consistently high risk behavior HHHH	91	17.3

behavior across the two-year period of observation. As shown in Table 12.2, sixteen possible combinations of lower- and higher-risk behavior were observed, falling into four broad categories: (a) consistently lower risk at each of the four assessments, (b) improving from higher- to lower-risk behavior without any subsequent recidivism, (c) inconsistent or deteriorating, and (d) consistently high-risk behavior at each of the four assessments.

The assessment of mental health and psychosocial variables in this cohort is based on use of both standard scales and either specially developed adaptations or new scales for use in populations of gay men. As described elsewhere, a year of preliminary work was devoted to focus group and individual interviews that led to the development of many of the indices described below (Joseph et al., 1984). This work was designed to take into account preexisting information concerning appropriate and reliable assessment as well as the special nature of this population and the AIDS crisis.

The 58-item Hopkins Symptom Checklist (HSCL) was used to assess psychological functioning in five domains during the preceding month: somatization, obsessive-compulsive behavior, interpersonal sensitivity or paranoialike ideation, depression, and anxiety (Derogatis, Lipman, Rickels, Uhlenhuth, & Covi, 1974). In addition, these items were summed to yield a total distress score. The content and distribution of the HSCL indices used are provided in Table 12.3. As suggested above, the social environment has been changed dramatically by the AIDS epidemic in ways that may provide unique stressors

TABLE 12.3

Assessment of Mental Health: Hopkins Symptom Checklist

Scales	Wave 1 X ± SD	Wave 4 X ± SD
Somatization (e.g., headaches; pains in heart)	10.4 ± 9.9	10.0 ± 10.7
Obsessive behavior (e.g., worrying about sloppiness; having to check and double-check what one does)	17.9 ± 16.8	16.4 ± 16.1
Anxiety (e.g., nervousness; being scared for no reason)	17.5 ± 15.4	16.1 ± 15.1
Interpersonal sensitivity (e.g., feeling shy or uneasy; feelings easily hurt)	20.8 ± 18.1	17.7 ± 16.6
Depression (e.g., feeling blue; feeling hopeless about the future)	21.2 ± 17.6	18.4 ± 16.1

capable of compromising the psychological well-being of gay men. Three such potential stressors were considered. The first was a simple dichotomy that contrasts those men who have experienced AIDS diagnoses among friends, acquaintances, or lovers with those who have not. The second assessment of a potential stressor is based on focus group results that resulted in a new inventory. This instrument examined experiences of discrimination or conflict associated with gay identity and the AIDS crisis. Eleven such items were assessed, ranging from workplace hostility to conflict in gay organizations. Both major events (such as violence or police harassment) and less extreme situations (for example, family disapproval) were included. With the exception of items dealing with conflicts with other gay men or within gay organizations regarding AIDS, the prevalence of such events was usually less than 10% for any given item. The occurrence of each of these items was summed and standardized to a 0–100 scale providing an aggregated, unweighted measure of experiences characterized by conflict or hostility.

An additional source of possible distress is that arising from receiving HIV serologic test results. As reported above, few men had sought their results prior to Wave 4; therefore, the impact of this event is less likely to explain the observed differences in mental health across behavioral groups. Nonetheless, the effect of notification regarding a positive serology was also examined.

Coping strategies were also examined for their relationship to the observed effect on mental health. Based on both standard scales (Folkman & Lazarus, 1980; Vitaliano, Russ, Carr, & Heerwagen, 1984) and focus group results, a coping inventory with four scales was developed specifically to describe responses to the AIDS crisis. The indices assessed four distinct coping strategies: health vigilance, collective involvement, spiritual approaches, and denial. These indices' scoring of the coping was also standardized to a 0–100 scale. It should be noted that alpha reliabilities were calculated and ranged from .59 to .75. Further description of these scales describing potential stressors and their distribution in the cohort is provided in Table 12.4.

In order to begin assessing the relationship between psychological distress and behavioral change, the mean level of each of the HSCL subscores as well as the total distress score at Wave 4 was plotted for each of the four behavioral patterns, as shown in Figures 12.1 and 12.2. It is important to remember that this is a distress score, with higher numbers indicating more distress.

It is apparent that for all scales, the lowest level of psychological distress was observed in those who maintained consistently higher-risk behavior in the preceding two years. Results of analysis of variance reveal that differences between the consistently high-risk group and the other groups usually achieve statistical significance. For example, with respect to the total HSCL score, the consistently high-risk group has lower scores than each of the other three behavioral groups ($p \leq$ .04), which do not differ from one another.

It is also possible to compare anxiety and depression scores to norms for the general population and psychiatric outpatient samples provided in validation studies of the HSCL. There are obvious difficulties in applying these norms to a cohort of well-educated and homosexual men. Nonetheless, this contrast makes it possible to develop at least some qualitative sense of what the observed HSCL scores "mean." The HSCL subscale scores in the cohort are intermediate between the two validation samples providing normative data, although closer to the general population mean value. This suggests that the cohort is typically experiencing distress rather than acute symptomatology.

The first question to ask regarding these provocative findings is whether the psychological differences precede rather than arise from the behavioral patterns. In order to examine this question, HSCL scores at entry (Wave 1) were examined in terms of their relationship to future behavioral patterns, as shown in Figures 12.3 and 12.4. There are no differences in psychological distress among the four groups defined by their future behavior. Put another way, those men

TABLE 12.4
Psychosocial Variables: Stressors and Coping Strategies

Social environmental stressors			
Network AIDS diagnosis	Personally know someone with AIDS? (single item)	yes = 33.3%	
Notified seropositive by W4		yes = 4.4%	

		Observed Range	X ± SD
Conflict/hostility experiences	Hostility or conflict: workplace, family, gay community, service providers (11 items)	0–80	26.3 ± 20.0
Coping strategies			
Health vigilance	Use of health care providers; attempts to improve health; pay attention to body (4 items; alpha = .59)	0–100	49.9 ± 22.8
Collective participation	Get involved and try to help; believe AIDS brings community together (3 items; alpha = .60)	0–100	35.1 ± 24.4
Spiritual responses	Seek spiritual comfort, approaches (2 items; alpha = .75)	0–100	22.0 ± 26.3
Denial	Avoid thinking, taking AIDS seriously; remind self most gay men healthy (3 items; alpha = .59)	0–100	24.9 ± 16.1

who subsequently had markedly different behavior did not differ from one another at the beginning of the study interval.

This, then, suggests that various patterns of behavior gave rise to differences in psychological functioning, rather than that differences

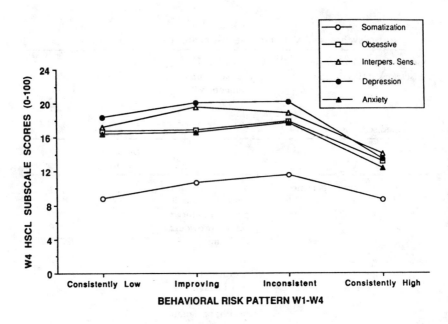

Figure 12.1 Relationship of Behavioral Pattern between Waves 1 and 4 to Subsequent HSCL Subscale Scores at Wave 4

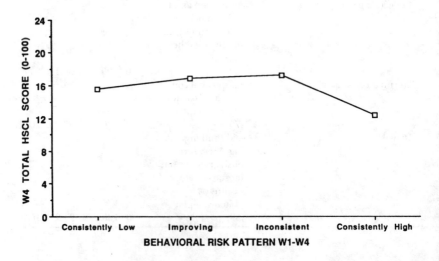

Figure 12.2 Relationship of Behavioral Pattern between Waves 1 and 4 to Subsequent HSCL Total Score at Wave 4

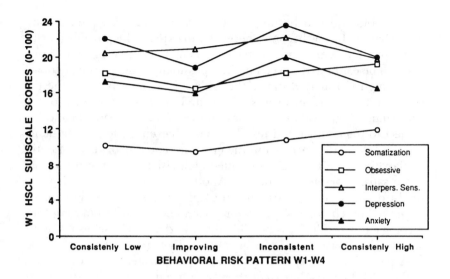

Figure 12.3 Relationship of Behavioral Pattern between Waves 1 and 4 to Preceding HSCL Subscale Scores at Wave 1

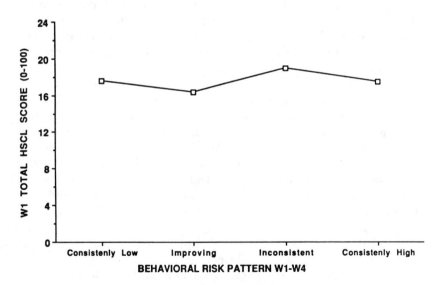

Figure 12.4 Relationship of Behavioral Pattern between Waves 1 and 4 to Preceding HSCL Total Score at Wave 1

in psychological functioning led to variability in subsequent behavioral change. It now becomes necessary to explore the possible mechanisms by which behavior may have such an effect. As suggested above, two will be examined here. The first possibility is that those at consistently high risk may distance themselves in some way from the gay community and from events within it. If this is the case, those at consistently high risk might be less aware of the toll of AIDS and less subject to the conflict and hostility that it has engendered. Maintaining this "social distance" from the epidemic could provide a potential explanation both for their continued high-risk behavior and for their more satisfactory mental health. Another way in which participants might distance themselves from the epidemic and thereby maintain improved psychological functioning would be to avoid obtaining HIV serologic test results. It is possible that avoidance of test result disclosure might characterize those at consistently higher risk.

A second possibility is that it is the coping strategies of consistently higher-risk men, rather than their circumstances, that contribute to the better mental health observed in that group. This explanation would lead to the hypothesis that even among those who are equally aware of the AIDS epidemic and its impact among other gay men, there may be marked differences in personal responses. As suggested above, use of denial might particularly be associated with improved psychological functioning, while at the same time encouraging maintenance of higher-risk behaviors.

In addition to these hypothesized psychosocial explanations, there are several confounders that may explain the observed relationship. It is possible, although unlikely, that health status may be better among those at consistently higher risk and would lead to improved mental health. This appears unlikely, as it is these men one would expect to become more rapidly infected and ill. Nonetheless, this explanation requires exploration. Additionally, more classical sociodemographic variables such as education or income might be unequivalently distributed across the four groups. This effect also needs to be examined.

An initial approach to the question of what characterizes those at consistently higher risk is to inspect differences in psychosocial or health variables among the four behavioral patterns. In analyses of variance not further reported there was little suggestion that those at consistently high risk are distinguished by differences in the AIDS-relevant social environment or their responses to it. Additionally, both serologic status and health status appeared to correspond poorly to

TABLE 12.5

Relationship of Behavioral and Psychosocial Variables to Total HSCL Score at Wave 4, Controlling for Mental Health at Wave 1: Results of Regression Analysis

	Coefficient	SE	P
High-risk behavior	−4.04	1.48	.007
Notification of positive serology	−3.12	2.99	.30
AIDS diagnosis in network	1.33	1.22	.27
Conflict/hostility experiences	1.81	0.33	<.001
Health vigilance	0.01	0.02	.62
Collective orientation	0.03	0.02	.23
Religious responses	0.00	0.02	.88
Denial	0.06	0.04	.10
Serologic status	0.52	1.36	.70
Health status	1.65	1.29	.20
Age	0.04	0.07	.56
Income	−0.63	0.15	<.001
Education	0.27	0.26	.29
Wave 1 HSCL total score	0.57	0.03	<.001

NOTE: N = 475; R^2 = 47.2%.

the differences observed in mental health. These preliminary, univariate analyses were then examined more rigorously in a multivariate regression approach.

A regression model was constructed that examined the relationship of behavioral and psychosocial variables to the total HSCL distress score at Wave 4. As shown in Table 12.5, the multiple linear regression includes a dummy variable describing membership in the group with consistently high-risk behavior. In addition, the other health, psychosocial, and sociodemographic variables discussed above were included in the regression analyses: receiving positive test results, AIDS diagnosis in one's network, experiences of conflict or hostility, the four coping strategies, positive HIV serology, health status, age, income, and education. In addition, to assess the effects of behavior on mental health at Wave 4 most rigorously, a covariate also described mental health at Wave 1. This is necessary because the strongest predictor of subsequent mental health is usually current mental health.

This analysis assesses whether the effects of being at consistently high risk are explained by covariates included in the model. As shown in Table 12.5, consistently high-risk behavior continues to be a significant predictor of better mental health after controlling for Wave 1 HSCL scores and all other covariates (B = −4.04, p = .007). Thus

neither the occurrence of stressors nor specific coping strategies explain the observed association. It is also true, however, that there
appears to be an independent relationship between experiences of
conflict or hostility and increased psychological distress (B = 1.81, $p <$
.001). In addition, a measure of socioeconomic status, income, is associated with better psychological functioning (B = -0.63, $p <$ .001).

Discussion

Results presented in this chapter help provide answers to a series of
important questions. The first and most fundamental is whether there
are psychological costs associated with behavioral risk reduction.
Based on both univariate and multivariate analyses, it appears that
there are psychological advantages associated with the maintenance of
higher-risk behavior and costs associated with behavioral change. The
second series of questions attempts to explain the benefits accruing to
those who are maintaining high-risk behavior. Two broad categories
of possible explanatory variables were suggested above. The first postulates that those at highest risk may be more peripheral to the gay
male community and to the epidemic itself. The second postulates
that those at higher risk participate in the community but are characterized by coping mechanisms that minimize both their distress and
the perceived need to change their own behavior. Multivariate findings demonstrated that the relationship of high-risk behavior to better
functioning persists after variables describing both possible explanations are controlled for. There is also an independent contribution of
negative experiences of conflict or hostility in the social environment
to adverse mental health.

The compelling reason for investigating any relationship between
behavior and mental health has to do with the maintenance of lower-
risk behaviors. The primary focus must be on behavioral risk reduction to prevent further HIV transmission. As reported above, if those
undertaking alterations of sexual behavior are experiencing increased
levels of psychological distress, this is extremely important to know.
Preventive educational messages might alert individuals to this possibility and assist them by providing resources for coping with such
adverse effects. In addition, more detailed analyses should be conducted to determine if there are specific behavioral changes that are
associated with decrements in psychological functioning. For example, is it men who are attempting to become celibate or those eliminat-

ing particular sexual practices who experience increased distress? We already know on the basis of previous work in this cohort that the majority of men are attempting to modify rather than eliminate their homosexual behavior. We have argued that such preferences, as well as epidemiologic information, might inform educational efforts so that reasonable changes are recommended. Analyses reported here suggest an extension of this strategy to determine if there are specific changes that are particularly stressful. If so, men might be apprised of this fact so that they can take it into account in selecting how they go about reducing their risk of AIDS.

There is yet another message that emerges from these results. It is well-recognized that the gay male community has experienced the devastation of untimely and ghastly death among too many of its members. The evidence is also overwhelmingly clear that in the face of this, both personal and community resources have been marshaled, leading to perhaps the most rapid and extensive (albeit still incomplete) change in human behavior ever observed. It is now possible to appreciate further that such behavioral changes may take their own toll and that those who are changing their lives do so in spite of concomitant depression, anxiety, and generalized distress. It may be that such psychological consequences are unavoidable. If so, they are nonetheless preferable to high-risk behavior and continued transmission of HIV. The second message of these analyses is that experiences of homophobia, hostility, and conflict further burden those who are attempting to deal successfully with this epidemic. These additional sources of distress are not a necessary or inevitable result of an individual's being at risk for AIDS, but instead arise from social and legal circumstances that are, in themselves, potentially modifiable.

References

Becker, M. H., & Joseph, J. G. (1988). AIDS and behavioral change to reduce risk: A review. *American Journal of Public Health, 78,* 394–410.

Centers for Disease Control. (1983). Prevention of AIDS: Report of interagency recommendations. *Morbidity and Mortality Weekly Report, 32,* 101–104.

Derogatis, L., Lipman, R., Rickels, K., Uhlenhuth, E., & Covi, L. (1974). The Hopkins Symptom Checklist (HSCL): A self-report symptom inventory. *Behavioral Science, 19,* 1–15.

Dohrenwend, B. S., & Dohrenwend, B. P. (Eds.). (1974). *Stressful life events: Their nature and effects.* New York: John Wiley.

Folkman, S., & Lazarus, R. (1980). An analysis of coping in a middle-aged community sample. *Journal of Health and Social Behavior, 21,* 219–239.

224   Joseph et al.

Friedman-Kier, A. E., et al. (1981). Kaposi's sarcoma and p. carinii pneumonia among homosexual men—NYC and California. *Morbidity and Mortality Weekly Report, 30*, 205–208.

Gottlieb, M. S., et al. (1981). P. carinii pneumonia and mucosal candidiasis in previously healthy homosexual men: Evidence of a new acquired cellular immunodeficiency. *New England Journal of Medicine, 305*, 1425–1431.

Institute of Medicine and National Academy of Sciences. (1986). *Confronting AIDS: Directions for public health, health care and research.* Washington, DC: National Academy Press.

Joseph, J., Emmons, C., Kessler, R., Wortman, C., O'Brien, K., Hocker, W., & Schaefer, C. (1984). Coping with the threat of AIDS: An approach to psychosocial assessment. *American Psychologist, 39*, 1297–1302.

Kasl, S. V. (1984). Stress and health. *Annual Review of Public Health, 5*, 319–341.

Kaslow, R. A., Ostrow, D. G., Detels, R., Phair, J., Polk, B. F., & Rinaldo, C. (1987). The Multicenter AIDS Cohort Study: Rationale, organization, and selected characteristics of the participants. *American Journal of Epidemiology, 126*, 310–318.

Koop, C. E. (1986). *Surgeon general's report on acquired immunodeficiency syndrome.* Washington, DC: U.S. Department of Health and Human Services, Public Health Service.

Lazarus, R. S., & Delongis, A. (1983). Psychological stress and coping in aging. *American Psychologist, 38*, 245–254.

Longue, J. N., Melick, M. E., & Hansen, H. (1981). Research issues and directions in the epidemiology of health effects of disasters. In N. Nathanson & L. Gordis (Eds.), *Epidemiologic reviews* (Vol. 3, pp. 140–162). Baltimore: Johns Hopkins University Press.

Martin, J. L., & Vance, C. S. (1984). Behavioral and psychosocial factors in AIDS: Methodological and substantive issues. *American Psychologist, 39*, 1309–1314.

Ostrow, D. G., Eller, M., & Joseph, J. G. (1987). Epidemic control measures for AIDS: A psychosocial and historical discussion of policy alternatives. In I. B. Coreless & M. Pittman-Linderman (Eds.), *AIDS: Principles, practices, and politics* (pp. 19–31). Washington, DC: Hemisphere.

Shiffman, S. (1982). Relapse following smoking cessation: A situational analysis. *Journal of Consulting and Clinical Psychology, 50*, 71–86.

Taylor, S. E., & Brown, J. (1988). Illusion and well-being: A social psychological perspective on mental health. *Psychological Bulletin, 103*, 193–210.

Vitaliano, P. P., Russ, J., Carr, J. E., & Heerwagen, J. H. (1984). Medical school pressures and their relationship to anxiety. *Journal of Nervous and Mental Disorders, 172*, 730–736.

13

Group Intervention to Reduce AIDS Risk Behaviors in Gay Men: Applications of Behavioral Principles

Jeffrey A. Kelly
Janet S. St. Lawrence
Ted L. Brasfield
Harold V. Hood

Since the start of the health crisis, cases of acquired immune deficiency syndrome in the United States and in most Western nations have been disproportionately concentrated among homosexual men. Approximately 63% of Americans with AIDS currently are gay or bisexual males, and an additional 7% of cases have occurred among gay men who are also users of intravenous drugs (Centers for Disease Control, 1988). It is now very clear that human immunodeficiency virus infection is also transmitted heterosexually, both from males to females and from females to males (Clumeck et al., 1984; Fischl et al., 1987; Redfield et al., 1985). However, the current prevalence of HIV infection is much higher among gay men than among most heterosexual populations in the United States, presumably due to the early introduction of HIV infection into this population and the efficiency of viral transmission among men who engage in anal intercourse with multiple partners. It is estimated that between 20% and 60% of nonmonogamous homosexual men are HIV infected, depending

Authors' Note: This research was supported by NIMH Grant R01-MH41800. Correspondence should be addressed to Jeffrey A. Kelly, Ph.D., Division of Psychology, Department of Psychiatry and Human Behavior, University of Mississippi Medical Center, 2500 North State Street, Jackson, MS 39216.

225

upon the city and the specific population surveyed (Anderson & Levy, 1985; Jaffe et al., 1985).

In response to the health crisis, aggressive grass-roots AIDS education programs have been implemented within the gay communities of many cities. These campaigns typically include widespread distribution of educational and "safer sex" materials, condoms, and information correcting misconceptions about risk. San Francisco's Stop AIDS program, one of the nation's first and most ambitious efforts, conducts education outreach programs in bars, community settings, and even in private homes. Several recent studies indicate that gay men in large AIDS epicenter cities such as San Francisco and New York have made substantial changes in sexual behavior over the past several years (Martin, 1987; McKusick, Horstman, & Coates, 1985; McKusick, Wiley, et al., 1985). Although highly promising, the changes occurred only after HIV infection prevalence became high and AIDS deaths became common among gay men in those cities. There is evidence that many persons still engage in risky behaviors at unacceptably high levels from a primary prevention perspective. One recent investigation found that homosexual men who live outside an AIDS epicenter continue to engage most frequently in unsafe sexual activities such as unprotected anal intercourse (St. Lawrence, Hood, Brasfield, & Kelly, 1988). Even in areas where significant reductions in AIDS risk behavior have been observed (see Martin, 1987; McKusick, Wiley, et al., 1985), it appears that many gay men engage in unsafe sexual practices, albeit less frequently than in the past. High-risk behavior, even at relatively low frequencies, still poses great danger given the increased prevalence of HIV infection and the now substantial likelihood that a male's nonmonogamous same-sex partner is infected.

Research from other areas of health threat behavior (such as cigarette smoking, obesity, drug use, cardiovascular risk, and teenage pregnancy) suggests that risk behaviors are most difficult to alter permanently when they are long-standing and highly reinforced, when they are socially coerced or prompted, and when the negative health consequence is temporally distant from the activity that creates the threat. Under such circumstances, cognitive awareness of risk alone may be insufficient to promote durable risk behavior change. Strategies most often used to amplify the effects of educational campaigns include (a) redefinition of norms and standards within an at-risk population to encourage safer behavior socially and to discourage health-threatening activities socially, (b) provision of community-based interventions that can assist individuals or groups in developing the skills needed to alter already-established high-risk patterns, or (c) some combination of these approaches.

Most research on AIDS prevention has examined naturalistically occurring changes in reported risk behavior practices and, less commonly, HIV seroconversion rates in large urban populations or cohorts. Few studies reported in the literature have used controlled experimental methods to evaluate the impact of AIDS risk behavior reduction approaches. The purpose of the current study was to examine the effectiveness of a community-based group intervention program to assist apparently healthy homosexually active men in altering those behaviors that create risk for HIV infection and for the transmission of HIV infection to others.

Project Setting, Environment, and Participant Recruitment

This project was conducted in mid-1987 in a city with a metropolitan population of approximately 400,000. The area has a moderate but increasing number of AIDS cases, and is probably representative of many medium-sized, nonepicenter cities with respect to HIV infection prevalence, demography, and level of AIDS awareness among gay men. Prevention activities prior to the start of the project primarily involved the distribution of AIDS education pamphlets and other materials in gay bars.

Following meetings with leaders of the local gay organization, bartenders and bar owners, and health department personnel, a participant recruitment campaign was developed. The program, popularly termed Project ARIES (an acronym for AIDS risk intervention series), was announced through brochures and posters distributed through bars, adult bookstores, health department HIV antibody test sites, college campuses, and health care providers. At the recommendation of bar owners, a 10-minute video describing the program was produced and was played in each club. Members of the research team visited bars and were occasionally invited to individuals' homes to establish visibility and to answer questions. Potential participants were asked to call the project's telephone number for an assessment appointment. Over a 2-month recruiting phase, an initial sample of 104 men entered the study. All reported some high-risk sexual activities during the previous 12 months. Table 13.1 summarizes major demographic and risk behavior characteristics of the recruited sample, which substantiate a high overall rate of risk activities. The sample was 87% White and 13% Black or Hispanic; 45% had finished college.

TABLE 13.1

Demographics and Risk Characteristics of Study Participants

Variable	M	SD
Age	31.0	8.3
Number of different same-sex partners in past year	16.2	30.4
Insertive unprotected anal intercourse occasions in past year	19.0	81.4
Receptive unprotected anal intercourse occasions in past year	18.3	97.6
Oral/anal sexual contact in past year	10.6	16.5
Insertive unprotected oral intercourse occasions in past year	19.1	55.4
Receptive unprotected oral intercourse occasions in past year	10.6	16.5

Assessment and Intervention Procedures

Assessment Measures

Upon entry to the study, each participant completed a battery of assessment measures and behavioral tasks. All materials were coded with a number rather than a name to protect confidentiality and encourage candor. The measures included a risk history survey, self-monitoring forms on which to record ongoing sexual activities, a measure of AIDS risk knowledge, role plays to assess assertiveness skills when confronted by coercive pressures to engage in unsafe sex, and paper-and-pencil psychological inventories.[1] The risk history survey asked the respondent to indicate the number of times and the number of different partners with whom various sexual activities occurred over the past 4 months and the past 12 months. The 4-month period was used as a retrospective baseline. Sexual practices assessed by the measure included receptive and insertive anal and oral intercourse, unprotected or protected with condoms; oral-anal contact; finger insertion; and other sexual practices.[2] To obtain a finer-grained measure of risk activity less susceptible to recall inaccuracy or bias, we also asked subjects to complete and return forms for self-monitoring the same behaviors on a biweekly basis over 4 baseline weeks.

Activities that create risk for HIV transmission are interpersonal in nature. If one member of a sexual dyad has the assertiveness skills needed to negotiate safer sex practices and, if necessary, refuse partner coercions to engage in dangerous practices, risk can be functionally lessened. To assess assertiveness in these areas, each subject role played responses in eight simulated interactions. Each scene included a brief narration of a situation followed by three verbal prompts of escalating coercion level, made by a research assistant who role played the coercive partner. Six of the scenes tapped assertiveness in refusing pressure from a sexual partner to engage in an unsafe activity, while two of the scenes assessed the subject's ability to initiate a discussion concerning the importance of taking AIDS risk precautions. All role plays were audiotape-recorded for later rating. Scenes in which the subject initiated discussion concerning risk precautions were rated on a single 7-point scale reflecting overall skill. Scenes in which the subject responded to coercive pressure to engage in a risky activity were rated for overall assertiveness on a 7-point scale. In addition, and based upon research on characteristics of effective assertion (see Eisler, Hersen, & Miller, 1973; Hersen & Bellack, 1976; Kelly, 1982), refusal scenes were also rated for the presence or absence of specific assertive verbal content. These content variables were acknowledgment or recognition of the partner's intention, specific refusal of the unreasonable (unsafe) request, provision of a reason for the refusal, statement of the need to be safe, and suggestion of an alternative. All ratings were made by a research assistant naive to whether a tape was from an experimental or control subject or from pre- or posttraining. A second assistant independently rated 25% of all role plays. Interrater agreements, based on Pearson product-moment correlation coefficients between the two judges' ratings, ranged from .75 to .95 for all assertiveness variables.

Finally, subjects completed four paper-and-pencil measures. A 33-item true/false test of practical knowledge concerning AIDS risk practices and transmission mechanisms was constructed based on current epidemiological and laboratory risk factors studies. The test is scored to yield a total number of items correctly answered (see Kelly, St. Lawrence, Hood, & Brasfield, 1988, for details on a revision of this measure). Each subject also completed the Beck Depression Inventory (BDI; Beck, Ward, Mendelson, Mock, & Erbaugh, 1961), the state version of the State-Trait Anxiety Inventory (STAI; Spielberger, Gorsuch, & Lushema, 1970), and the Health Locus of Control Inventory (HLOC; Wallston, Wallston, & Devellis, 1978). When all participants had been individually assessed, the sample was randomly divided into an immediate intervention experimental group (N = 51) and a waiting list control group (N = 53). Multivariate analyses of variance confirmed that the two groups did not differ initially on demographic or risk behavior variables. Persons assigned to the experimental condition participated in a series of 12 weekly group sessions. After the conclusion of the intervention, all subjects from both groups were reassessed with all measures including another 4-week period of self-monitoring. In addition, persons in the experimental group self-monitored risk behavior throughout the intervention and completed self-monitoring, risk history survey, and AIDS risk knowledge test measures at an 8-month postintervention follow-up. For ethical reasons, persons who had been initially assigned to the waiting list control group were offered the same intervention immediately after the experimental group's posttraining assessment, eliminating the possibility of a comparison group only at the long-term follow-up point.

Intervention Procedures

Group sessions were conducted in a small but quiet officelike location in the city. The setting was chosen for its privacy as well as its central and accessible location. Because 51 persons constitutes a group too large for effective discussion and training, the experimental group was subdivided into three smaller groups that met on different evenings of each week but were identical in content. Sessions lasted 60–90 minutes and were always led by two clinical psychologists and two project assistants.

The conceptual foundation underlying the intervention was that altering sexual risk behavior, especially when it has been long-standing, requires accurate knowledge about risk but also behavioral skills for changing high-risk patterns. These skills include applications of behavioral self-management, sexual assertiveness, and the development of social supports, relationships, and health beliefs conducive to safer life-styles (Kelly, St. Lawrence, Hood, & Brasfield, 1989). The intervention's content was structured around these areas.

Accurate information about AIDS and risk reduction. Following an initial program introduction and group discussion about health concerns, information was presented concerning AIDS risk behaviors and risk-reduction steps. The presentation reviewed basic medical and virological characteristics of HIV infection, transmission mechanisms and the rationale for each transmission route, and sexual practices that carry high, moderate, or low risk for viral transmission. Sexual behaviors were conceptualized along a risk-level continuum, from highest to lowest, based upon epidemiological studies of HIV risk and public health recommendations for prevention. Examples of highest-risk practices were unprotected anal intercourse, "fisting," and activities involving "fluid exchange." Lowest-risk practices included mutual masturbation, frottage, and other nonpenetrative activities, especially when condoms are used or when no contact with fluids occurs. To encourage responsibility for the health of others as well as oneself, activities were defined as risky if they might pose risk for either partner; distinctions between insertive and receptive roles were not stressed. Participant misconceptions about AIDS, HIV infection, and risk practices were also identified and corrected. Three sessions of the intervention addressed educational topics.

Self-management to alter risk antecedents. Three group sessions taught participants to identify and alter functional antecedents to personal high-risk behavior. Subjects were asked to prepare written descriptions of past situations when a risky sexual contact occurred and to identify factors such as setting, intoxicant use, mood state, cognitive intentions, and sexual partner characteristics that preceded or accompanied the encounters. Although patterns differed across individuals, most participants were able to identify personal antecedents or "triggers" to past risky behavior. The most common were intoxicant overuse, visiting settings where anonymous sex occurred, or feeling the need to please one's sexual partner by consenting to unsafe sexual practices.

The group leaders and other participants presented self-management strategies of several kinds that could be used to alter such risk antecedents. These included practical environmental strategies (keeping condoms readily available if sexual activity might occur, practicing condom use while alone, establishing limits for alcohol use, or avoiding settings associated with casual sex) and cognitive modification strategies (developing explicit self-reinforcement patterns for taking risk-reduction steps, developing intentions to socialize rather than casually "cruise," and, if needed, generating AIDS-related visual images and cognitive self-statements that could be used to interrupt high-risk sexual activity). These strategies were related only to high-risk practices, not to sexual expression in general or to low-risk practices. Participants chose several of the techniques for in vivo practice and were encouraged during subsequent sessions to discuss success and problems encountered.

Sexual assertiveness training. Over three group sessions, participants rehearsed ways to initiate discussion of AIDS precautions and ways to refuse coercive pressures from a sexual partner to engage in unsafe practices. Following standard paradigms for assertiveness training (see Eisler et al., 1973; Hersen & Bellack, 1976; Kelly, 1982), the group leaders first outlined characteristics of effective social/assertive skill and modeled for the group skillful ways to handle such situations. Elements of assertiveness in sexually coercive situations were defined to include acknowledgment of the partner's wish but refusal to engage in the unsafe practice, provision of a reason for the refusal, statement of the need to be safe, and suggestion of an alternative.

After discussion of various ways that coercive pressures and initiation of AIDS risk precaution discussion could be handled, the group was divided into role-play practice triads. Each triad was given written descriptions of situations requiring assertiveness. One member of the triad first role played the partner, one first role played himself in the situation, and the third was an observer/trainer. The members of each triad practiced and alternated roles until each was proficient in assertiveness skills. Group leaders monitored the behavior rehearsed and offered feedback as needed. The same general procedure was used in each assertion training session, but sessions focused on different situations, and assignments were made to practice the skills in vivo if situations requiring assertiveness arose.

Social supports, relationships, and health beliefs. Successful implementation of effective risk-reduction steps may be facilitated by the presence of positive personal relationships and life-style goals, social supports, and beliefs concerning health, the efficacy of risk behavior change, and pride (Coates et al., 1987; Joseph et al., 1987; Kelly & St. Lawrence, 1988a; McKusick, Coates, Wiley, Morin, & Stall, 1987). For that reason, participants were encouraged, through discussion, peer feedback, and problem solving, to evaluate issues including the quality of life produced by frequent casual, high-risk sexual encounters; constructive versus maladaptive responses to the threat posed by AIDS; the development and maintenance of stable relationships and health-oriented social supports; and involvement in community activities that affirm personal pride and health interest. Although such issues alone are not necessarily sufficient to alter risk behavior, they may establish "context" supports and motivations relevant to the implementation and maintenance of behavior change. In the final group session, each participant identified for the group specific steps he had taken to reduce risk and how the changes were made. This exercise was intended to expose each member to multiple coping strategy models, and to reinforce the efficacy and desirability of risk reduction.

Of the 51 subjects assigned to the experimental condition, 47 (92%) began the intervention and 42 (82%) completed training and the postintervention assessments. Participants attended an average of 10.3 of the 12 intervention sessions. Of the 53 subjects who were assessed and assigned to the control group, 43 (81%) also completed assessments at the point when the experimental group had finished the intervention. Only subjects who completed assessments at the pre- and posttraining points were included in any result analyses.

TABLE 13.2

Pre- and Posttraining Scores on AIDS Risk Knowledge Test and
Assertiveness Role Plays

	Experimental Group		Control Group		
	Pre M	Post M	Pre M	Post M	F, p-value
AIDS risk knowledge test score	26.2	29.4	25.3	25.4	34.3, $p < .0001$
Initiation role play scores overall skill rating	3.2	5.1	2.9	3.3	41.2, $p < .0001$
Refusal of sexual coercion scenes					
overall skill rating	2.6	5.1	2.5	2.7	118.2, $p < .0001$
acknowledge partner	0.1	0.3	0.0	0.0	29.2, $p < .0001$
refusal	0.5	1.0	0.4	0.5	30.5, $p < .0001$
rationale for refusal	0.4	1.0	0.4	0.4	77.1, $p < .0001$
need to be safe	0.3	1.0	0.2	0.6	63.2, $p < .0001$
alternative	0.3	0.8	0.2	0.3	36.8, $p < .0001$

NOTE: F-values are for ANCOVAs on each variable. All MANCOVAs were also significant; df = 2.82 for knowledge test and 1.76 for role play variables. Overall skill ratings were based on a 1–7 scale. Frequency values for verbal components reflect mean frequency of occurrence in subject response per role-played scene.

Impact of the Intervention

Risk Knowledge, Assertiveness Skill, and Risk Behavior

To evaluate the effectiveness of the intervention, data for all measures except behavior self-monitoring records were analyzed with multivariate analyses of covariance (MANCOVAs) using pretest scores as covariates. Univariate analyses of covariance (ANCOVAs) were performed for individual variables when a significant multivariate effect was found. Behavior self-monitoring data differences between experimental and control subjects were analyzed with univariate analyses of variance for repeated measures, and within-group changes for the experimental group with univariate ANOVAs.[3]

Table 13.2 presents pre- and posttraining results for the experimental group and for the control group assessed at the same points in time on the AIDS risk knowledge test and on skill ratings of performance in the assertiveness role plays. As these data show, persons in the experimental group became more knowledgeable about AIDS risk-reduction steps following intervention. Role-play results indicate that experimental group participants were judged as more behaviorally skillful overall after training in their handling of situations that required initiation of discussion about AIDS precautions and in situations that required assertiveness to refuse high-risk coercions from a sexual partner. Posttraining improvements for experimental participants in overall assertion skill were accompanied by consistent increases in appropriate verbal assertive content such as refusing the high-risk coercion, explaining that a practice is dangerous, noting the need to be safe, and proposing an alternative.

Analyses of covariance did not reveal significant changes on the BDI, STAI, and HLOC inventories. The absence of change on these measures may have been due to the fact that subjects in the study scored near the general adult norms even before intervention (BDI M = 8.1, STAI M = 39.4, HLOC M = 32.5).

Risk Behavior over 4-Month Retrospective Periods

The MANCOVA comparing experimental and control subjects' reported frequencies of risk behaviors during the 4-month period prior to intervention and a 4-month period postintervention was significant (Hotelling T2 = .52, df = 6.72, $p < .0001$). Univariate tests indicated that experimental group participants significantly reduced their frequency of unprotected anal intercourse ($F = 8.83$, df = 1.77, $p < .004$), increased the frequency of condom use during intercourse ($F = 14.56$, df = 1.77, $p < .0001$), and had a higher proportion of all intercourse occasions protected by condoms ($F = 18.11$, df = 2.47, $p < .0001$).[4] These effects are depicted graphically in Figure 13.1. At 8-month follow-up, frequency of anal intercourse had decreased to near-zero levels and condoms were used in 77% of those few anal intercourse occasions that took place. The absolute frequency of condom use shown in the graph's middle panel suggests some nonsignificant decrease at follow-up. However, this is apparently due to the rare occurrence of anal intercourse activity at follow-up and the correspondingly lessened need to use condoms. Other sexual activities assessed on the risk history survey did not show significant change.

Self-Monitored Risk Behavior

When biweekly self-monitoring records for experimental and control subjects were compared, experimental subjects after training significantly decreased their frequency of unprotected anal intercourse ($F = 5.13$, df = 3.81, $p < .002$) and increased the proportion of all intercourse occasions when condoms were used ($F = 4.14$, df = 3.81, $p < .002$) relative to control group subjects. These changes are depicted

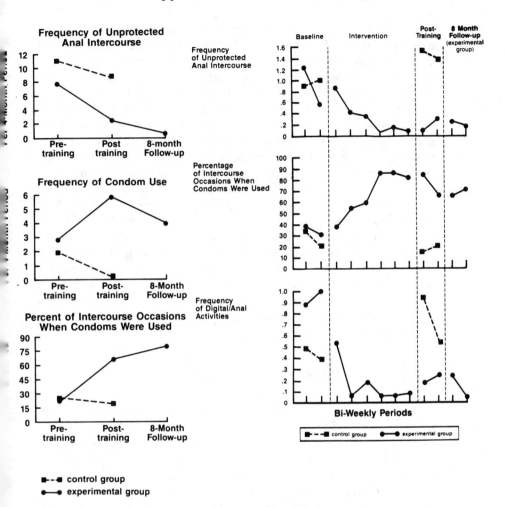

Figure 13.1 (left) Frequency of unprotected anal intercourse, frequency of condom use, and proportion of all intercourse occasions protected by condoms among experimental group (circle, solid line) and control group (square, broken line) subjects during four month periods before and after intervention.

Figure 13.2 (right) Self-monitored frequency of unprotected anal intercourse, proportion of all intercourse occasions protected by condoms, and frequency of digital/anal contacts by experimental group (circle, solid line) and control group (square, broken line) subjects. Each point represents the group mean frequency per two-week monitoring period.

in Figure 13.2. In addition, evidence was found suggesting decreased oral-anal contacts ($F = 2.97$, df $= 3.81$, $p < .03$) and a trend for fewer sexual partners ($F = 2.39$, df $= 3.81$, $p < .07$) among experimental participants.

Because participants in the experimental group self-monitored risk behavior throughout the intervention and again for 4 weeks at 8-month follow-up, univariate analyses were also performed to examine within-group change over time. Significant changes within the experimental group were found for unprotected anal intercourse ($F = 3.46$, df $= 11.486$, $p < .0001$), proportion of intercourse occasions protected by condoms ($F = 2.95$, df $= 11.158$, $p < .002$), and finger-rectal insertion activity ($F = 4.01$, df $= 11.485$, $p < .0001$). As Figure 13.2 shows, these changes were all in the direction of decreased risk and all were well maintained at long-term follow-up.

Finally, experimental group participants were asked to evaluate the intervention's utility anonymously, using 10-point scales. Participants assigned the program a mean value rating of 9.8 and a mean rating of 8.9 for the degree to which the intervention was perceived as personally useful. All participants indicated they would recommend the program to others.

Implications for AIDS Primary Prevention

Gay men in apparently good health but at very high behavioral risk for HIV infection and AIDS made substantial and well-maintained changes in risk activities following participation in a community-based group intervention. The magnitude of change shown by participants in the experimental intervention was great relative to the risk behavior levels of a control group assessed at the same points in time, especially for unprotected anal intercourse, the practice most strongly predictive of HIV transmission among homosexual males (Kingsley et al., 1987). This practice declined to near-zero levels after intervention and at 8-month follow-up. The effects of training were further confirmed by changes across a number of different assessment modalities, including AIDS risk knowledge, assertiveness skill for refusing risky sexual coercions, frequency of high-risk sexual behavior over successive 4-month periods, and frequency of high-risk sexual behavior over fine-grained self-monitored intervals. Taken together, these changes confirm the robustness of a risk-reduction intervention that combines educational, self-management, assertiveness training, and other health-promotion components.

Because the intervention tested in this project incorporated multiple training elements, it is not possible to determine which aspects of the program were most responsible for the observed changes. We suspect that frequent AIDS high-risk behavior is influenced by a variety of situational, cognitive, perceived vulnerability, self-control, relationship, and reinforcement history factors. This suggests the importance of employing multifactorial prevention approaches (see Coates et al., 1987; Kelly & St. Lawrence, 1988a, 1988b). The current study did not attempt to compare the relative impact of different types of prevention efforts. However, all subjects in the study, including those in the control group, were members of a gay community that had routinely received standard AIDS educational materials, and all subjects scored relatively high on the AIDS risk knowledge test measure even before intervention. In that sense, the project functionally compared the impact of a structured, skills-training-based approach with a control group having a level of educational AIDS awareness that might be considered "typical" for gay men in many cities. Experimentally controlled comparative studies evaluating different kinds of community-based AIDS prevention strategies are needed.

Participants in this project described frequencies of high-risk behavior prior to intervention that were considerably greater than those recently reported from surveys of homosexual men in San Francisco, New York City, and other epicenter areas. These geographical risk behavior differences may be due to variations in the intensity and effectiveness of ongoing community educational programs, the presence of a highly organized gay community for focused intervention in cities like San Francisco, social norms that sanction only certain forms of sexual activity, or the immediacy of perceived threat from AIDS. The long latency between the introduction of HIV infection in a population and an increased, visible presence of AIDS raises significant problems for primary prevention efforts. We are impressed by the possibility that different types of intervention may be needed to promote substantial risk behavior change among gay or bisexual men depending upon AIDS prevalence in a geographical area, perceived degree of personal threat and contact with friends who have AIDS, duration of high-risk behavior history, race and ethnicity, and age (Kelly & St. Lawrence, 1988a; McKusick et al., 1987; Siegel, Mesagno, Chen, & Christ, 1987). Each of these variables has been shown to predict compliance with risk-reduction recommendations. Although some individuals may eliminate high-risk practices following sustained educational campaigns, especially when perceived personal threat is high, other individuals may require involvement in more structured behaviorally based interventions and support systems to acquire the skills needed to reduce level of risk meaningfully. The already high prevalence of HIV infection in the homosexual male population means that, for gay men in particular, there is now very little room for delay, error, or inconsistency in making risk-reduction changes. The speed and magnitude of change produced by AIDS prevention interventions for gay men are now essential criteria of effectiveness.

Intervention of the kind described here could be provided to people in a number of primary and secondary prevention settings. Group intervention based on behavioral principles could be offered to focused at-risk populations by community AIDS prevention organizations, public health department HIV testing and counseling programs, clinics that specialize in the treatment of sexually transmitted diseases, schools, and similar facilities. Programs that require the constitution of organized groups of "help-seeking" individuals are usually not sufficient to meet wide primary prevention objectives. However, the inclusion of risk behavior change group interventions within wide-scale community-based outreach/education AIDS prevention programs would afford a mechanism to reach the many people who still engage in risky patterns. In an effort to make behavioral interventions of this kind accessible to larger numbers of people, our research team is currently studying the effects of a more abbreviated version of the same intervention, the conduct of group sessions in community settings such as gay bars, and training key, socially influential gay men to serve as risk behavior trainers for their own peers.

The HIV serostatus of participants in this study was not assessed and behavior change data relied primarily upon self-report and self-monitoring measures. To gain accurate and unbiased information, confidential subject-generated number codes rather than names were used on all measures, all forms employed clear and behaviorally referenced risk behavior items, and brief self-monitoring and retrospective intervals were used. Establishing reductions in HIV seroconversion rate following intervention would further validate program impact. Because probability of seroconversion in gay men is highly predicted by the occurrence of unprotected anal intercourse (Kingsley et al., 1987), the near-absolute cessation of this practice by experimental group participants indicated greatly diminished likelihood of seroconversion for persons who were initially HIV negative. Even if some individuals were asymptomatic but HIV positive upon study entry, the intervention also functioned to modify behaviors that would otherwise result in the transmission of HIV infection to others.

Research on AIDS prevention requires the development and evaluation of education approaches and delivery mechanisms, methods to redefine social norms within population subgroups to favor reduced-risk conduct, and means to promote behavior change before persons have immutable personal proof that they are threatened. The results of this project indicate that behavioral intervention principles similar to those employed in other health risk areas can also be used to assist individuals in reducing their own levels of risk.

Notes

1. For purposes of brevity, descriptions of assessment measures, certain aspects of the intervention's content, and statistical analyses are presented in summary fashion in this chapter. More detailed information is available upon request from the first author.

2. Few subjects reported heterosexual contacts, and some high-risk practices were reported rarely or never by subjects in this study. These behaviors were not included in the analyses. Only one subject reported any history of intravenous drug use. Risk factor studies most clearly implicate unprotected anal intercourse as a strong predictor of HIV infection among gay men, although other sexual practices that might involve "fluid exchange" are also believed to carry a degree of risk.

3. For a detailed discussion of the rationale of these analyses, see Kelly et al. (1989). On the risk history measure, subjects had idiosyncratic profiles with high frequencies of certain risk behaviors but low frequencies of others. This produced positively skewed distributions for each variable. As recommended by Winer (1971) and Kirk (1968), these data were linearly transformed using a $\log 10$ $(x + 1)$ formula before analysis.

4. In this chapter, insertive and receptive anal intercourse occurrences have been consolidated to reflect a single combined variable. Analyses were also performed on insertive and receptive intercourse occurrences separately. In all cases, the same patterns of significance and change following intervention were found.

References

Anderson, R. E., & Levy, J. A. (1985). Prevalence of antibodies to AIDS-associated retrovirus in single men in San Francisco. *Lancet, 1*, 217.

Beck, A. T., Ward, C. H., Mendelson, M., Mock, J., & Erbaugh, J. (1961). An inventory for measuring depression. *Archives of General Psychiatry, 4*, 561–571.

Centers for Disease Control. (1988, June 27). *Acquired Immunodeficiency Syndrome (AIDS) weekly report: United States AIDS program.* Atlanta: Author.

Clumeck, N., Sonnet, J., Taelman, H., Mascart-Lemone, F., DeBruyere, M., Van de Perre, P., Dashnoy, J., Marcelis, L., Lamy, M., Jonas, C., Eycksmans, L., Noel, H., Vanhaverbeek, M., & Butzler, J. P. (1984). Acquired Immunodeficiency Syndrome in African patients. *New England Journal of Medicine, 310*, 492–497.

Coates, T. J., Stall, R., Mandel, J. S., Boccellari, A., Sorenson, J. L., Morales, E. F., Morin, S. F., Wiley, J. A., & McKusick, L. (1987). AIDS: A psychosocial research agenda. *Annals of Behavioral Medicine, 9*(2), 21–28.

Eisler, R. M., Hersen, M., & Miller, P. M. (1973). Components of assertive behavior. *Journal of Clinical Psychology, 29,* 295–299.

Fischl, M. A., Dickinson, G. M., Scott, G. B., Klimas, N., Fletcher, M. A., & Parks, W. (1987). Evaluation of heterosexual partners, children, and household contacts of adults with AIDS. *Journal of the American Medical Association, 257*(5), 640–644.

Hersen, M., & Bellack, A. S. (1976). Social skills training for chronic psychiatric patients: Rationale, research findings, and future directions. *Comprehensive Psychiatry, 17,* 559–580.

Jaffe, H. W., Darrow, W. W., Echenberg, D. F., O'Malley, P. M., Getchell, J. P., Kalyanaram, V. S., Byers, R. H., Drennan, D. P., Braff, E. H., Curran, J. N., & Francis, D. P. (1985). The Acquired Immunodeficiency Syndrome in a cohort of homosexual men. *Annals of Internal Medicine, 103,* 210–214.

Joseph, J. G., Montgomery, S., Kessler, R. C., Ostrow, D. G., Emmons, C. A., & Phair, J. P. (1987, June). *Two-year longitudinal study of behavioral risk reductions in a cohort of homosexual men.* Paper presented at the Third International Conference on AIDS, Washington, DC.

Kelly, J. A. (1982). *Social skills training: A practical guide for interventions.* New York: Springer.

Kelly, J. A., & St. Lawrence, J. S. (1988a). AIDS prevention and treatment: Psychology's role in the health crisis. *Clinical Psychology Review, 8,* 255–284.

Kelly, J. A., & St. Lawrence, J. S. (1988b). *The AIDS health crisis: Psychological and social interventions.* New York: Plenum.

Kelly, J. A., St. Lawrence, J. S., Hood, H. V., & Brasfield, T. L. (1988, June). *A test of AIDS risk knowledge: Scale development, validation, and norms.* Paper presented at the Fourth International Conference on AIDS, Stockholm.

Kelly, J. A., St. Lawrence, J. S., Hood, H. V., & Brasfield, T. L. (1989). Behavioral intervention to reduce AIDS risk activities. *Journal of Consulting and Clinical Psychology.*

Kingsley, I., Detels, R., Kaslow, R., Polk, B. F., Rinaldo, C. R., Chmiel, J., Detre, K., Kelsey, S. F., Odaka, K., Ostrow, D., Van Raden, M., & Visscher, B. (1987). Risk factors for seroconversion to human immunodeficiency virus among male homosexuals. *Lancet, 1*(8529), 345–349.

Kirk, R. E. (1968). *Experimental design: Procedures for the basic sciences.* Belmont, CA: Brooks/Cole.

Martin, J. L. (1987). The impact of AIDS on gay male sexual behavior patterns in New York City. *American Journal of Public Health, 77,* 578–581.

McKusick, L., Coates, T. J., Wiley, J. A., Morin, S. F., & Stall, R. (1987, June). *Prevention of HIV infection among gay and bisexual men: Two longitudinal studies.* Paper presented at the Third International Conference on AIDS, Washington, DC.

McKusick, L., Horstman, W., & Coates, T. J. (1985). AIDS and sexual behavior reported by gay men in San Francisco. *American Journal of Public Health, 75*(15), 493–496.

McKusick, L., Wiley, J. A., Coates, T. J., Stall, R., Saika, G., Morin, S., Charles, K., Horstman, W., & Conant, M. A. (1985). Reported changes in sexual behavior of men at risk for AIDS, San Francisco, 1982–1984: The AIDS Behavioral Research Project. *Public Health Reports, 100*(6), 622–628.

Redfield, R. R., Markham, P. D., Salahuddin, S. Z., Wright, D. C., Sarngaharan, M. G., & Gallo, R. C. (1985). Heterosexually acquired HTLV-III/LAV disease (AIDS-related complex and AIDS): Epidemiologic evidence for female-to-male transmission. *Journal of the American Medical Association, 254*(15), 2094–2096.

Siegel, K., Mesagno, F., Chen, J. Y., & Christ, G. (1987, June). *Factors distinguishing homosexual males practicing safe and risky sex.* Paper presented at the Third International Conference on AIDS, Washington, DC.

Spielberger, C. D., Gorsuch, R. L., & Lushema, R. E. (1970). *Manual for the State-Trait Anxiety Inventory.* Palo Alto: Consulting Psychologists.

St. Lawrence, J. S., Hood, H. V., Brasfield, T. L., & Kelly, J. A. (1988, June). *Patterns and predictors of risk knowledge and risk behavior across high- and low-AIDS prevalence cities.* Paper presented at the Fourth International Conference on AIDS, Stockholm.

Wallston, K. A., Wallston, B. S., & Devellis, R. (1978). Development of the Multi-dimensional Health Locus of Control (MHLOC) scales. *Health Education Monographs, 6,* 160–170.

Winer, B. J. (1971). *Statistical principles in experimental design.* New York: McGraw-Hill.

14

Implications of the AIDS Risk-Reduction Model for the Gay Community: The Importance of Perceived Sexual Enjoyment and Help-Seeking Behaviors

Joseph A. Catania
Thomas J. Coates
Susan M. Kegeles
Maria Ekstrand
Joseph R. Guydish
Larry L. Bye

This chapter reviews the San Francisco gay community's prevention efforts in response to the AIDS epidemic. In addition, we discuss a model that conceptualizes the processes that may influence changes in high-risk sexual behavior (ARRM; Catania, Kegeles, & Coates, in press). The prevention implications of two elements of this model are discussed in depth: perceived sexual enjoyment and help-seeking behavior. Finally, we expand on the help-seeking findings to suggest that community-based intervention strategies provide a viable prevention approach.

A Brief History

In 1978, Bell and Weinberg described the sexual practices of over 600 gay men in San Francisco. They found relatively high levels of

Authors' Note: This research was supported in part by NIMH Grant MH39553, NIMH/NIDA Center Grant MH42459, NIAID Grant NO1-AI-82515, and the San Francisco AIDS Foundation.

sexual activity. For instance, 75% of White males (n = 575) reported more than 100 lifetime sexual partners, with 57% having had 10 or more partners in the prior year. Moreover, 78% of White men and 90% of Black men (n = 111) were performing insertive anal inter-course, and 67% and 78%, respectively, were practicing receptive anal intercourse.

The high levels of multiple-partner sex for some gay men had serious health consequences before AIDS. For instance, 70% of the syphilis cases in the 1970s were found in gay or bisexual men (Centers for Disease Control, 1987). There were also epidemics of hepatitis, gonorrhea, and parasitic infections among gay men.

In the decade following Bell and Weinberg's report, over 48,000 AIDS cases have been identified by the CDC, with gay or bisexual men representing 65% of those cases. In San Francisco, 4,411 AIDS cases (1981–1988) and 2,521 AIDS-related deaths have been reported (California State Office of AIDS, personal communication, June 1988). In response to this crisis, the San Francisco gay community implemented a massive behavior change effort.

The Community Responds

Intervention Efforts

The diversity of interventions conducted in the San Francisco gay community has been astounding. Programs such as Bartenders Against AIDS and Stop AIDS were developed to intervene at the grass-roots level. Stop AIDS, for example, trained people from the community to provide educational-motivational programs in their homes for friends, lovers, acquaintances, and friends of friends. Since July 1985 anonymous HIV antibody test sites have been operating citywide to provide free HIV testing, AIDS education, individual brief counseling, and referrals for further help. Newspapers have provided nearly daily coverage of the many facets of the epidemic, posters and pamphlets saturate the gay community, and "safe sex" videos adorn the shelves of major video shops. There has been a continuous bar-rage of television and radio programs on AIDS issues; public forums, church and school programs, and self-help books have proliferated. The sum total of these intervention modes represents what has been termed a "community-level intervention" (Coates & Greenblatt, 1988).

Unfortunately, the San Francisco intervention effort has not been evaluated formally at the level of specific programs. However, a number of studies have been conducted that provide an evaluation in terms of the overall community response. These large-sample longitudinal studies were initiated in 1983 and 1984 and have charted the shifts in gay men's sexual behavior in San Francisco. They include the following projects: the San Francisco Behavior Cohort (SFBC; McKusick, Coates, Wiley, Morin, & Stall, 1984; McKusick, Horstman, & Coates, 1985), which recruited 824 volunteers from bars, bathhouses, and advertisements to complete self-administered questionnaires and mail-return them (current N = 580); the San Francisco Men's Health Study (SFMHS; Winkelstein et al., 1987), for which the cohort was selected in 1984 using multistage household probability sampling (face-to-face interviews) from the 19 San Francisco census tracts with the highest cumulative incidence of AIDS, and which has reassessed these men at semiannual intervals (current N = 641); and Communication Technologies (Com Tech; Bye, 1987), which, using phone interviews and random-digit dialing techniques, has interviewed a longitudinal sample of gay men at yearly intervals since 1984 (current N = 190) and has drawn new cross-sectional samples each year since then.

Changes in Sexual Behavior: Anal Intercourse

The three studies described above provide a consistent picture of the changing sexual patterns in San Francisco's gay community. Indeed, the results concerning sexual behavior change converge across studies despite differences among surveys in sampling strategies and data collection methods. In fact, the methodological differences among studies underscore the reliability of the observed changes. However, the majority of respondents in these studies are White and well educated (see Becker & Joseph, 1988), thereby limiting generalizations.

The dramatic changes in sexual behavior in the San Francisco gay community have occurred to a degree that exceeds anything previously documented in the public health education field (Coates, Stall, Catania, Dolcini, & Hoff, 1989). For example, 57% of men in the SFBC have maintained zero levels of unprotected anal sex (receptive or insertive) for two to three consecutive years (1984–1986). Reductions in unprotected anal sex by SFBC respondents have been most notable for HIV-positive men (Coates, Morin, et al., 1988). A small percentage of SFBC men relapsed (13.4%) at some point between 1984 and 1986, and 20% have continued to practice unprotected anal sex over those years. Considerable work is needed to understand why some men relapse and why a sizable minority continue to practice unsafe sex.

The SFMHS has reported reductions of 59.7% (receptive) and 66.4% (insertive) in unprotected anal intercourse (Winkelstein et al., 1987). Guydish and Coates (1988) report that the number of men in the SFMHS having unprotected anal intercourse (receptive or insertive) has reduced significantly from 1985 to 1987. For example, unprotected anal insertive behavior was reported by 38% in 1985, but only 4% in 1987. In contrast, 90% of single men in the heterosexual community have continued to have unprotected vaginal intercourse at each of the three assessment dates (Guydish & Coates, 1988; note that the SFMHS includes a random sample of single heterosexual men). These findings underscore the point that San Francisco's intervention efforts have perhaps targeted and have had greater impact on gay than on heterosexual men.

Significant declines in anal sex were also observed in the Com Tech survey (Bye, 1987). This longitudinal study demonstrated 100% (receptive) and 80% (active) declines in unprotected anal intercourse by gay men over three years (a fourth longitudinal study of San Francisco gay men—the Hepatitis B Cohort—showed 90+% declines in anal sex over a seven-year period; Doll, Darrow, Jaffe, O'Malley, & Bodecker, 1987; see also Coates et al., 1989).

Corroborating the behavioral findings are recent data from the SFMHS (Winkelstein et al., 1987). They show that the decline in annual HIV infection rates, from a high of 18.4 in 1982–84 to a low of 4.2 in 1986, was associated with a 60% reduction in the prevalence of high-risk sex among gay men. In addition, it should be noted that rates for other sexually transmitted diseases have also dropped; for example, there has been a 63% decline in gonorrhea among gay men in San Francisco (Zenilman, Cates, & Morse, 1986; see also Coates et al., 1989).

Studies of gay communities in other areas of the country (e.g., New York, Chicago, Los Angeles) have also shown declines in high-risk sexual behavior over time (for reviews, see Becker & Joseph, 1988; Coates et al., 1989; Coates, Stall, & Hoff, 1988). However, the findings are not as dramatic. For example, Fox et al. (1987) report only a 28% decline in anal intercourse (receptive) in the MACS longitudinal cohort study (N = 3,581 gay men from Chicago, Baltimore, Pittsburgh, and Los Angeles). Moreover, in the MACS Pittsburgh site 65% of gay men reported having unprotected anal intercourse in recent months (Valdiserri, Lyter, Callahan, Kingsley, & Reynaldo, 1987). Thus in other major cities, aside from New York (Martin, 1987), there have been fewer changes in gay men's high-risk sexual behavior (Coates, Stall, & Hoff, 1988; Valdiserri et al., 1987).

Other Social and Behavioral Changes

Reductions in risk for HIV exposure may also be achieved by avoiding sex or by limiting one's sexual behavior to a mutually monogamous relationship. Thus some gay men have opted for becoming sexually celibate or mutually monogamous. Men in the SFMHS did evidence modest increases from 1985 to 1987 in percentages who were celibate (8.3% to 19.8%) or monogamous (25.6% to 30.9%) (Ekstrand & Coates, 1988). However, as is also apparent from the SFBC's 1986 survey, celibacy (14.5%) and mutual monogamy (23%) are not modal events. Moreover, a sizable minority of those who initially select one of these routes later abandon it. For instance, of men in the SFBC who had tried monogamy or celibacy from 1984 to 1986, 40% and 50% (respectively) later discontinued those practices.

Another interesting, and creative, shift in sexual practices is represented by J.O. (jack off) clubs or parties. That is, sex club participants have modified their behavior to include only self- or mutual masturbation in a group situation. Thus some gay men are modifying the behavioral content of their sexual repertoires, but retain the original social contexts in which their sexual interactions occur.

In brief, the San Francisco gay community has been flooded with intervention programs. Data from three independent studies suggest that the goals of those interventions have been met. However, we cannot specify which particular programs were most efficacious. Reductions in high-risk sexual behavior have been accomplished through modification of specific sexual behaviors as opposed to opting for celibacy or mutually monogamous relationships. Despite the good news, it should not be forgotten that the tragedy of the AIDS epidemic will continue for years to come. Indeed, 50% of the San Francisco gay community may currently be seropositive (Winkelstein et al., 1987). Moreover, future cohorts of gay men (i.e., those still in the developmental pipeline) will need to be socialized to safe sex. Consequently, there is a continuing need for intervention (and evaluation) particularly among gays in their teens and early 20s (see Stall, Catania, & Pollack, 1989).

Epidemics or Interventions

A very important question remains to be asked of the behavioral results. Are the behavioral changes a consequence of prevention efforts, or are they related to influences of an "epidemic psychology" that reflects the growing visibility and concern with AIDS at all levels of society? Both factors may be operating. A growing body of research indicates that many of the psychosocial factors that predict changes from unhealthy to healthy behaviors in other health contexts also predict changes in sexual behavior among gay men (e.g., knowledge, self-efficacy, social skills; see Catania, Kegeles, & Coates, in press). Moreover, these predictors (e.g., knowledge) represent psychosocial conditions on which most AIDS intervention programs were designed to have an impact. This argument for the effectiveness of AIDS interventions is of course inconclusive, since we lack an adequate control community to compare with San Francisco. It is also apparent that a crisis of epidemic proportions may have some unique effects on behavior. For example, one early predictor of reducing high-risk sex was knowing someone with AIDS (McKusick et al., 1984). Obviously, as the epidemic grows, more and more people will have personal contact with someone who has AIDS. Clearly, an epidemic creates a context different from that in which we typically conduct research on health issues. Further work is needed to flesh out the unique qualities of the AIDS epidemic for any given community, and gay communities provide a salient arena in which to conduct this work currently.

The AIDS Risk-Reduction Model

We have developed the AIDS risk-reduction model (ARRM) as a conceptual framework for organizing the factors that may influence people's abilities to change high-risk sexual behaviors (Catania, Kegeles, & Coates, in press). ARRM builds on several related models of behavior change: the health belief model (Becker, 1974; Janz & Becker, 1984; Maiman & Becker, 1974), self-efficacy theory (Bandura, 1977), diffusion theory (Rogers, 1983), help-seeking models (Fischer, Winer, & Abramowitz, 1983; Gross & McMullen, 1983), and decision-making models (Fishbein & Ajzen, 1975). We believe ARRM provides a useful framework for directing research on the predictors of high-risk sexual behavior. That is, ARRM organizes predictors of health behavior in general (e.g., susceptibility beliefs) and sexual behavior specifically (e.g., sexual enjoyment), and also incorporates some unique influences created by the AIDS epidemic (e.g., personal contact with an AIDS victim).

ARRM: An Integration

ARRM is seen as complementary to, but broader in scope than, a number of other models discussed in this volume. Most of the models presented emphasize cognitive determinants of health behaviors (health belief model, Kirscht & Joseph, Chapter 8; theory of reasoned action, Fishbein & Middlestadt, Chapter 7; perceptions of personal susceptibility to harm, Weinstein, Chapter 10; decision-making models, Fischhoff, Chapter 11). Although we agree that cognitive factors are important to the change process, there is still need for greater specification of where in the change process particular cognitions have their initial or most important impact. For example, it is unclear whether the same beliefs or attitudes that influence the onset of behavior change will also affect maintenance of new behaviors over time.

Further, high-risk sexual activity is social in nature. Thus it is useful to have an understanding of the dynamics of the social context in which sexual behaviors occur. In our view, sociosexual contexts are not understandable solely in terms of a set of beliefs or attitudes. For instance, skills necessary for negotiating safe sex may rely on important factors such as timing, effective communication skills, verbal tone, and assertiveness abilities.

Finally, it is important to consider the processes that underlie changes at the community level. The relevance of this issue is obvious when we consider that only a fraction of all people practicing high-risk behavior will ever directly contact our intervention programs. However, many people may benefit indirectly from intervention programs as a function of other social processes (e.g., help seeking). The extent to which intervention programs can modify or utilize these social processes is dependent on having complete knowledge of how they operate in a given community. ARRM also considers indirect avenues to change that occur "naturally" within a community.

In short, ARRM integrates many of the models presented elsewhere in this volume. The details of those models provide important refinements on a number of ARRM components. ARRM, however, adds additional elements that accent the fact that the contexts in which sexual behavior occurs and in which our interventions are expected to penetrate are social in nature.

Stages of the Change Process

Figure 14.1 provides an overview of the change processes relevant to the onset of actions directed at reducing the risk of sexually contracting HIV. This process is broken into several stages that reflect (a) recognizing and labeling one's sexual behavior as high risk for contracting HIV, (b) making a commitment to reduce high-risk sexual contacts and increase low-risk activities, and (c) seeking and enacting strategies to obtain these goals.

In brief, ARRM posits that to avoid HIV infection people exhibiting high-risk activities must first perceive that their sexual behaviors place them at risk for HIV infection. Further, they must be willing to make a strong commitment to changing their activities; this may require deciding if the behaviors can be altered and whether the benefits of change outweigh the costs. In addition, they need to be willing to seek help with obtaining solutions. In this regard, people may make multiple efforts at seeking solutions through self-help, informal social support, and professional helpers before success is achieved (Catania, Pollack, McDermott, Qualls, & Cole, in press). Finally, enactment of solutions may require complex negotiations with sexual partners, who may not have the same degree of commitment to pursuing change.

The processes represented by labeling, commitment, and enactment are neither unidirectional nor irreversible. For instance, some people may face great difficulty in changing their behavior, and come to relabel their activities as nonproblematic or reduce their commitment to change. In addition, the hypothesized stages may not be invariant. For example, some very compliant individuals may not perceive their behavior as problematic, but, nonetheless, come to change their activities because of the proddings of highly motivated sexual partners.

Influences on Stage Outcomes

Figure 14.2 summarizes a number of hypothesized cognitive, emotional, and social influences on the various stage outcomes and provides some general examples of how stage outcomes might be operationalized (see Catania, Kegeles, & Coates, in press). The complexity of the relationships cannot be adequately detailed by this type of summary depiction. For instance, perceptions of sexual enjoyment are hypothesized to have their initial impact on an individual's commitment to initiate new sexual behaviors, but this hypothesis does not

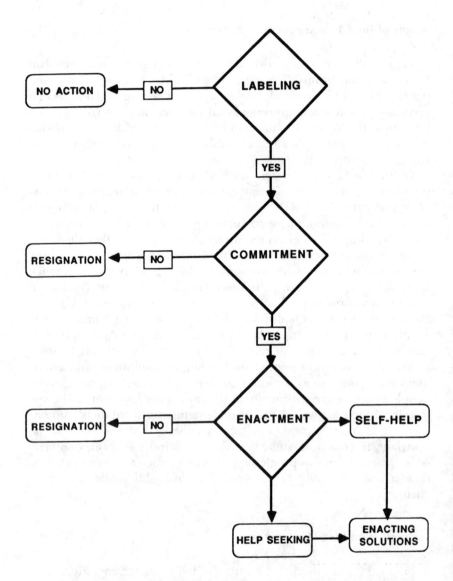

Figure 14.1 Stages of the Change Process

Stage	Some [Hypothesized] Influences	Outcome Indicators
One: Labeling	Susceptibility Trans. Know. Aversive Emotions	Is your sexual behavior putting you at risk for HIV infection?
Two: Commitment	Aversive Emotions Perceptions of: enjoyment risk reduction Self-Efficacy Condom Attitudes	Do you expect to do "x" in the next 4 weeks?
Three: Enactment	Aversive Emotions Communication Primary New Partners Informal Networking Formal Help-Seeking	What have you done?

General Model

Enactment = Stage 3 Influences + Commitment + Labeling

Figure 14.2 AIDS Risk Reduction Model Influences

preclude the obvious importance of perceived enjoyment to maintenance of these behaviors over time. Space considerations limit explication of the numerous relationships we currently consider relevant. Consequently, we will focus on four topics that our prior work has only touched on and that have major implications for intervention content and delivery (emotions, sexual enjoyment, social norms and networks, and help-seeking behavior).

Emotions and Sexual Enjoyment

Without venturing into the "causation debate" between cognitive and emotion theorists (Izard, 1982), we consider it necessary to include both elements. From our perspective, aversive and positive emotions serve important functions in attempts to alter high-risk sexual behavior. In the context of AIDS, some people may be influenced by fear, others may be motivated by love, and many will be affected by sexual pleasure considerations.

Aversive emotions are particularly salient, given that AIDS is an incurable disease that exacts an excruciating toll before it kills. Aversive emotions are hypothesized to motivate continued movement

TABLE 14.1

Relationship of Perception of Enjoyment and Risk to
Frequency of Protected Anal Intercourse

Variables	R	Beta	df
Enjoyment	.25*	.25*	1,545
Enjoyment	.26*	.25*	2,544
Health risk		−.09**	

$*p = .00001; **p = .03$

across all stages of our model. This view is based on the observation
that both labeling a situation as problematic and efforts to obtain
solutions to problems are typically motivated by moderate to high
levels of distress (Catania, in press; Gross & McMullen, 1983; Mechanic, 1978). With respect to HIV transmission, high levels of distress are related to more frequent use of condoms by IV drug users
(Gibson et al., 1988) and lower numbers of sexual partners among
heterosexual college students (Baldwin & Baldwin, 1988). Consumption of alcohol and drugs, which blunt aversive emotional states, facilitates relapse from low- to high-risk sexual behaviors among gay men
(Stall, McKusick, Wiley, Coates, & Ostrow, 1986; Stall & Ostrow, in
press). Unclear from past studies is whether aversive emotions are
important to both initiating reductions in high-risk behavior and long-
term maintenance of safe sex. Moreover, the impact of AIDS interventions that attempt to elicit aversive emotions is unknown. Further,
serious consideration needs to be given to research on the potential
long-term harm such interventions may have on the sexual development of adolescents who learn to equate sex with death.

Although work has accumulated on the effects of aversive emotions
on health actions (Job, 1988), much less work has been devoted to
understanding how positive emotions influence healthy behavioral
changes. Positive emotions are an obvious consideration when talking
about sexual behavior. Indeed, with regard to AIDS prevention, people are being asked to avoid behaviors perceived as extremely pleasurable and to increase less enjoyable activities. It is not surprising, then,
that people who view condoms as unenjoyable are less likely to use
them during high-risk sex (Bye, 1987; also see Table 14.1). In short, a
key component to practicing safe sex may be an individual's ability to
achieve and maintain a satisfying sex life within the context of safe
sex.

The issue of perceived enjoyment has not gone entirely unrecognized by those who have developed AIDS intervention programs

(Bye, 1987; D'Eramo, Quadland, Shattis, Schuman, & Jacobs, 1988). The key concept in this area is "eroticizing safe sex." From a prevention standpoint two issues are reflected in this concept: (a) use of "hot sex" to make safe sex messages more appealing, and (b) the development of techniques to make safe sex physically pleasurable for the participants.

Hot messages. Eroticizing safe sex messages makes considerable sense, given that adults at high risk for HIV infection through sexual routes are those who enjoy sex often and with multiple partners (e.g., Bell & Weinberg, 1978). In Bullough's (1980) terms, these individuals are highly sex positive. To make safe sex messages appeal to highly sex positive individuals, we need "sexy-hot presentations" to get their attention and hold it, and to strengthen cognitive-affective associations between hot sex and safe sex. The importance of this issue is documented by several results indicating that "hot safe sex" presentations increase positive attitudes toward condoms (Solomon & DeJong, 1986; Tanner & Pollack, in press) and initiation of safe sex activities (D'Eramo et al., 1988).

Hot action. Maintenance of safe sex behavior over time is particularly problematic if people do not enjoy the physical result. Condom use, in particular, raises a number of "enjoyment" problems for people. It is not uncommon to hear men complain that condoms decrease penile sensitivity. However, some men may derive sexual benefits from condom use (e.g., delayed orgasm for men who typically find that they come sooner than they want), but such bonuses cannot be shared by everyone. Indeed, since penile sensitivity differs among men (Solnick, 1978; Solnick & Birren, 1977), it is reasonable to expect that men in the lower half of the penile sensitivity distribution may experience sexual dissatisfaction when using condoms. Many of these problems may have solutions. For instance, better condom materials might be developed. However, no one, to our knowledge, is conducting research to develop latex materials that would increase penile sensitivity more than current products. Adding lubricants to the inside and outside of a condom may enhance sensitivity, but there is a great deal of imprecision about this advice, as well as potential hazards (e.g., increased condom slippage). Considerable work is needed to resolve problems in enhancing condom pleasure, and studies are needed to demonstrate the efficacy of current advice in this area. The importance of these issues is underscored by data from the San Francisco Behavioral Cohort indicating that frequency of condom use is more strongly predicted by its perceived enjoyment ratings than by its health ratings (i.e., ability to inhibit HIV transmission; see Table 14.1).

Social Networks and Norms

Not depicted in Figure 14.2 are the roles social networks and norms are hypothesized to play in the change process. These social factors may have important consequences for adoption of prevention messages, particularly by those in the community who never attend prevention programs. These individuals may be indirectly influenced, however, as a function of social diffusion processes. Diffusion of new ideas (e.g., safe sex) throughout a community has been found to be dependent on social networks and norms that facilitate acceptance of new behaviors or ideas (Rogers, 1983). For health behaviors, social networks and norms may (a) guide the labeling of health problems (Gross & McMullen, 1983) by influencing health knowledge (Berkman, 1985; Kaplan, Johnson, Bailey, & Simon, 1987), (b) funnel people toward an appropriate health decision, (Berkman, 1985), and (c) influence health-relevant beliefs (e.g., self-efficacy beliefs).

Group norms have been shown to influence contraceptive behavior (Condelli, 1986; Nathanson & Becker, 1986). In addition, recent studies of gay respondents have shown that the degree of social support and strength of group norms prescribing safe sex practices are inversely related to the frequency of unprotected receptive anal intercourse (San Francisco AIDS Foundation, 1987; two papers—same study sample—did not find this relationship: Emmons et al., 1986; Joseph et al., 1987), have a negative correlation with the number of sex partners (Emmons et al., 1986; Richardson, Schott, McGuigan, & Levine, 1987), and predict avoidance of anonymous sex partners (Joseph et al., 1987). Social networks, however, may also inhibit labeling high-risk behaviors as a problem (i.e., through social stigmatization; Fischer et al., 1983).

Help-Seeking Behavior

A key process underlying social network and norm influences on high-risk sexual behavior is that of help seeking (see Catania, in press; Catania, Pollack, et al., in press). ARRM posits that help seeking is a major social pathway by which people come to initiate changes in high-risk sexual behavior (Catania, Kegeles, & Coates, in press). With respect to HIV prevention, seeking help from others is hypothesized to be integral to solving what is essentially a social problem. That is, the first step in initiating safe sex is seeking the assistance of one's sexual partner in meeting this goal. Obviously, verbal communication and problem-solving skills are needed to engage one's partner successfully in safe sex behavior. Sexual communication abilities, as several studies have shown, are important to achieving success in changing sexual behaviors (Everaerd, 1977; Tullman, Gilner, Kolodny, Dornbush, & Tullman, 1981) and in facilitating contraceptive use (including condom use; see Polit-O'Hara & Kahn, 1985; Schinke, Gilchrist, & Small, 1979). A recent survey of urban heterosexuals suggests that approximately 40% are unable to communicate about safe sex with a potential sexual partner (San Francisco AIDS Foundation, 1986). Moreover, even among those who report being able to talk about safe sex with a new partner, it is still unclear how adequate their communication skills are with regard to asserting desires for safe sex with an uncooperative partner. Thus some individuals may need skills training if they are to adopt safe sex practices successfully in a satisfying fashion.

Help seeking also underlies the process by which people contact formal prevention programs. Consequently, help seeking may function to facilitate the diffusion of intervention efforts throughout a given community (see Rogers, 1983). Thus people who seek help from formal programs may be able to render aid to those who seek their help but do not attend programs. In general, if a large segment of a community seeks help with solving safe sex issues, then rapid diffusion of innovations directed at reducing HIV risk may result. Consequently, for community-based interventions to be successful, they may need to identify and train the major help sources in a community in addition to creating new sources of aid. This tactic requires studies to characterize existing patterns of help seeking and determine what new patterns would be acceptable within particular communities.

Help-seeking processes also have obvious implications for maintenance of safe sex. That is, an individual may continue to seek help as additional problems arise around the issue of incorporating safe sex into a satisfying sexual relationship.

Help Seeking and Sexual Problems

Prior work has shown that, in general, people with sexual problems utilize a wide variety of problem-solving responses in coping with their concerns (Catania, Pollack, et al., in press). These responses include doing nothing about the problem, using self-help, and seeking help from others, with the majority of people employing self-help and help-seeking activities (Catania, Pollack, et al., in press). With respect to problems concerning safe and high-risk sexual be-

TABLE 14.2

San Francisco Behavioral Cohort, 1986 Wave: Where People Sought Help (%)

	HIV+	HIV-	Untested	Total
Informal help: lovers and friends				
friends	94	90	90	91
primary partner	69	75	66	69
secondary partner	72	61	58	62
Informal help: relatives				
siblings	47	55	44	49
parents	47	51	44	48
Formal help				
medical professionals	70	66	51	59
psychological professionals	61	57	43	49
testing center staff	69	69	26	43
clergy/spiritual leaders	44	45	28	36
N	69	72	245	412

NOTE: Of 564 gay men, 412 (73%) sought some form of help. Total sample includes people who declined to answer question regarding HIV antibody testing. Mean numbers of help sources utilized are as follows (total sample): informal M = 3.1, SD = 1.5; formal M = 1.8, SD = 1.6; overall M = 5.0, SD = 2.9.

havior, gay men in San Francisco have been seeking informal and formal sources of help in relatively large numbers (Bye, 1987; Catania, Kegeles, & Coates, 1988). From Table 14.2, it is apparent that, for gay men in the SFBC study, informal help seeking was the dominant coping response, though formal help seeking was also much in evidence. Surprising is the large number of people who sought help from psychologists (49%). This figure is nearly double that observed nationally for help seeking from psychological sources for all types of psychosocial problems (see Veroff, Kulka, & Douvan, 1981).

In terms of grass-roots programs, Com Tech found that some 20% of their longitudinal respondents had participated in Stop AIDS programs between 1984 and 1987, and 12% had attended San Francisco AIDS Foundation programs. In comparison to gays, heterosexuals in San Francisco have done little help seeking. Com Tech's survey of 402 heterosexuals in 1986 indicated that only 20% had sought any form of help for problems in reducing HIV risk behavior, and of these the major source of help was a medical care provider (33%; friends were a distant second at 18%).

In general, when large segments of a community seek help with solving safe sex issues, rapid diffusion of intervention messages may result. Considerable work needs to be done in order to understand the community characteristics that inhibit or facilitate the diffusion of safe sex messages. The diffusion process may be inhibited by political prudery and antisex religious values, as well as the tendency of some people to view sex as so private that they never discuss it with anyone.

The help-seeking data also underscore the importance of community-level interventions. That is, the help-seeking results suggest that no single formal intervention delivery method can be expected to have a direct impact on each community member. Thus interventions need to utilize multiple sources of delivery that build on existing avenues of help seeking, and identify and utilize new help sources that will be acceptable to the community. As mentioned before, this approach requires a complete understanding of a community's existing help-seeking behaviors.

Since community-level interventions have an important role to play in AIDS prevention efforts, we will end our discussion with a brief overview of this approach. Additional discussion of community-based interventions can be found in Chapter 22 of this volume, by Flora and Thoreson.

Community-Based Interventions

Coates and Greenblatt (1988) build upon the above idea in deriving several of their basic principles for community-based interventions. These principles can be summarized as (a) pragmatic—use all avenues and types of helpers indigenous to that community; (b) sympatico—the interventions and methods of delivery must be consistent with the dominant values of the community; (c) persistent—interventions need to occur and reoccur frequently over time to maximize the diffusion process and shape new community norms; and (d) grass roots—special care must be taken to include community leaders (help sources) in planning (and delivering) interventions. It is clear that community-level interventions require having a considerable understanding of the formal and informal help-seeking processes in a given community and knowledge of how prevention programs need to be shaped in order to coincide with local customs.

Is the community-based intervention approach effective? From our perspective, the effectiveness of community-based interventions is firmly reflected in the tremendous behavioral changes observed in the San Francisco gay community. Unfortunately, we do not have appropriate comparison communities by which to judge those changes.

However, more rigorously designed studies concerning a different problem, teen pregnancy, found the community-based intervention approach to have a powerful effect—reducing teen pregnancies from 54 to 25 per 1,000 in the target community while matched control communities maintained relatively constant rates of between 46 and 60 per 1,000 (Vincent, Clearie, & Schluchter, 1987).

Summary

Evidence from San Francisco's gay community clearly indicates that these men have taken substantial strides in reducing the risk of HIV transmission. Two key elements that may have facilitated the change process in this community are preventions aimed at eroticizing safe sex and the extensive amount of help seeking that has taken place. Help seeking is viewed here as an underlying social process that facilitates diffusion of innovative practices and beliefs throughout a community. In this respect, help seeking may underlie the community-based intervention approach. This approach is suggested to be an important method for preventing the spread of HIV among gay, heterosexual, teen, adult, and minority populations.

References

Baldwin, J. D., & Baldwin, J. I. (1988). Factors affecting AIDS related sexual risk taking behavior among college students. *Journal of Sex Research, 25*, 181–196.

Bandura, A. (1977). Self-efficacy: Toward a unifying theory of behavioral change. *Psychological Review, 84*, 191–215.

Becker, M. H. (1974). The health belief model and personal health behavior. *Health Education Monographs, 2*, 220–243.

Becker, M. H., & Joseph, J. (1988). AIDS and behavior change. *American Journal of Public Health, 78*, 394–410.

Bell, A., & Weinberg, M. (1978). *Homosexualities: A study of diversity among men and women.* New York: Simon & Schuster.

Berkman, L. (1985). The relationship of social networks and social support to morbidity and mortality. In S. Cohen & S. Syme (Eds.), *Social support and health* (pp. 241–262). New York: Academic Press.

Bullough, V. (1980). *Sexual variance in society and history.* Chicago: University of Chicago Press.

Catania, J. (in press). Help-seeking associated with sexual problems: An avenue for adult sexual development. *Dissertation Abstracts International.*

Catania, J., Kegeles, S., & Coates, T. (1988, June). *Seeking help for problems in reducing high risk sexual behavior.* Paper presented at the Fourth International Conference on AIDS, Stockholm.

Catania, J., Kegeles, S., & Coates, T. (in press). Towards an understanding of risk behavior: An AIDS risk reduction model (ARRM). *Health Education Quarterly.*

Catania, J., Pollack, L., McDermott, L., Qualls, S., & Cole, L. (in press). Help-seeking behavior of people with sexual problems. *Archives of Sexual Behavior.*

Centers for Disease Control. (1987). Increases in primary and secondary syphilis—United States. *Morbidity and Mortality Weekly Report, 36*, 393–397.

Coates, T., & Greenblatt, R. (1988). Behavioral change using interventions at the community level. In M. K. Holmes et al. (Eds.), *Sexually transmitted diseases.* New York: McGraw-Hill.

Coates, T., Morin, S., McKusick, L., Hoff, C., Catania, J., Kegeles, S., & Pollack, L. (1988, June). *Long-term consequences of AIDS antibody testing on gay and bisexual men.* Paper presented at Fourth International Conference on AIDS, Stockholm.

Coates, T., Stall, R., Catania, J., Dolcini, P., & Hoff, C. (1989). Prevention of HIV infection in high risk groups. In P. Volberding & M. Jacobson (Eds.), *1989 AIDS clinical review.* New York: Marcel Dekker.

Coates, T., Stall, R., & Hoff, C. (1988). *Changes in sexual behavior of gay and bisexual men since the beginning of the AIDS epidemic* (Report to the U.S. Office of Technology Assessment). (Available from T. Coates, UCSF-CAPS, 74 New Montgomery St., Suite 600, San Francisco, CA 94105).

Condelli, L. (1986). Social and attitudinal determinants of contraceptive choice: Using the health belief model. *Journal of Sex Research, 22*, 478–491.

D'Eramo, J., Quadland, M., Shattis, W., Schuman, R., & Jacobs, R. (1988, June). *The 800 men study: A systematic evaluation of AIDS prevention programs.* Paper presented at the Fourth International Conference on AIDS, Stockholm.

Doll, L., Darrow, W., Jaffe, H., O'Malley, P., & Bodecker, T. (1987, June). *Self-reported changes in sexual behaviors in gay and bisexual men from the San Francisco City Clinic Cohort.* Paper presented at the Third International Conference on AIDS, Washington, DC.

Ekstrand, M., & Coates, T. (1988, June). *Prevalence and change in AIDS high risk behavior among gay and bisexual men.* Paper presented at the Fourth International Conference on AIDS, Stockholm.

Emmons, C., Joseph, J., Kessler, R., Wortman, C., Montgomery, S., & Ostrow, D. (1986). Psychosocial predictors of reported behavior change in homosexual men at risk for AIDS. *Health Education Quarterly, 13*, 331–345.

Everaerd, W. (1977). Comparative studies of short term treatment methods for sexual inadequacies. In R. Gemme & C. Wheeler (Eds.), *Progress in sexology.* New York: Plenum.

Fischer, E., Winer, D., & Abramowitz, S. (1983). Seeking professional help for psychological problems. In A. Nadler, J. Fisher, & B. DePaulo (Eds.), *New directions in helping: Vol. 3. Applied perspectives on help seeking and receiving.* New York: Academic Press.

Fishbein, M., & Ajzen, I. (1975). *Belief, attitude, intention and behavior: An introduction to theory and research.* Reading, MA: Addison-Wesley.

Fox, R., Ostrow, D., Valdiserri, R., Van Raden, M., Visscher, B., & Polk, B. (1987, June). *Changes in sexual activities among participants in the Multicenter AIDS Cohort Study.* Paper presented at the Third International Conference on AIDS, Washington, DC.

Gibson, D., Sorensen, J., Lovelle-Drache, J., Catania, J., Kegeles, S., & Young, M. (1988, June). *Psychosocial predictors of AIDS: High risk behaviors among intravenous drug users.* Paper presented at the Fourth International Conference on AIDS, Stockholm.

Gross, A., & McMullen, P. (1983). Models of the help seeking process. In B. DePaulo, A. Nadler, & J. Fisher (Eds.), *New directions in helping: Vol. 2. Help seeking.* New York: Academic Press.

Guydish, J., & Coates, T. (1988, June). *Changes in AIDS related high-risk behavior among heterosexual men.* Paper presented at the Fourth International Conference on AIDS, Stockholm.

Izard, C. E. (1982). Comments on emotion and cognition: Can there be a working relationship? In M. S. Clark & S. T. Fiske (Eds.), *Affect and cognition: The seventh annual Carnegie Symposium on Cognition.* Hillsdale, NJ: Lawrence Erlbaum.

Janz, N. K., & Becker, M. H. (1984). The health belief model: A decade later. *Health Education Quarterly, 11*, 1–47.

Job, R. (1988). Effective and ineffective use of fear in health promotion campaigns. *American Journal of Public Health, 78*, 163–167.

Joseph, J., Montgomery, S., Emmons, C., Kessler, R., Ostrow, D., Wortman, C., O'Brien, M., & Eshleman, S. (1987). Magnitude and determinants of behavioral risk reduction: Longitudinal analysis of a cohort at risk for AIDS. *Psychology and Health, 1*, 73–96.

Kaplan, H., Johnson, R., Bailey, C., & Simon, W. (1987). The sociological study of AIDS: A critical review of the literature and suggested research agenda. *Journal of Health and Social Behavior, 28*, 140–157.

Maiman, L. A., & Becker, M. H. (1974). The health belief model: Origins and correlates in psychological theory. *Health Education Monographs, 2*, 336–353.

Martin, J. (1987). The impact of AIDS on gay male sexual behavior patterns in New York City. *American Journal of Public Health, 77*, 578–581.

McKusick, L., Coates, T., Wiley, J., Morin, S., & Stall, R. (1984, June). *Prevention of HIV infection among gay and bisexual men: Two longitudinal studies.* Paper presented at the Third International Conference on AIDS, Washington, DC.

McKusick, L., Horstman, W., & Coates, T. (1985). AIDS and the sexual behavior reported by gay men in San Francisco. *American Journal of Public Health, 75*, 493–496.

Mechanic, D. (1978). Sex, illness, illness behavior and the use of health services. *Social Science and Medicine, 12B*, 207–214.

Nathanson, C., & Becker, M. (1986). Family and peer influence on obtaining a method of contraception. *Journal of Marriage and the Family, 48*, 513–525.

Richardson, J., Schott, J., McGuigan, K., & Levine, A. (1987). Behavior change among homosexual college students to decrease risk for acquired immune deficiency syndrome. *Preventive Medicine, 16*, 285–286.

Rogers, E. M. (1983). *Diffusion of innovation.* New York: Free Press.

Polit-O'Hara, D., & Kahn, J. (1985). Communication and contraceptive practices in adolescent couples. *Adolescence, 20*, 33–42.

San Francisco AIDS Foundation. (1986). *Designing an effective AIDS risk reduction program for San Francisco: Results from the first probability sample of multiple/high-risk partner heterosexual adults.* San Francisco: Research and Decision Corporation, Communication Technologies.

San Francisco AIDS Foundation. (1987). *Designing an effective AIDS risk prevention campaign strategy for San Francisco: Results from the fourth probability sample of an urban gay male community.* San Francisco: Research and Decision Corporation, Communication Technologies.

Schinke, S. P., Gilchrist, L. D., & Small, R. W. (1979). Preventing unwanted adolescent pregnancy: A cognitive-behavioral approach. *American Journal of Orthopsychiatry, 49*, 81–88.

Solnick, R. (1978). Sexual responsiveness, age and change: Facts and potentials. In R. Solnick (Ed.), *Sexuality and aging*. Los Angeles: University of Southern California Press.

Solnick, R., & Birren, J. (1977). Age and male erectile response and sexual behavior. *Archives of Sexual Behavior, 6*, 1–9.

Solomon, M., & DeJong, W. (1986). Recent sexually transmitted disease prevention efforts and their implications for AIDS health education. *Health Education Quarterly, 13*, 310–316.

Stall, R., Catania, J., & Pollack, L. (1989). *AIDS as an age-defined epidemic*. In M. Riley, M. Ory, & D. Zablotsky (Eds.), *AIDS in an aging society: What we need to know*. New York: Springer.

Stall, R., McKusick, L., Wiley, J., Coates, T., & Ostrow, D. (1986). Alcohol and drug use during sexual activity and compliance with safe sex guidelines for AIDS: The AIDS Behavioral Research Project. *Health Education Quarterly, 13*, 259–371.

Stall, R., & Ostrow, D. (in press). IV drug use, the combination of drugs and sexual activity and HIV infection among gay and bisexual men: The San Francisco Men's Health Study. *Journal of Drug Issues*.

Tanner, W., & Pollack, R. (in press). The effect of condom use and erotic instructions on attitudes toward condoms. *Journal of Sex Research*.

Tullman, G., Gilner, F., Kolodny, R., Dornbush, R., & Tullman, G. (1981). The pre- and post-therapy measurement of communication skills of couples undergoing sex therapy at the Masters and Johnson Institute. *Archives of Sexual Behavior, 10*, 95–109.

Valdiserri, R., Lyter, D., Callahan, C., Kingsley, L., & Reynaldo, C. (1987, June). *Condom use in a cohort of gay and bisexual men*. Paper presented at the Third International conference on AIDS, Washington, DC.

Veroff, J., Kulka, R., & Douvan, E. (1981). *Mental health in America: Patterns of help seeking from 1957 to 1976*. New York: Basic Books.

Vincent, M., Clearie, A., & Schluchter, M. (1987). Reducing adolescent pregnancy through school and community based education. *Journal of the American Medical Association, 257*, 3382–3386.

Winkelstein, W., Samuel, M., Padian, N., Wiley, J., Lang, W., Anderson, R., & Levy, J. (1987). The San Francisco Men's Health Study: III. Reduction in HIV transmission among gay and bisexual men, 1982–86. *American Journal of Public Health, 76*, 685–689.

Zenilman, J., Cates, W., & Morse, S. (1986). Neisseria gonorrhoeae: An old enemy rearms. *Infectious Diseases Medical Letter of Obstetrics and Gynecology, 7*, 2.

Commentary

Stephen F. Morin

Remarkable behavior change has been reported among gay and bisexual men in response to the AIDS epidemic. This behavior change has resulted in greatly reduced numbers of newly infected people, particularly in urban centers such as San Francisco, where comprehensive prevention campaigns have been mounted. The chapter by Jill Joseph and her associates indicates quite clearly that this change in behavior is associated with increased levels of psychological distress. It may be that the extent of behavior change could be even greater if change were not so closely related to level of distress. Alternatively, the research findings may suggest that inducing psychological distress is a key ingredient in promoting behavior change.

Knowledge of AIDS risk-reduction guidelines or information about how the AIDS virus is transmitted appears to be a necessary but not sufficient condition to produce behavior change. Understanding how specific sexual practices allow the virus to move from an infected person to an uninfected sexual partner allows an individual to assess the extent to which he or she is taking risks. This in turn allows an individual to label certain behaviors as problematic. Even if the individual simply ceases the practice creating risk, it is easy to imagine how concern about past risk taking could produce distress. For those who continue with sexual practices that they themselves label as problematic, it is easy to see how this would produce even more distress.

Personal efficacy, or a belief that one is personally capable of making necessary changes to prevent infection, is a major predictor of initial behavior change. This sense of personal efficacy is also related to self-esteem. Again, labeling oneself as incapable of making the necessary changes is a perception that one has a problem. This perception, in turn, causes distress.

Distress, however, may be helpful. It can lead a person to seek help, either informally from friends or formally from groups and professional providers. Help seeking in this situation is healthy, and can lead to both a reduction in risk taking and an alleviation of distress. Service organizations to assist people seeking such help have been formed in many metropolitan areas. Generally these service organizations have been formed by gay community groups responding to a perceived need.

Social support is perhaps the best predictor of long-term change in behavior. One reason for the unparalleled extent of behavior change reported among gay men is the change in gay community standards over the years since the AIDS epidemic began. Many gay men have made a personal commitment to do whatever is possible to stop the AIDS epidemic. The prevailing community norm is something like "We do not do anything that would transmit this virus." This creates peer pressure for change and a perception of social support for avoidance of high-risk activity.

The perception that one must make changes is probably inherently distressing. Successfully making and maintaining those changes can be a source of pride and increased self-esteem. The gay community and thousands of gay men across the country deserve much credit for responding in positive ways to the challenge of the AIDS epidemic. Many believed that the extent of change now observed in the gay community could never be obtained. There is no reason to believe that the same basic principles that have been used in prevention campaigns within the gay community could not be adapted to other target populations. This gives us hope.

15

AIDS Prevention in Black Populations: Methods of a Safer Kind

Vickie M. Mays

Epidemiology of AIDS in Black Americans

The earliest cases of AIDS that aroused physicians' concern involved White gay men who had unexpected opportunistic infections. This led initially to the perception that AIDS was a disease of White America. However, as we now know, that perception is wrong. As of January 2, 1989, 21,929 of the more than 82,764 reported cases were Blacks, or 26% of cases. This is so even though Blacks represent only 12% of the population. An additional 15% of cases involve Hispanics, although Hispanics represent only approximately 6% of the American population (U.S. Department of Commerce, 1983). Asians and Native Americans, categorized as "other ethnic groups" by the CDC, account for 1% of AIDS cases and 2% of the population.

In 1987, using the Centers for Disease Control surveillance data, it was estimated that 1% to 1.4% of the Black population was then HIV infected, an incidence rate three times that of Whites (Mays & Cochran, 1987). Using the Centers for Disease Control model that estimated both a stable 25% proportion of Blacks among reported cases and the 270,000 cases in 1991 estimate that is so often quoted in the popular press, my colleague and I suggest that about 67,500 of these cases will be Black Americans (Mays & Cochran, 1987).

Author's Note: This chapter was partially funded by a National Institute of Mental Health grant (1 R01 MH 42584–02) and a National Research Services Award (T32 HS 00007) from the National Center for Health Services Research and Health Care Technology Assessment. This work was completed while Dr. Mays was a National Center for Health Services Research Fellow at the RAND Corporation, Santa Monica, CA.

In that article the point is made that the Public Health Service speculates that the empirical model used to derive these estimates may *underestimate* by at least 20% the serious mortality and morbidity (Mays & Cochran, 1987). A variety of factors are responsible for this underreporting. Limited access to health care facilities and early deaths may diminish accurate reporting of AIDS-related symptoms. In addition, biases in surveillance data reporting by health care personnel and organizations to the Centers for Disease Control may differentially affect the accuracy, including the reporting of AIDS cases in Black Americans. Already, cases in Blacks have risen to 26% of the total and, currently, nearly 36% of all newly reported AIDS cases are among Blacks (AIDS Program, Center for Infectious Disease, 1988).

A second issue is that although AIDS is a catastrophic illness for everyone affected by it, for Blacks and Hispanics length of survival following diagnosis is significantly shorter than that for Whites. It has been estimated that the mean survival time for Blacks is 8 months, while for Whites it is 22 months. This is the result of several factors. First, Blacks are more likely to seek treatment later in the disease process, and hence diagnosis may occur later in the disease progression cycle. Second, it has been reported that large numbers of Blacks have not participated in experimental drug trials that would affect their length of survival after diagnosis. Thus, among reported AIDS cases, Blacks and Hispanics are more likely to be deceased.

AIDS and HIV infection have been described as a set of overlapping epidemics, each with its own particular characteristics. Generally, when AIDS in the Black population is discussed, the discussion begins and ends with the citation of the 26% statistic. However, this obscures some very important epidemiologic and methodological issues in AIDS prevention.

AIDS in Gay Men

In cases where male homosexual sexual contact is thought to be the risk behavior that led to HIV infection, 13% were Blacks and 10% Hispanic. However, even here Blacks and Hispanics are overrepresented. For example, 10.6% of the male population over age 12 are Black males. In contrast, Whites represent 85% of males over age 12, but only 77% of AIDS cases in homosexual men (Centers for Disease Control, 1989).

Recent articles note the drop in sexually transmitted disease infection rates and the major behavioral changes that have occurred in the gay community. However, though incidence rates of syphilis and gonorrhea have markedly decreased in the population as a whole, the rates in Black and Hispanic communities have *increased* in the last two years (Centers for Disease Control, 1988). Even among gay men, Black gay men are not showing the deceleration of syphilis incidence noted among White gay men (Landrum, Beck-Sague, & Kraus, 1988).

We have little empirically based knowledge of behavioral changes among ethnic gay and bisexual men. This status of knowledge is so because ethnic gay men have not participated in large numbers in the NIMH or NIH studies. Those Black gay men who may have been participants may also not be representative of the overall Black gay community. One of the points of investigation in our national study of AIDS-related information in Black gay and bisexual men is the distinction between Black gays and gay Blacks. This distinction is best described by M. C. Smith (1986):

> Gay Blacks are people who identify first as being gay and who usually live outside the closet in predominantly White gay communities. I would estimate that they amount to roughly ten percent of all Black homosexuals. Blacks gays, on the other hand, view our racial heritage as primary and frequently live "bisexual front lives" within Black neighborhoods. (p. 226)

We also contend that there is another group of Black gays who are a part of the emerging Black gay male community (Cochran & Mays, 1988). The importance of these distinctions for prevention efforts and research methodology are enormous. The various groups are probably quite different in their social activities, social support systems, access to AIDS-related information, and, potentially, in their sexual behaviors. In addition, prevention programs for Black gay men must interface with the overall Black community since many of these men are hidden within the social, economic, and community-based activities of the broader, predominantly heterosexual community.

AIDS in Bisexual Men

The fact that Black males are dramatically overrepresented among bisexual men, accounting for 28% of cases, may reflect the issue of maintenance of ties to the Black heterosexual community. The incidence of bisexual behavior in the Black community has often been interpreted negatively. One rationale is that the Black community does not support homosexuality. This is a very simplistic explanation. For those of us knowledgeable about the Black community, openly gay men have always been a part of the community. Acceptance of bisexuality and homosexuality in the Black community as identities or instances of sexual behavior is complicated (Cochran & Mays, 1988). There are a multitude of factors that may account for bisexuality in the Black community.

First, we know less about the behavior of Black men who identify as bisexual than we know about Black gay men. We know even less about the bisexual behavior of those Black men who identify as heterosexual. Yet we do know that Black men are imprisoned in greater numbers than are other ethnic males. While in prison, these men may engage in homosexual activities but not consider this sexually activity more than situationally determined (Cochran & Mays, 1988).

Second, much of our thinking about bisexuality has been shaped by Kinsey's bipolar representation, with heterosexuality on one side and homosexuality on the other, with bisexuality somewhere in the middle. This orientation to bisexuality does not include ethnicity, culture, class, and economics as interactive factors influencing the expression of sexual behavior or sexual orientation. While Blacks and Whites may engage in the same sexual behaviors, it is not necessarily true that they perceive these sexual acts in the same way or come to the same conclusion regarding sexual orientation.

Third, given the differences in experiences between the two populations, it would seem important that our prevention and research efforts use frameworks that incorporate the cultural, ethnic, and economic realities of our target groups. For example, in a national study currently being conducted we are interested in recruiting Black men who have had sex with other Black men regardless of whether they identify as bisexual or gay (Mays & Cochran, 1988). Some of our recruitment efforts look no different from efforts of approximately two years ago in the recruitment of lower-SES Black women into a smoking cessation project. Black women, in their roles as mothers, siblings, and friends, are sometimes aware of same-sex behavior in some Black men, and we expect these women will tell those men about our study.

AIDS in Intravenous Drug Users

Intravenous drug users are classified by the Centers for Disease Control into one of four categories: homosexual males, bisexual males, heterosexual males, and females. Even here, the overrepresentation of Blacks and Hispanics continues, with Blacks accounting for 22% of homosexual male intravenous drug users and

32% of bisexual intravenous drug users. Hispanics account for 13% and 18%, respectively. In prevention efforts, this is sometimes a group that falls between the cracks. Their needs are not well met in gay-oriented programs that do not focus on their intravenous drug use. On the other hand, drug treatment programs have in some cities been reluctant to take seropositive individuals. Also, some drug programs embrace philosophies that are at times homophobic. What is important here is not to forget that some Black intravenous drug users may be gay or bisexual (Mays & Cochran, 1988a).

When we look at cases of intravenous drug users among females and heterosexual males, the impact of this epidemic on the Black and Hispanic communities becomes even more apparent. Blacks account for nearly half of cases among heterosexual men and 58% of cases among women. Hispanics, too, are dramatically affected, accounting for 32% of heterosexual male cases and 19% of female cases.

AIDS and Heterosexual Transmission

Although among Whites AIDS is most frequently found in gay and bisexual men, Blacks show a very dispersed epidemiologic infection pattern. It has been suggested that current heterosexual transmission cases represent the second wave of an epidemic among heterosexuals (Redfield, 1987). The first occurred in IV drug-using individuals; the second, in their sexual partners. According to CDC classification techniques, heterosexual transmission is coded if (a) there are no other risk factors and (b) the person has had sex with a known or suspected HIV carrier, or (c) the individual comes from a Pattern II geographic region. Pattern II refers to individuals from certain parts of central, eastern, and southern Africa or some countries in the Caribbean where HIV transmission is thought to be nearly exclusively due to heterosexual contact (Centers for Disease Control, 1989).

The vast majority of heterosexual transmission cases in men are in Blacks, accounting for 81% of cases. Among women, 53% are in Blacks and 22% in Hispanics. Figure 15.1 illustrates the importance of looking at data by ethnic group and by gender. Surgeon General Koop and others state that AIDS is not a profound problem for heterosexuals. While this may be true for the U.S. population as a whole, this is not the case in some ethnic communities. Using the Centers for Disease Control data examining the number of cases of AIDS in ethnic women as a function of their percentage in the population reveals that Black women are approximately 13.2 times more likely than White women to contract AIDS. For Hispanics, the risk ratio is ap-

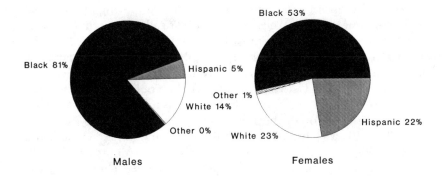

Figure 15.1 Heterosexual Sexual Transmission of HIV by Ethnic Group as of January 2, 1989
SOURCE: Data are from Centers for Disease Control (1989).

proximately 9 times greater than that for White women (Mays, Cochran, & Roberts, 1988; Selik, Castro, & Pappaioanou, 1988). Thus the risk is not the same. In our prevention efforts it is important that we present information with its appropriate caveats.

One of the implications of increasing numbers of female AIDS cases is, of course, the growing number of pediatric cases. Currently 52% of all pediatric cases are Black and 23% are Hispanic.

From this quick look at the epidemiology of AIDS in ethnic minorities, we can see that AIDS in these populations is a much more diverse epidemic than among Whites. There are many reasons this is so. Let me focus now on some issues that are often overlooked when we think about AIDS in Black Americans, particularly when we are concerned with prevention issues.

Migration and the Transmission and Prevention of HIV Infection

It has often been said that international travel sets the stage for the AIDS epidemic. Migration of subpopulations also occurs within the United States. This has potential implications for the future of AIDS in this country, particularly if these migratory subpopulations maintain an ethnic identification with attendant social structure serving to restrict sexual contacts and drug-use behavior to within the subpopulation.

For some Blacks, achieving the dream of a better life requires migration in order to take advantage of better opportunities or to escape political or racial oppression. The people who move geographically are often those with expectations and dreams of moving up the social and economic ladder (Wells, 1985). Historically, between 1910 and 1960 there was a mass exodus of Blacks from the South. Between 1910 and 1940 an estimated 1.5 million Blacks left the South, migrating primarily to New York, Pennsylvania, Ohio, Illinois, Michigan, and Washington, D.C. (Robinson, 1986). The pull for Blacks was the attraction of jobs in northern industries. This migration outward continued steadily through the 1960s. Through the 1940s an estimated 1.6 million Blacks left the South, in the 1950s another 1.6 million, and in the 1960s 1.4 million, all in search of jobs. The proportion of Blacks who lived in the Northeast and the Midwest from 1940 to 1970 rose from 22% to 39%.

The decade of the 1970s was a time in which the hopes of many Blacks, particularly those who had moved from the South, turned to frustration, disappointment, and bitterness (Jordan, 1980). The simultaneous recession and double-digit inflation hit the Black community particularly hard. Unemployment rates increased to 61% among Black teenagers while increasing to 40% among White teenagers (Hill, 1981). One study that sought to determine why so many young Black men in the ghetto did not work found that they believed that their education (graduation from high school) qualified them for jobs better than those that were actually available—cleaning floors, washing cars, or delivering packages (Anderson, 1979). These young men also knew Black men in their 40s and 50s who had worked at low-paying jobs all of their lives. They felt that if they accepted menial jobs they would be dead-ended careerwise. Employers, when interviewed, did not want to hire these young men because they felt they would steal and not work hard. For some, an economic alternative to low-paying jobs came from criminal pursuits. The marketing of women, drugs, and stolen goods led to the financial success and status that they desired.

Starting in the 1970s there began a reversal of the migration patterns. Many of the deteriorating social and economic conditions for Blacks in the Northeast and Midwest led to a migration out of the North, back to the South. Black migration to the South accounted for 11% of the 1.8 million migrants the South gained between 1975 and 1980 (Robinson, 1986). Results of the 1985 Current Population Survey indicate that while this trend has slowed, Blacks, particularly in the 25 to 34 age group, are still moving to the South. Since 1980, the South has gained 87,000 Blacks. The Northeast has lost a net of 30,000, and the Midwest 67,000. At the same time, the West has gained 10,000.

Given what we know about the epidemiologic patterns of the virus in ethnic minorities, one step toward prevention may be to determine more about the migrants who are moving permanently to the South, as well as any increases in transitory migration as a result of the arrival of the new migrants. For example, my research project recently completed a focus group in a major southern city, and out of ten Black gay men who participated, two were recent arrivals. Prior to their permanent move, these two men, one from Los Angeles and the other from New York, had visited this southern city and stayed for extended periods. These visits subsequently led to their permanent relocation. For individuals with little disposable income, vacation sites are often chosen according to where friends and relatives reside who can provide housing and transportation. Then, if an individual is able to get the means to arrive in the city and a little bit of cash to spend, the vacation is possible.

It is important in our prevention efforts that we not lose sight of the behavioral and social issues that may drive the HIV epidemic. Changes in social and economic conditions in an area resulting from a large influx of individuals from high-prevalence regions indicate a site for primary prevention.

Cultural Context of AIDS and HIV Transmission and Prevention

It is important to understand the cultural context of AIDS and HIV prevention in the Black community in order to develop effective prevention strategies. The lesson of the importance of cultural context has been clearly demonstrated by the successes of the gay community. Prevention efforts and risk-reduction activities occur within a framework that incorporates norms, tastes, preferences, shared language, and the like within large segments of that community. Culture and context are equally important dimensions for prevention efforts in Black populations.

Religion

Religion is a backbone of the Black community. It is important that as researchers and intervention planners we understand something about the different religions most prevalent in Black populations. Religion influences attitudes and behaviors concerning sex, specific sexual practices, contraceptive use, and premarital, extramarital, and other intimate relationships. Methods of education or interventions involving fundamentalist Christians, such as Jehovah's Witnesses, may and should differ radically from those targeting liberal Episcopalians. For example, it has been estimated that approximately 90% of fundamentalists and Baptists believe in an afterlife. For many, the afterlife is a place of reward or punishment for actions on earth. One strategy for addressing groups with this orientation is that of asking them not to judge, but to leave God to judge the actions of individuals. Instead, they can focus on the role that they can play in ministering to and helping those suffering from AIDS through house visits, food drives, and providing child care or respite care to families. This service, regardless of the sin of the person served, will be rewarded by God. The language and the method of intervention used in working with fundamentalists become appropriate in the context of their belief system. In working with individuals from this group, the focus on the use of condoms is not primarily as protection against AIDS; rather, the emphasis is on the fact that medical science has found that condoms offer some protection against the transmission of the virus. This latter statement is accepted more as a fact and less as a value or moral statement.

Of the various religions, fundamentalists and Baptists seem most likely to condemn homosexuality as well as extramarital and premarital sex (T. W. Smith, 1984). According to a study by T. W. Smith (1984), 86% of fundamentalists judged extramarital relations to be always wrong, as did 82% of Baptists, 76% of Lutherans, 75% of Methodists, 70% of Presbyterians, 59% of Catholics, and 50% of Jews. Among those with no religious affiliations, only 40% believed extramarital relations were wrong.

A second important factor in understanding the nature of Black religious affiliations is that they provide some clue to sources of support, social networks, and potential organizing structures for prevention activities. Fundamentalists often take part in church activities on a regular basis. For some this may involve attending church functions several days a week for several hours at a time. On Saturdays, Jehovah's Witness families may be found walking door to door, passing out literature. Muslim brothers can be seen on some street corners on Saturdays selling bean pies. We can better understand who may be a source of peer influence, how to approach the development of norms, and how realistic our expectations for our programs are if we are sensitive to the spiritual and emotional lives of Black Americans.

Following is an example of how insensitivity to the role religion plays for some ethnic groups can actually damage future prevention efforts. In the Los Angeles area last year, an outreach project of a predominantly White gay male organization targeted to the Hispanic community openly advocated condom use as a prevention strategy for

HIV infection for Hispanics. This led to a confrontation with the Catholic church. As a result of the confrontation that occurred, the church issued an official statement against the use of condoms. While AIDS education had previously been conducted through church groups and on church property used by community groups, after the public statement neither the parish priests nor the church members were willing to violate openly the recommendations issued by the church. Hispanic AIDS educators felt they lost a great deal of ground with individual churches after this cultural blunder.

Communication of Risks

While the relationship between attitudes and behaviors has been debated for years (e.g., Ajzen & Fishbein, 1980; Fishbein, 1967), presenting the Black community with specific information and education to assist them over time in their attitude formation about HIV-related risk behaviors may be one of the influencing factors in behavior change. If the information is presented in a manner that engages the attention of the Black community and is believed, then the prevention or protective influence has a greater chance of occurring. Yet, in communicating the risk of HIV infection we have used little of our available knowledge about influencing the attitudes and behaviors of Blacks.

Television. Certain facts about the use of television and credibility of media messages are well established (see Bales, 1986, for a review). Television has a greater impact on Blacks when compared to Whites (Allen & Bielby, 1979; Bogart, 1972). Blacks on the average watch more television (Allen, 1981; Comstock, 1980), have less hostility toward television as a medium (Durand, Teel, & Bearden, 1979), and view its contents as more believable (Bower, 1973). Not only do Blacks give greater credibility to television as a source of information, when compared to Whites, Blacks are more likely to rely on it as their primary source for news and information (Johnson, 1984).

Based on the characteristics of the segment of the Black community with the most watching hours (which seems also to be associated with having limited means and resources to engage in other leisure outlets; Comstock, 1980) and the literacy level, it would appear that television would serve as an ideal medium for disseminating information and influencing attitudes of particular segments of the Black community. Television commercials have been shown to be an effective means for the delivery of information (Davis, 1987).

Currently, several different 30- and 60-second public service an-

274   Vickie M. Mays

nouncements are airing about AIDS; many are delivered by
nonminority actors. Very few are delivered by Blacks. Even worse are
the AIDS specials. In fact, one half-hour special on heterosexuals and
AIDS that originated in Los Angeles focused almost exclusively on the
concerns of White Americans. At the end of the show, when the
members of the audience were asked to raise their hands if they knew
someone who had gotten AIDS through heterosexual contact, two
Blacks but no Whites raised their hands. The newscaster commented
that the sight of hands raised was unexpected, because AIDS is not a
major problem for heterosexuals yet—not so if you are Black.

Koop, Mason, Curran, and Morgan Fairchild will seldom elicit attention from, achieve credibility with, or influence large segments of
the Black population most at risk. Often, simply because such programs lack Black faces, they will be switched off by Blacks. The first
step in using the media is getting the target group to attend to the
message. Several studies have documented the role of social comparison in media use of Blacks (Allen & Bielby, 1979; Fairchild, Stockard,
& Bowman, 1986; Graves, 1980; Poindexter & Stroman, 1981; Roberts & Bachen, 1981). Blacks, like other groups, seek programming
that includes representatives of their own ethnic group or portrays
ethnically relevant life experiences (Fairchild et al., 1986). This was
clearly demonstrated in data analyzed from the National Survey of
Black Americans, a national probability sampling of Black Americans
in the United States, on their viewing preferences and satisfaction
with the epic story *Roots* (Fairchild et al., 1986). *Roots* was watched by
approximately 87% of the sample. The epic increased Black viewers'
knowledge about slavery; indeed, Blacks absorbed greater knowledge
than Whites (Hur, 1978) and were emotionally involved in the story
(Howard, Rothbart, & Sloan, 1978). Clearly, if we are interested in
getting Blacks to attend to the message, social science and communication research have demonstrated the importance of ethnic relevance.

The second step is to get Blacks to view the delivery of the message
as credible and to believe the information. In a study of Blacks' perceptions of credibility of Black versus White male and female newscasters,
Black male newscasters were rated as the most credible, followed by
White male, Black female, and, lastly, White female newscasters (Johnson, 1987). What most often comes through in this line of research is
that most people want to listen both to some experts and to some
people like themselves. If Koop wants to deliver an effective message
to the Black community regarding AIDS, role playing with Susan Dey
rather than a member of the Cosby show would be better.

But there are also other ways of enlisting attention and increasing credibility among Black viewers. Credibility in the Black community can come in the form of Whoopi Goldberg, who has expressed the mood of some in the Black community with her remarks about AIDS (Christon, 1988). Goldberg has her character Fontaine, who is now an ex-junkie, mystified as to why national TV channels are locked on the Baby Jessica incident but appallingly indifferent to the Florida family whose home was bombed and gutted because their kids were HIV infected. The Black community identifies well with this. In fact, similar remarks were made by colleagues working with Black pediatric AIDS cases when they saw the stuffed bears and gifts sent to Baby Jessica but knew, in spite of appeals, that nothing would be forthcoming for the AIDS babies. Goldberg's comment that Nancy Reagan's "Just Say No" antidrug campaign doesn't hold much water for a welfare mother whose 13-year-old son makes $13,000 a month dealing drugs expresses an important point relevant to AIDS risk reduction in the Black community. The Centers for Disease Control and many of us would do well to remember it.

Print and radio media. Early studies have found that Blacks are less likely than Whites to use newspapers as sources of information (Warren, 1972). A study of Black women's media usage compared to that of White women found interesting differences (Darden & Darden, 1981). In the area of periodicals, White women were heavier readers of *Time, Newsweek, U.S. News & World Report, Reader's Digest, Family Circle, Women's Day, Ladies' Home Journal, McCall's,* and *National Geographic.* Black women, on the other hand, read *TV Guide* in greater numbers and, of course, the Black publications *Ebony* and *Jet.* Black women were also more likely than White women to tune in to AM radio, listening to radio news, sports, talk shows, and talk-and-call-in shows proportionately more. This study supports others that conclude that White women may be more likely than Black women to trust sources other than television and radio for news (Darden & Darden, 1981; Warren, 1972). Equally revealing here is that Blacks rely on word of mouth more than printed sources for their information and news (Warren, 1972).

It has been stated consistently in the last couple of years at numerous Black health conferences that R. J. Reynolds, Reeboks, Anheuser-Busch, and others have the technology to influence smoking, alcohol consumption, shoe brands, or car models purchased by Black Americans. When Anheuser-Busch wants to get Blacks to drink its brand of beer or wine coolers, it purchases billboard, magazine, and ethnic newspaper advertising. It sponsors community events and gives away free caps, T-shirts, and, in some instances, samples of its product.

These strategies have not been exploited by the Centers for Disease Control in their efforts to change behavior. In spite of our knowledge from other health-based prevention programs (e.g., hypertension, CHD, smoking cessation, nutrition) that some of these strategies coupled with other interventions do increase knowledge, change attitudes, and sometimes change behaviors, little emphasis has been given to the virtues of social marketing in the AIDS epidemic. The gay community entertained the notion of social marketing for condoms, but the response to condom use has gone so well that no major campaigns were launched. Those interested in prevention efforts in the Black community may find that our colleagues in the fields of social psychology, marketing, and communications should be some of the primary collaborators for a successful fight against the spread of HIV infection.

Underclass Economics

There are other issues here as well, one of which is relevant to a subgroup of the Black population, particularly those in the Northeast and some parts of the Midwest. Members of this group cannot move in search of a new life—they are the underclass. This is also a very difficult-to-reach population. Many are probably already infected. Some are highly resistant to our primary prevention efforts after already experiencing years of frustration and anger at their treatment by society. Some of these individuals have found ways to support themselves relatively well, but in illicit careers which we suddenly want them to discontinue. Our advice is perceived by some members of the underclass as not that easy; nor, in many ways, does it make sense to them. This story helps to illustrate the problem. A teenage son of someone I know sold crack and cocaine. This young man had several people working for him, all adult Black males who otherwise would be marginally employed. Many of the young children in the neighborhood looked up to the teenage son, as he often bought them candy or sodas or took them for rides in his jeep. He always encouraged the kids to stay in school and protected them from gang violence or gang involvement. When around and not busy, he always had time to listen to the kids' problems and dreams, trying to fix one and encourage the other. His father was very supportive of his activities for several reasons. First, his son's income provided him with the kind of security that a Ph.D. or tenure provides. He knew that if racism at his job got out of hand he would merely quit and work for his son. Second, the son bought him a new truck and supported his mother, who was the mistress of the father. There are many who profit positively from the son's drug dealing. While drug dealing, in itself, is an illicit activity with many negative social costs, it provides some people with benefits. Some of the factors that facilitate spread of the virus in the Black community require complex prevention efforts that may need to focus not just on the Black community but on our social policies.

Summary

It is important that we not fool ourselves about the task of prevention in the Black community. AIDS has exposed some of the worst of societal ills, and we can hope to begin to see the best of what society is only by instituting sensitive and comprehensive prevention efforts. It is important that in designing prevention efforts for the Black community we recognize the richness and value of the support networks, culture, and tradition that have helped that community to mount successful efforts against many other ills.

References

AIDS Program, Center for Infectious Disease. (1988). Quarterly report to the Domestic Policy Council on the prevalence and rate of spread of HIV and AIDS—United States. *Morbidity and Mortality Weekly Report, 37*, 551–554, 559.

Ajzen, I., & Fishbein, M. (1980). *Understanding attitudes and predicting social behavior.* Englewood Cliffs, NJ: Prentice-Hall.

Allen, R. L. (1981). The reliability and stability of television exposure. *Communication Research, 8*(2), 233–256.

Allen, R. L., & Bielby, W. T. (1979). Blacks' relationship with print media. *Journalism Quarterly, 52,* 488–496.

Anderson, J. E. (1979). Measurement of welfare cost under uncertainty. *Southern Economic Journal, 45*(2), 1160–1171.

Asante, M., & Davis, A. (1985). Black and White communication: Analyzing work place encounters. *Journal of Black Studies, 16*(1), 77–93.

Bales, F. (1986). Television use and confidence in television by Blacks and Whites in four selected years. *Journal of Black Studies, 16*(3), 283–291.

Bogart, L. (1972). Negro and White media exposure: New evidence. *Journalism Quarterly, 49,* 15–21.

Bower, R. (1973). *Television and the public.* New York: Holt, Rinehart & Winston.

Centers for Disease Control. (1989, January 2). *Public information data use tape* (AIDS Program, Center for Infectious Disease). Atlanta: Author.

Christon, L. (1988, July 9). Whoopi puts truths on the laugh track. *Los Angeles Times,* Part VI, pp. 1, 10.

Cochran, S. D., & Mays, V. M. (1988). Epidemiologic and sociocultural factors in the transmission of HIV infection in Black gay and bisexual men. In M. Shernoff & W. A. Scott (Eds.), *The sourcebook on lesbian/gay health care* (2nd ed.). Washington, DC: National Gay and Lesbian Health Foundation.

Comstock, G. (1980). *Television in America*. Beverly Hills, CA: Sage.

Darden, D. K., & Darden, W. R. (1981). Middle-class females' media usage habits. *Journal of Black Studies, 11*(4), 421–434.

Davis, R. A. (1987). Television commercials and the management of spoiled identity. *Western Journal of Black Studies, 11*(2), 59–63.

Fairchild, H. H., Stockard, R., & Bowman, P. (1986). Impact of *Roots*: Evidence from the National Survey of Black Americans. *Journal of Black Studies, 16*(3), 307–318.

Fishbein, M. (1967). Attitudes and the prediction of behavior. In M. Fishbein (Ed.), *Readings in attitude theory and measurement* (pp. 447–492). New York: John Wiley.

Graves, S. B. (1980). Psychological effects of Black portrayals on television. In S. B. Withey & R. P. Abeles (Eds.), *Television and social behavior: Beyond violence toward children*. Hillsdale, NJ: Lawrence Erlbaum.

Hill, R. (1981). Whither family research in the 1980's: Continuities, emergents, constraints, and new horizons. *Journal of Marriage and the Family, 43*(2), 255–257.

Howard, J. G., Rothbart, G., & Sloan, G. (1978). The response to "Roots": A national survey. *Journal of Broadcasting, 22*, 279–287.

Hur, K. K. (1978). Impact of "Roots" on Black and White teenagers. *Journal of Broadcasting, 22*, 289–298.

Johnson, E. R. (1984). Credibility of Black and White newscasters to a Black audience. *Journal of Broadcasting, 28*, 365–368.

Johnson, E. R. (1987). Believability of newscasters to Black television viewers. *Western Journal of Black Studies, 11*(2), 64–68.

Jordan, V. E. (1980). The state of Black America in the 1970's. *Urban League Report, 5*(1), 4–6.

Landrum, S., Beck-Sague, C., & Kraus, S. (1988). Racial trends in syphilis among men with same-sex partners in Atlanta, Georgia. *American Journal of Public Health, 78*, 66–67.

Mays, V. M., & Cochran, S. D. (1987). Acquired immunodeficiency syndrome and Black Americans: Special psychosocial issues. *Public Health Reports, 102*, 224–231.

Mays, V. M., & Cochran, S. D. (1988a). Black gay and bisexual men coping with more than just a disease. *Focus, 4*(1), 1–3.

Mays, V. M., & Cochran, S. D. (1988b). Issues in the perception of AIDS risk and risk reduction activities by Black and Hispanic/Latina women. *American Psychologist, 43*(11), 949–957.

Mays, V. M., Cochran, S. D., & Roberts, V. (1988). Heterosexuals and AIDS. In A. Lewis (Ed.), *Nursing care of the person with AIDS/ARC*. Rockville, MD: Aspen.

Poindexter, P. M., & Stroman, C. A. (1981). Blacks and television: A review of the research literature. *Journal of Broadcasting, 25*, 103–122.

Roberts, D. F., & Bachen, C. M. (1981). Mass communication effects. *Annual Review of Psychology, 32*, 307–356.

Robinson, I. (1986). Blacks move back to the South. *American Demographics, 8*(6), 40–43.

Selik, R. M., Castro, K. G., & Pappaioanou, M. (1988). Racial/ethnic differences in risk of AIDS. *American Journal of Public Health, 78*, 1539–1545.

Smith, M. C. (1986). By the year 2000. In J. Beam (Ed.), *In the life: A Black gay anthology*. Boston: Alyson.

Smith, T. W. (1984). America's religious mosaic. *American Demographics, 6*(6), 19–23.

U.S. Department of Commerce, Bureau of the Census. (1983). *Characteristics of the population: General population characteristics, part I.* Washington, DC: Government Printing Office.

Warren, D. I. (1972). Mass media and racial crisis: A study of the New Bethel Church incident in Detroit. *Journal of Social Issues, 28*(1), 111–131.

Wells, R. V. (1985). *Uncle Sam's family: Issues in and perspectives on American demographic history.* Albany: State University of New York Press.

16

Pulling Coyote's Tale: Native American Sexuality and AIDS

Terry Tafoya

There is a grim irony in the difficulty of providing adequate resources for AIDS preventive care among Native American communities. Native Americans have not been seen as a priority population, literally invisible within ethnic minority statistics that profile Blacks and Hispanics, but list Native Americans as "other," if at all. And yet it is the original exposure to European diseases through contact with Caucasians that has successfully reduced Native Americans to such a minority status. For example, it is estimated that within two generations of White contact, over 80% of the Native population of the Pacific Northwest died of infection from European diseases to which American Indians had no acquired immunity. Lewis and Clark describe in their journals passing by Columbia River Indian villages with populations of over 3,000, only to pass by them on their return voyage to discover fewer than 300 remaining alive. This pattern of devastation remains consistent with American Indians experiencing White contact. For example, before Spanish contact with the Pueblos of what is now New Mexico, there were over 90 villages, compared to 19 today; in the Southeast, over 30,000 Natives died of infectious European diseases.

There are indeed a number of interesting parallels within the Native American historical experience of Whites and their diseases and the gay and bisexual experience of AIDS. In both instances, church and government organizations identified elements of sexual behavior and gender orientation as "bad" and "deviant." In the case of the religious bodies, those who developed illness were informed that this was a direct punishment from God for their "unnatural" sins. Specific sexual behaviors were condemned, and sexual/social behavior changes were demanded.

For the majority of Native American communities, for whom extended family networks make up the very foundation of activity and

280

self-identity, the rapid loss of lives was overwhelming, and the effects are still noted today. Some researchers have compared the experience to that of Holocaust survivors, but even such a comparison pales when one realizes genocide is a literal term for the experience of a number of different tribal groups. For those who did manage to live through the first generations of illness and build up some degree of immunity to European-introduced disease, there has often been a tremendous loss of language, culture, and religion, hampering a sense of continuity and self-efficacy.

To this one must add the direct attempts of the federal government to regulate, control, and destroy Native American behavior patterns. Reservations were established by the American government and turned over to Christian missionaries to administer, since *Christianity* and *civilization* were considered to be synonymous. Indians were allowed to leave the reservation only with passes provided by the reservation superintendents, and noncompliance with White rules and regulations meant withholding of food supplies, vital to many tribes now "trapped" on reservations and unable to use their usual and accustomed hunting and fishing territories. Native American religions were regularly persecuted by White authorities, resulting in legal challenges to religious freedoms that culminated in both the Indian Reorganization Act in 1934 and the Native American Religious Freedom Act of 1978. Native American children were regularly removed from their homes as early as the age of 5 (sometimes at gunpoint by federal troops) to attend federal Indian boarding schools, where they would be isolated from parental influences (and thus, in the eyes of the federal government, more easily "civilized") and physically abused to prevent them speaking their Native languages or practicing their traditional religions.

American Indians and Alaskan Natives are unique from other racial/ethnic minorities in that they possess a legal relationship with the American federal government, created by the treaties between the United States and the various Indian nations. Because of this treaty relationship, it is estimated that there are more than 2,000 laws and regulations that apply only to American Indians and Alaskan Natives and not to other American citizens. American Indians did not even become citizens of the United States until 1924. All this combines to create massive confusion regarding local, state, tribal, and federal concepts of jurisdiction and financial responsibilities immediately relevant to Native American AIDS care and prevention.

Given the historical reality, Native Americans are often suspicious of bureaucrats, interviews, and health care facilities. For many Native

Americans, health care facilities are difficult to reach, often minimally staffed, and, as a result, are underutilized. For some traditional elders, White hospitals are places one goes to die; this becomes a self-fulfilling prophecy, since many people will not seek preventive care, but wait until the advanced stages of illnesses, resulting in a poorer chance of successful treatment.

It should also be emphasized that it is misleading to conceptualize Native Americans as belonging to one culture, language, religion, and so on. In reality, there are more than 300 American tribes, and over 250 Indian languages, excluding the many tribes of Canada and Central and South America. Health beliefs vary among tribes, with differences increased by the degree of acculturation of individuals. Complicating matters further is the estimate that over 25% of Native American children were being reared in non-Indian homes prior to the Indian Child Welfare Act of 1977, which attempted to halt the wholesale removal of Native children for the purpose of White adoptions.

Tracking Native American demographics is so difficult that, having attempted to trace Native American infant mortality rates and failed, some government agencies despair of ever really having an accurate count of Native American AIDS cases. There are at least nine legal definitions of *Native American*, including having one-fourth blood of a federally recognized tribe. It should be mentioned here that American Indians and Alaskan Natives (a category that includes Alaskan Indians, Eskimos, and Aleuts) remain the only American ethnic group tracked by blood quantum by the federal government. This is, of course, of advantage to the government, which can deny economic resources to those tribes (federally unrecognized) or individuals who do not meet federal standards of identity.

It is estimated that there are at least 1.6 million Native Americans, with about a 60/40 split between urban and reservation dwellers. In the 1950s, a massive effort called "relocation" was undertaken by the federal government to move Indians off their reservations into major urban centers, such as Los Angeles, New York, Seattle, and Chicago. This was an attempt to use a loophole within treaty obligations, which stated that Indians must live "on or near" their reservations to receive federal services. By moving them to cities, they were no longer "on or near" their reservations. This has further disrupted traditional child rearing, as access to extended family networks is restricted.

Without some sense of Native American historical reality, listing AIDS demographics would make little sense. For example, the Centers for Disease Control originally relied totally on Indian Health Services (IHS) to provide reports of Native American AIDS cases. This resulted in a jurisdictional issue, since IHS could report only on those individuals who used IHS facilities. For those Native Americans who used private, city, or state health care facilities, there would be no cross-referencing to IHS or CDC. Up until 1988, most states had no official category for reporting Native American AIDS cases, listing them as "other" or, in some instances, mislabeling Native Americans as Hispanic, Black, or even Asian. Depending on the first Whites to invade their territories, Native Americans often have French, English, or, in the case of the American Southwest, Spanish surnames. (Many tribes had no concept of a paternal surname, but rather named people as individuals. Such names might change during an individual's lifetime. Needless to say, this did not sit well with White bureaucrats, who demanded easier bookkeeping, and forced White surnames or "Indian names" to be used as surname equivalents.) There has been a slightly higher death rate due to AIDS among Native Americans than among non-Indians, resulting in coroners, incorrectly identifying Native Americans.

In preparation for the international AIDS symposium "A Biosocial/Biomedical Integrated Approach," sponsored by the Kinsey Institute and various federal agencies, a call was made to CDC and IHS to determine the number of reported Native American AIDS cases. For the three-state area of Washington, Oregon, and Idaho, Indian Health Services reported no cases of AIDS, and three HIV-positive cases out of the urban areas, as of July 1987. When further questioned, IHS had no ethnic breakdown of the HIV-positive cases. This was at best awkward, since urban-based clinics in Seattle and Portland do not restrict their services to Native American clients, and there was no way of determining whether these three instances represented American Indians or Alaskan Natives. A call to the Northwest AIDS Foundation based in Seattle uncovered eleven Native American AIDS cases, three of whom had died. This difficulty of tracking AIDS cases in the Native American communities is typical; some health professionals feel there may be at least two to four times the number of reported AIDS cases.

There is also an additional concern that IHS providers may have misdiagnosed AIDS/ARC cases. Dr. Ben Muneta, past medical director of the Navajo Nation Department of Health, has stated that the average life span of his Navajo patients with AIDS between diagnosis and death was six weeks. He reported five deaths from AIDS at Na-

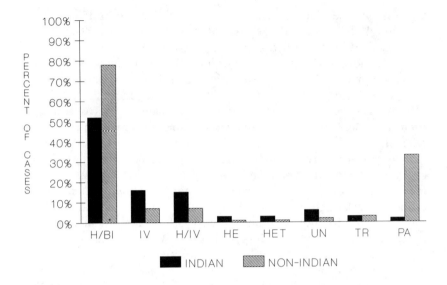

Figure 16.1 AIDS Transmission Categories, Indian versus Overall United States, as of January 2, 1989
SOURCE: Centers for Disease Control, *AIDS Weekly Surveillance Report.*

vajo in 1987. Dr. Muneta has expressed concern that this may indicate that Indians wait until they are critically ill before seeking care, but it could also indicate prior misdiagnosis.

Because of the small number of reported Native American AIDS cases, IHS has been reluctant (i.e., it refuses) to give a breakdown of geographic and tribal cases, and provides little information on pediatric Native American AIDS, due to a concern for confidentiality.

As of May 24, 1988, 64 Native American AIDS cases in 22 states had been identified. Figure 16.1 indicates a comparison between Indian and non-Indian AIDS transmission categories. The significantly higher percentage of cases among IV drug users (combined homosexual/heterosexual) among Indians than among the non-Indian population should be noted.

Unpublished preliminary studies of American Indians and Alaskan Natives tested for HIV antibodies by the Seattle AIDS Information Project indicate a significantly higher percentage of this population (over 40%) showing HIV positive than any other ethnic group tested. Having so stated, it should be realized that virtually all the data are questionable, since they are based on such a small sample. For example, the 6% hemophiliacs among Native Americans actually translates to 3

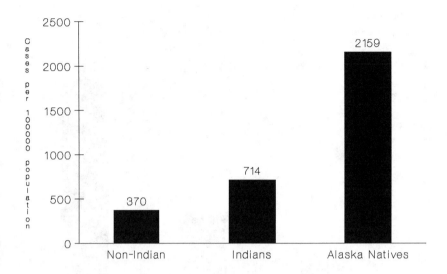

Figure 16.2 Gonorrhea Rates in Alaska, Arkansas, North Carolina, New Mexico, Oklahoma, Oregon, South Dakota, and Washington
SOURCE: Centers for Disease Control data from 1985.

individuals; 50% of the Alaskan Natives in Seattle tested who have HIV antibodies translates to 4 of 8 individuals tested. Most epidemiologic studies are based on a population of 100,000, a minimum number that would eliminate all but 1% or so of tribal groups from being fairly compared without making major statistical adjustments.

One exception to this is a rather disturbing CDC study conducted in 1985 on sexually transmitted diseases among some Native groups. Gonorrhea rates among Native Americans in eight states with sizable Indian populations were found to be 714 per 100,000, compared to 370 per 100,000 for the non-Indian population (see Figure 16.2). In Alaska, Natives had rates of 2,159 per 100,000. Indian primary and secondary syphilis rates were 26.5 per 100,000, compared with 7.1 per 100,000 for non-Indians. In Arizona, Indian people had syphilis rates of 79.1 per 100,000 (Figure 16.3). Obviously, these extreme rates of sexually transmitted diseases may be an indication of a corresponding danger of HIV transmission.

Females make up 15% of the reported Native American AIDS cases (see Figure 16.4). There is a greater percentage of pediatric AIDS among Native Americans, but, again, the percentages are greatly misleading due to the extremely small sample size.

Much has been written about Native American problems with alco-

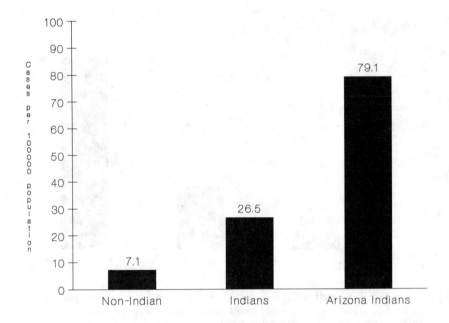

Figure 16.3 Primary and Secondary Syphilis Rates in Alaska, Arkansas, North Carolina, New Mexico, Oklahoma, Oregon, South Dakota, and Washington
SOURCE: Centers for Disease Control data from 1985.

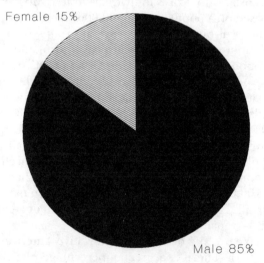

Figure 16.4 Native American AIDS Cases by Sex, as of December 20, 1988

hol abuse. The majority of the ten most frequent causes of death among Natives are related to high rates of alcohol and substance abuse. More than one-third of all Indian people die before the age of 45 from diseases directly related to "drinking and drugging." In an unpublished study conducted by Dr. Kathleen Toomey in the San Francisco Bay Area, 30 out of 60 gay American Indian men being tested for HIV antibodies were IV drug users. The issue of IV drug abuse among Indians has been ignored while health care providers have focused on the more visible alcohol abuse. Anecdotal evidence from California Indian treatment programs and comments from tribal leaders indicate that growing numbers of Indian youth are shooting drugs, especially amphetamines, intravenously. Indian shooting galleries have been described in Los Angeles and Minneapolis by IV drug users and health providers. In addition to drug abuse, there is concern regarding high incidence of diabetes among Native Americans, who risk a potential health problem of shared needles among diabetics.

Finally, there is the issue of epistemological differences in Native American concepts of gender and sexual behaviors. There is evidence that a number of tribal groups have traditionally had more than two concepts of gender, that is, male and female. At least 135 tribes have specific terms for individuals who are not exactly male or female. *Berdache* is commonly used in the anthropological literature as a general term to describe such people. In some instances, these individuals may share some of the characteristics Western society identifies as gay or lesbian, but the homosexual categories are White constructs that may overlap, but not include, some Native American concepts of gender. For example, there is some documentation that indicates a berdache might have been available not only as a sexual outlet for men whose wives were unavailable to them (for example, when they were pregnant or having their periods), but as a sexual outlet for women who were lacking male partners. For some tribal groups, however, a berdache would not be able to have sex with another berdache, since this would be seen as "unnatural."

This has immediate application in AIDS outreach to Native communities. A death by AIDS of a member of one of the pueblo villages has caused a problem in identifying this individual's sexual partners. As a member of a "third gender," this person's male sexual partners would not conceptualize themselves as bisexual or gay, since they were not having sex with another man. This is somewhat different from some other tribes, and Hispanic groups, where a male in the active (i.e., insertive) role in anal intercourse would not be considered homosexual, but the male in the passive (i.e., receptive) role would be.

It should be remembered that the term *homosexual* came into use only in 1869, and then as a medical term. Although Western influence has forced a "gay overlay" on tribes, for many Native Americans, there was never the rigid classification typical of Western polarity that divides the world into straight and gay. Determination of an individual's identity on the basis of sexual behavior makes no conceptual sense to many American Indians.

The stress among Native Americans is on the function of extended families. To achieve adulthood, one must have the experience of parenting, even if children are not biologically one's own. If one is responsible in meeting the obligations of the extended family network, what one does in one's own time is one's choice. As long as the family is not threatened, personal sexual behavior is no one else's business.

While this is a traditional way of behaving for members of many tribes, there are more urbanized Indian people who strongly identify with the gay movement. Any attempts at preventive AIDS care must therefore include gay and lesbian Native Americans as well as Indians who would not identify themselves as gay. Unpublished data from the American Couples work of Phillip Blumstein and Pepper Swartz indicate that Native Americans have a much higher percentage of bisexuality than any other ethnic group, even though all the Natives in the study were in gay or lesbian relationships at the time of the study. This may reflect the more fluid concepts of sexual behavior representative of the historical berdache.

Due to Western-influenced homophobia, some tribal groups that traditionally accepted berdache people now find their behavior unacceptable, encouraging many individuals to lead "double lives," one on reservation and one off. This can allow the transmission of HIV infection, as an individual can engage in high-risk behavior in an urban area and then expose reservation neighbors to the virus. An additional concern is with Native American street youth in urban areas who may be affected. Many prostitutes will no longer engage in unsafe sex, but johns will offer twice the money for unsafe sex to street youth. Outreach and education need to be provided to young Native Americans before they drop out of school and attempt to support themselves by prostitution.

Recommendations

(1) The federal government should require AIDS surveillance reporting in a uniform format from states that includes American Indians/Alaskan Natives as an ethnic category. Failing that, the CDC should undertake a special study to determine the true number of AIDS cases among American Indians.

(2) Congress should consider language in future IHS funding legislation that requires IHS to provide AIDS-specific training to all its clinical personnel, from physicians to community health representatives, in order to ensure clinical competence in dealing with seropositive patients and in diagnosing ARC/AIDS cases.

(3) IHS should implement desperately needed research on the extent of intravenous drug use among Native Americans nationwide, both in urban areas and on reservations, and report to Congress, detailing its plan for addressing identified problems.

(4) It is critical that Native American sex research be conducted, since it is meaningless to suggest alterations in sexual behavior if one has no idea what the sexual behavior may be.

(5) Since financial support through Indian tertiary care is appallingly low (for example, in 1986, IHS spent an average of only $7.00 per eligible Indian per year in California), it is vital that a catastrophic care fund adequate to cover the cost of providing care to Indian people with AIDS/ARC who are eligible for IHS services be made available through appropriate legislation.

(6) The need for multicultural approaches should be stressed and made a requirement for funding to any organization providing services or assistance to individuals or communities affected by AIDS. It should also be required that any state or federally funded curriculum materials be reviewed by appropriate members of ethnic communities, with adequate compensation provided for such reviewers.

17

AIDS Prevention Models in Asian-American Communities

Bart Aoki
Chiang Peng Ngin
Bertha Mo
Davis Y. Ja

Epidemiology of AIDS among Asians

AIDS is an invisible disease in the Asian community. It is invisible to most members of the community and it is invisible to public health officials on local, state, and federal levels, even though AIDS has affected Asian-Americans since the first case was diagnosed in the United States in 1981. To date, resources available for research, training, prevention, and education for the Asian community are scarce and difficult to find.

Review of Previous Research

Currently there are extremely few studies of AIDS transmission among Asians. A Medline search produced two references, both of which discuss the linkages between HTLV-I, a subgroup of the AIDS virus (HTLV-III), and adult T-cell leukemia (ATL). ATL is a condition endemic to southern Japan and the Caribbean basin. HTLV-I has been implicated epidemiologically as the causative agent in ATL. Bartholomew and his colleagues (1985) reported on the characteristics of human T-cell leukemia/lymphoma (HTLV-I) and AIDS (HTLV-III) in Trinidad. HTLV-III, a subgroup of HTLV-I, has recently been isolated from many patients with the Acquired Immunodeficiency Syndrome and pre-AIDS, thus indicating that this variant is the primary cause of AIDS. Yim, Hayashi, Yanagihara, Kardin, and Nakamura (1986) describe a case of HTLV-I-associated T-cell leukemia in a Nisei (second-generation Japanese-American) resident of Hawaii. The dis-

290

ease was initially indolent, then clinically explosive, characterized by cutaneous lesions, leukemic lymphocytes with convoluted nuclei of T-cell phenotype, and hypercalcemia, and resulted in an infection that proved terminal. These two articles hint at the possibility of a genetic association between the Japanese and AIDS. However, research is needed to test this hypothesis.

In a study by Winkelstein and Samuel (1987), prevalence data of HIV infection according to ethnicity from the San Francisco Men's Health Study indicated that of 391 infected homosexual and bisexual men, 3 were Asians. The cohort had a total of 11 Asian subjects; thus the 3 represent a 27.3% infection rate.

Dr. Gisella Schecter of the San Francisco Department of Health at San Francisco General Hospital is studying the association of tuberculosis with AIDS. She hypothesizes that a person with TB who later contracts AIDS would be likely to exhibit pronounced TB due to the compromised immune system caused by the AIDS virus. Thus far, Dr. Schecter has found 50 individuals from San Francisco who have both TB and AIDS. Of this 50, 3 individuals are Asian—2 were born in the Philippines and 1 was born in China. In San Francisco, 50–60% of TB cases are found among Asian-born individuals, mainly from the Philippines and China. Asian countries, in general, have a high prevalence of TB. Given the high number of Asian immigrants in San Francisco and the low number of Asians with TB and AIDS in her study, Dr. Schecter theorizes that there may not be much HIV infection in Asian countries.

Although plausible, this hypothesis requires further investigation. Dr. Schecter's research does not specifically target Asians. In addition, biases due to selection, small sample size, and insufficient time frame underestimate the problem. The sampling frame or scheme might exclude Asian immigrants because of cultural and socioeconomic factors. The assumed high prevalence of TB among Asian countries is not true of all Asian countries; for example, Japan does not have a high TB rate.

Finally, focus groups were conducted by the Asian AIDS Project, which completed a report for the San Francisco Department of Public Health in June 1987. The report summarized the conclusions of focus groups from the Chinese, Japanese, Korean, and Pilipino communities. Each group assessed AIDS issues for its own community in San Francisco, and the report lists options and a process for needs assessment in these Asian communities. The report is unique in its attempts to delineate the problems of AIDS education and research in each of these communities.

TABLE 17.1

Asian AIDS Cases Nationwide, by Transmission Category as of January 2, 1989

Transmission Category	Number	Percentage
Homosexual or bisexual male	360	73.8
Homosexual/bisexual IV drug user	8	1.6
IV drug user	16	3.3
Transfusion recipient	43	8.8
Hemophiliac/coagulation disorder	12	2.5
Heterosexual contact	15	3.0
None of the above	34	7.0
Total	488	100.0

SOURCE: Data extracted from *AIDS Weekly Surveillance Report*, U.S. AIDS Program, Center for Infectious Diseases, Centers for Disease Control.

TABLE 17.2

U.S. Asian AIDS Cases by Age Group

Age Group	Number of Cases	Percentage
12 and under	6	1
13-19	5	1
20-29	84	17
30-39	204	42
40-49	122	25
50 and over	67	14
Total	488	100

SOURCE: Data extracted from *AIDS Weekly Surveillance Report*, U.S. AIDS Program, Center for Infectious Diseases, Centers for Disease Control.

The Statistics and Data Management Branch at the Centers for Disease Control provided national statistics for Asian AIDS cases. As of January 2, 1989, there were 488 cases of AIDS among Asians in the United States. The transmission categories indicate that the highest number of cases of AIDS in the Asian community occurs among homosexual and bisexual men. Tables 17.1 and 17.2 show the distribution of the transmission categories and age groups of the cases.

Although the number of Asian AIDS cases has been relatively low, a review of existing data indicates that the number of reported cases is increasing. The extent of the epidemic among Asians is not well understood. This is primarily due to several factors.

First, the method by which surveillance data on AIDS are being collected and reported gives an incomplete picture of the epidemic among Asians. In a few surveillance programs, linguistically, racially,

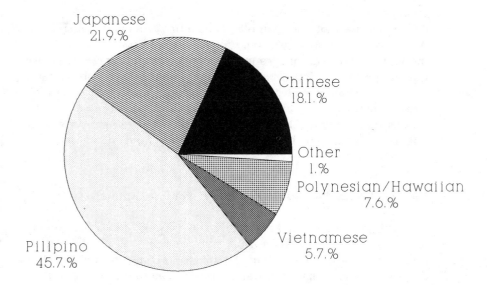

Figure 17.1 Asian AIDS Cases in San Francisco, January 1982 Through January 1989
SOURCE: San Francisco Department of Public Health (1989).

and culturally different Asian groups are placed in the general category of Asians. In most, Asians are combined with Pacific Islanders or placed with Native Americans in an "other" category. It is therefore difficult to detect patterns in rates, modes of transmission, or other variables in each ethnic group. Second, there is a lack of any epidemiological research conducted on the Asian population, with the prime focus of research so far having been on the homosexual and bisexual White population.

While seroprevalence and incidence figures show that AIDS has had an impact on the Asian community as a whole, they say little about the impact the epidemic has had on various Asian subcommunities (see Figure 17.1). Data from the San Francisco HIV Antibody Counselling and Testing Program show that of the 969 Asian who were tested between 1985 and 1988, 11% tested positive.

Asians are an extremely heterogeneous group, with 32 distinct ethnic groups with different languages, attitudes, traditions, and behaviors. There exists no single "Asian community"; it consists of Chinese, Japanese, Koreans, Pilipinos, Vietnamese, Samoans, Laotians, Cambodians, Hawaiians, and so on. There are fifth-generation, immigrant, and refugee Asian-Americans. They reside in both urban and rural areas and in all parts of the country. Many live in "ghettos," yet many others are part of the "yuppie" subculture. In planning effective AIDS prevention strategies, questions about differential rates among the various Asian ethnic groups become important. Is the incidence rate higher among Japanese than among Pilipinos? Are foreign-born Asians overrepresented compared to second- and third-generation Asian-Americans? To answer these questions we need to see the groups that make up the Asian/Pacific Islander community as separate communities with specific sociocultural and historical backgrounds.

Cultural Issues Around AIDS in the Asian Communities

In this section, we will focus on the diversity and similarities among the three groups of Asian-Americans currently most affected by AIDS—Pilipinos, Chinese, and Japanese—keeping in mind the fact that within each Asian subgroup there exists another range of differences based upon nativity, number of years in the United States, social class, and education. First, we will briefly look at the philosophical and cultural norms of the homeland; next, we will describe the different subgroups within each of the three Asian groups; finally, we will discuss beliefs about health, illness, death, sexuality, and homosexuality. Of these three ethnic subgroups the Chinese- and Pilipino-Americans are probably the most diverse and the Japanese-Americans the most homogeneous.

Cultural Roots

The cultural roots of Pilipino-Americans are Malayo-Polynesian (carried from Java via Malaysia and Thailand), Chinese (from Chinese merchants and sailors), Spanish, and American. In 1521, the islands were colonized by Spain, which established the Catholic church in the Philippines. Today, approximately 90% of all Pilipinos are Catholic. In 1898, after the Spanish-American War, the Philippines became a territory of the United States. The Unites States developed a free public education system that included medical schools promoting allopathic medicine.

The values of China and Japan, unlike those of the more Western-influenced Pilipino culture, are rooted in Confucian ethics. High value is placed on duty, obedience, filial piety, and ancestor worship. In Japan, *bushido* (the way of the warrior) was grafted onto the Confucian values. The extended family is the primary unit of social, legal, and political organization. The family is thought to be continuous through time, including the past, present, and future members of the family.

The most important expression of filial piety, at least for male children, is to marry and have children (particularly boys) who will in turn worship the ancestors and perpetuate the family and its name. In both China and Japan this was so important in the past that if a wife should be barren, a mistress or concubine might be found to bear an heir for the family. In Japan, if a family had only daughters, a son-in-law might be adopted into the family who would take on the surname of his in-laws. This was not a practice in China. In all three cultures a person is not viewed as an individual but as a representative of his or her family (and, in the case of Japanese-Americans, the entire community). Maintaining "face," the public persona, dignity, or self-esteem, is all-important. Loss of face has serious repercussions because it reflects negatively on the individual's entire family and community and not just on the individual. One maintains face by fulfilling culturally appropriate responsibilities and acting in accordance with norms with respect to one's social role. For example, all children of a certain age are expected to marry and have families of their own.

Asian Communities in America

The immigration of Pilipinos to the United States can be divided into three distinct waves: (a) During the 1920s and 1930s, single males with little education came as laborers in agriculture and service industries; (b) next, single males with a basic elementary education who served in the U.S. Navy or Philippine Scouts found work in the better-paying sectors of service industries, as factory workers, and the better educated entered government service; (c) after 1965, professionals who were highly trained entered, but because of discrimination and licensing laws, they found it difficult to obtain positions commensurate with their training. In addition, large numbers of women and the families of Pilipino ex-servicemen entered the United States after 1965 under the family reunification category. Most Pilipinos are bilingual in English and in a Pilipino dialect.

Japanese-Americans are a fairly homogeneous group. Most first-generation (Issei) Japanese-Americans came in the 1890s as sojourners, intent on making money and then returning home. They earned minimal wages as domestic servants and farm laborers. Discrimination and personal preference led a majority of them to return to Japan to marry or to choose a "picture bride." Although some Issei are bilingual, many prefer to speak Japanese, and there are Japanese-language newspapers, community services, and Japantowns that cater to their needs.

The Nisei (the American-born children of Issei) and the Sansei and Yonsei (who are their children and grandchildren) are primarily English speaking and, compared to other Asian-Americans, are very acculturated. This acculturation may be traced to the wholesale incarceration of Japanese-Americans during World War II and the confiscation of all Japanese material culture as subversive evidence. Nonetheless, this has not obliterated some very basic cultural beliefs and practices related to the family and illness.

Chinese-Americans can be divided into the following categories: (a) elderly bachelors who came as sojourners who are bilingual, but usually prefer to speak their native language; (b) reunited families consisting of an older male who has been joined by spouse and children (in some cases, adult children and their families) who came after 1965—largely monolingual; (c) Chinese refugee families from Southeast Asia who speak a variety of Chinese dialects and Southeast Asian languages; (d) Chinese families from Hong Kong, mainland China, and Taiwan who in the main are minimally bilingual, usually preferring to speak their native language; and (e) American-born Chinese and their families, who fall within a wide bicultural spectrum.

Cultural Beliefs and AIDS

In considering culture and AIDS, it is probably useful to bear in mind that most Asian-Americans are to a greater or lesser degree bicultural, but that in situations of perceived threat or vulnerability these individuals have a tendency to revert to traditional, familiar Asian cultural norms. Education for preventing AIDS is particularly challenging in the Asian-American community because it brings to the fore several topics—illness, death, sex, and homosexuality—that are difficult if not taboo to discuss in public. As in many societies, there exists among some Asians the belief that discussing illness is bad luck and can even bring about an occurrence of the illness. Concern with daily health practices stands, for example, in sharp contrast to the strict taboo within most Asian cultures against discussion of serious and terminal illness. Physicians in contemporary Japan, as part of standard practice, do not disclose a cancer diagnosis to the patient (Ohnuki-Tierney, 1984). Cancer is such a taboo topic in Asian cultures that past health education efforts among Asians in San Francisco to increase cervical cancer screening and breast self-examination have had to be couched in the language of health promotion rather than cancer detection and have been held in nonmedical settings.

The notion of the self-fulfilling prophecy also contributes strongly to the prohibition against discussions about death and related topics. In addition, Japanese Shinto beliefs and Chinese folk beliefs define everything related to death and blood as polluting (DeVos & Wagatsuma, 1966). An ethnic minority multicultural study of death states that while there is a general taboo against discussing death among all generations of Japanese-Americans, the Issei are particularly knowledgeable about and practice numerous avoidances and positive acts to keep harm and death away. For example, the character for the number four, *shi*, is also a homophone for the word for death. Therefore, the word *yon* is substituted. There is also an avoidance of serving or selling four of anything (Kalish & Reynolds, 1981).

Among Asian immigrants and to a lesser extent among succeeding generations, naturalistic, metaphysical, and spiritual beliefs about the origins of illness exist alongside varying degrees of understanding and acceptance of Western models (Koo, 1982). Within the context of an array of differing beliefs regarding the prevention, transmission, and treatment of illness in Asian communities, standard prevention models may have limited utility.

Asian notions about how contagious diseases are spread need to be examined and addressed, because spurious connections between diseases endemic at one time to Asian countries—such as TB, smallpox, and malaria—may make it difficult for Asian-Americans to see the efficacy of AIDS prevention methods.

The myth that AIDS is spread by mosquitoes is quite widespread in the Chinese- and Japanese-language press in the United States. Because TB, endemic to most Asian countries, is spread easily through the air, sputum, and saliva, it is difficult for Asians to accept that AIDS, another contagious disease, is not spread the same way. Finally, because smallpox, that scourge of the entire world that was practically eliminated less than a decade ago, can be spread via the personal belongings of the infected individual, many Asians expect that the same is true of AIDS. These deep-seated beliefs about contagious diseases when generalized to AIDS make it difficult for Asians to accept as authoritative the information that AIDS is not spread in the same manner and understandably also lead to skepticism about proffered prevention methods.

To illustrate, a contract for completing construction of an AIDS hospice was recently awarded to an Asian-American building firm. The firm, with the support of its Asian attorneys, withdrew at the last minute because of the refusal by the Chinese construction crew to work on a project that they perceived would jeopardize their health. Despite attempts by a bilingual health worker to dispel their fears, the workers stood firm in their refusal and furthermore burned their "contaminated" work clothes. Among the host of factors operating in this situation was probably a generalized notion of how AIDS is spread based on previous knowledge about other contagious diseases.

There is enormous complexity in the way different Asian cultures integrate issues of sexuality into their lives. This may be partly due to the Confucian edicts that seek to sanction sexuality only as it serves to perpetuate the family line. Unharnessed sexual expression outside marriage is a threat to the integrity of the family and, by extension, to the community and to the state. In contrast, there exists a certain naturalness about sexuality in rural, agricultural Asian societies and in the extreme a certain preoccupation and romantic notion of sexuality among the literate upper classes and literati. In general, among Asian-Americans public expression of sexuality is inhibited, and the issue itself is particularly difficult for most Asians to discuss or even to acknowledge openly (Abramson, 1986; Coleman, 1983).

Homosexuality is a difficult subject to discuss in Asian society partly because it often precludes fulfillment of the most important expression of filial piety—marriage and the procreation of heirs to carry on the family name. As mentioned above, almost 80% of Asians with AIDS identify themselves as either homosexual or bisexual. Being both Asian and gay, these individuals have probably already had to grapple with reconciling their own sexuality with being socialized in a subculture in which the family is valued as the primary social unit throughout life. In this cultural context, one's behavior reflects upon the entire family and one's primary obligation, especially as a son, is the continuation of the family through marriage and the bearing of children. When a family produces a child who is homosexual, it implies that the parents have failed in their role and that the child is rejecting the importance of both family and culture. In effect, especially if the child is the only son, his homosexuality is seen as the end of the family (Jue, 1987).

Evidence exists that homosexuality is more accepted in Pilipino society, and consequently it appears that Pilipino gays exhibit less psychological conflict (Hart, 1968; Sechrest, 1969; Sechrest & Flores, 1969).

The interrelationship between death and homosexuality is a highly charged topic, particularly in the Confucian-dominated cultures. The very traditional Chinese believe that the child who dies before his or her parents is unfilial. In some cases this may preclude parents' mourning publicly for their children. In addition, the spirits of children who do not marry are feared because, according to traditional definitions of happiness and fulfillment, they have led incomplete lives. Unfortunately, dying young, unmarried, or without children characterizes most Asians who have died of AIDS.

Health Behavior Change Models

Self-Efficacy Model

In bridging the gap between knowledge about AIDS and risk-reducing behavior, Bandura's self-efficacy theory has both powerful explanatory capability as well as certain limitations. The core of the model, that self-perception of efficacy influences thought patterns, actions, and emotional arousal, is broadly applicable to many populations and situations. However, in using the model to conceptualize and develop AIDS prevention within Asian-American communities, it would seem that many of the specific social constraints or cultural norms discussed earlier affect its direct application to this population.

No substantial research has been published evaluating the explanatory value of self-efficacy as it relates to health promotion among Asian-American individuals. Sue (1977) has proposed that the concept of learned helplessness when applied to Asian-Americans explains the prevalence of alienation, anxiety, and anger among these groups despite objective indices of achievement and success in American society. He argues that rather than developing out of identity conflict, the sense of alienation and depression more likely develops when Asians experience the lack of control and choice inherent in a society that overtly limits cultural plurality. In his recommendations for counselors, Sue suggests that the psychological well-being of Asian-Americans can be enhanced by facilitating a better sense of self-control in certain life situations. He points out that in American culture the ability to verbalize needs and desires appropriately is highly functional and enhances the individual's sense of control, particularly over the surrounding social environment. Although it contradicts the Asian cultural value of restraint, he proposes that development of this skill would have direct and positive implications for psychological well-being among Asian-Americans.

In his discussion of learned helplessness, Sue also raises issues pertinent to the closely related self-efficacy model in its application to Asian-Americans. Like other American minority groups experiencing discrimination within the society, Asian-Americans often experience a limited sense of control over certain areas of life and a limited sense of self-efficacy. Given the cultural underpinnings that predispose Asians to a fatalistic view of the world, the application of the model in directly explaining and predicting health-inducing behavior becomes complicated. Are preventive interventions differentially effective due partly to the necessity of overcoming societally induced lower levels of self-efficacy and/or a culturally determined fatalistic attitude present despite high levels of personal efficacy?

When we seek to promote risk-reducing behavior among Asian-Americans, it becomes more apparent that culturally based motives may intervene and affect the experience of the individual. One particular factor that may intervene is the high value placed upon interdependence among Asian cultures. It is important to recognize that those within the Asian ethnic communities who are most likely engaged in high-risk behaviors are often at the periphery of the culture because of sanctions within Asian cultures. In those situations, the desire for acceptance and the effort to achieve culturally valued outcomes, though submerged or consciously denied, may be even more intense, superseding personal concerns about health. Unlike the self-efficacy model, both the theory of reasoned action and the health belief model address the effect of social or subjective norms upon health behavior change, a component essential to understanding behavior change among Asian-American communities.

The self-efficacy model is also limited in providing conceptual guidance in addressing the issue of "felt need." Independent of levels of self-efficacy as it relates to other important areas of their lives, many within the different Asian ethnic communities across the country would probably feel distant from the threat of HIV infection, due partly to the absence of Asian faces in media campaigns. A model with the most utility for this population would help conceptualize and focus interventions aimed at increasing the felt need to implement behavior changes in this area. The self-efficacy model could then be applied in the actual development of interventions once the need is experienced as immediate and necessary.

Among Asian communities in urban areas where HIV infection is high and visible in the broader population, felt need may be experienced at the other extreme, with fear of contagion distorting individuals' perceptions of personal capability to avoid infection. In this situation, the self-efficacy model would be more relevant and central to preventive efforts aimed at enhancing realistic perceptions of self-efficacy.

Theory of Reasoned Action

Aspects of Fishbein's theory of reasoned action may have relatively more utility as we seek to prevent AIDS within Asian communities. In particular, this model accounts for the effects of attitudes and subjective norms under individuals' intentions to perform health-promoting behaviors. Understanding these effects would enable educators to intervene in components of behavior likely to influence Asian-Americans.

Beliefs about the consequences of adopting or ignoring AIDS risk-reduction behaviors probably vary extremely within different segments of the Asian-American community, dependent partly upon general knowledge and partly upon culturally based beliefs about the transmission of disease. Thus, although protecting oneself from disease would be a highly valued attribute across Asian ethnic groups, beliefs about the specific consequences of behavior vis-á-vis HIV infection are probably culturally influenced and interact to distort a given Asian individual's intention to change behavior. Beliefs about AIDS and, more important, about the transmission of disease in general are critical foci in any intervention effort within Asian-American communities.

The expectations of significant others and the importance of conformity constitute the subjective norms within the family and community that contribute greatly to determining behavior across many Asian cultures. The fact that the theory of reasoned action incorporates these factors also critically increases its applicability to Asian communities. Given the culturally defined and valued interdependence among individuals, it is less likely that an Asian individual will act against subjective norms to institute health-promoting behavior. Indeed, as in the case of AIDS, if the community and family share the belief that initiating risk-reducing behavior implies membership in a stigmatized group, whether intravenous drug user or homosexual, further subjective cultural norms may constrain the individual from acting in the interest of personal health.

This model would then suggest that in order for any effort to be effective with this population, education needs to focus both upon changing beliefs about the direct personal consequences of adopting or ignoring protective behavior and upon affecting the community norms so as to integrate such behavior into the subjective standards and practices of the community as a whole. If Asians believe that other Asians are susceptible, that their own behavior is identified as at risk, and, critically, that their significant others share their concern and support behavioral changes, the intention to institute these changes should be affected greatly within these communities.

Health Belief Model

The health behavior change model that seems most comprehensive in identifying the underlying process through which cultural norms and experiences may affect health behavior is the health belief model (Becker, 1974). According to the model, behavior to prevent a disease is a function of the individual's perception of susceptibility to the disease and the severity of the consequences. These aspects combine to constitute a perception of personal threat. This threat will vary and, depending upon its level (it should ideally be moderate), will affect positively the motivation to change behavior. In addition to personal threat as a significant component, the health belief model underscores the importance of perception of the effectiveness of the proposed health-related behavior, including its simplicity and convenience. Last, the fact that social group influence and situational modifiers are recognized as necessary factors in understanding health behavior ultimately expands the theory's comprehensiveness and applicability to specific subpopulations and ethnic groups.

As discussed earlier, the perceived level of the threat of AIDS is a critical issue among different segments of the Asian community. In a recent study of the correlates of AIDS-associated high-risk behavior among Chinese and Pilipino gay men (Kitano, 1988), the critical predictor of such behavior was found to be "denial," or a lack of acknowledgment of realistic levels of personal and community threat. In other segments of the Asian community, particularly recent immigrants in urban settings, level of threat may be perceived as so high based upon culturally ingrained beliefs about transmission of disease that it leads to irrational behaviors aimed at protection while having little effect upon more central sexual behaviors. Thus, as posited by the health belief model, it is important within Asian communities to plan preventive interventions that will help "titrate" the perceived level of threat. In addition, as the model also suggests, the perception of the actual usefulness of risk-reduction methods, often mediated by cultural assumptions, needs to be addressed directly by intensive education.

Kitano's (1988) ground-breaking survey of 123 gay-identified Pilipino and Chinese men, while admittedly limited in its generalizability, also resulted in findings that support the importance of social group influence and situational modifiers upon the adoption of risk-reducing behavior. In particular, she found differences in high-risk behavior between Asian ethnic groups and suggests that AIDS information may not currently be "culturally sensitive" to Pilipinos. We also speculate that social group and cultural norms regarding sexuality and more specifically homosexuality differ greatly between the two groups. Another of Kitano's relevant findings was the difference in risk behavior between subgroups of foreign-born Asians depending upon the number of years they have been in the United States. Interestingly, although she expected that high-risk sexual behavior would be highest among the most recently immigrated, the pattern seemed to suggest that those in the United States at the height of the gay liberation movement, with its concomitant sexual freedoms, were most likely to be engaged in high-risk sexual behavior currently.

As posited by the health belief model and suggested by these findings, both social group influence and situational modifiers appear to be additional important factors when attempting to understand the adoption of risk-reduction behaviors among Asian-Americans. In addition, the health belief model begins to incorporate and highlight the extreme complexity and diversity of influences that must be considered in planning targeted preventive interventions within minority communities.

Current Prevention Efforts Targeting Asian-Americans

Although there were AIDS cases in the Asian community early in the epidemic (the first Asian case in San Francisco was in 1982), it was only after 1986 that any prevention efforts targeting Asians were established. Predictably, most of these efforts were initiated in metropolitan areas with high concentrations of Asians, such as New York, Los Angeles, and San Francisco.

AIDS Project Los Angeles has developed written material on AIDS transmission and HIV antibody testing in Chinese, Japanese, Tagalog, Korean, and Vietnamese. The project also instituted an information telephone line with recorded AIDS information in several Asian languages. In New York, the Chinatown Health Clinic cosponsored a daylong community forum on AIDS early in 1988. Asian Health Services in Oakland plans during 1989 to develop educational material in various Asian languages in order to train Asian health providers. Currently they provide presentations on an ad hoc basis to their predominantly Asian clients. The Department of Health Services in Hawaii has produced basic AIDS educational material in several Asian languages.

The Asian AIDS Project in San Francisco is engaged in preventive efforts targeting Asian-Americans in a programmatic way. This project's interventions include providing culturally sensitive basic AIDS presentations and producing AIDS education messages in the media to the general population of the various ethnic groups, developing AIDS education brochures in several Asian languages targeting both the general and gay communities, providing training to Asian health and human service professionals, implementing an Asian model of a successful interactive prevention program targeting gay and bisexual men (the Stop AIDS Project), and providing one-on-one education to Asian clients at drug rehabilitation programs. Much of the work at the Asian AIDS Project is subcontracted to community agencies in the various Asian ethnic groups.

Newcomer Health Services in San Francisco, which deals primarily with Southeast Asian refugees, includes an AIDS-specific educational session in its presentations in outreach to adult classes in English as a second language. This session is given by an English-speaking health educator aided by an interpreter. A one-page handout, available in Chinese, Vietnamese, Cambodian, and Laotian, is given to participants.

All the AIDS prevention programs described above are recent, and so their eventual effectiveness remains unknown. However, a few generalizations can be made about their intent. First, most of the education efforts, such as brochures, hotlines, presentations, and media publicity, are focused on information dissemination. The Stop AIDS Project of the Asian AIDS Project is the only program in which the clients interact actively during the education process. Most of the sources of information described above emphasize the fact that Asians are not protected from AIDS. At the same time, this message is carefully phrased to prevent hysteria. Second, most of the AIDS education programs targeting Asians are sensitive to the heterogeneity of the Asian community. Educational materials produced by AIDS Project Los Angeles, Asian AIDS Project, and Hawaii Department of Health Services are in several languages. However, some of the materials are merely translations of English versions, while others were developed specifically for a particular audience and tested via focus groups. Utilization of written educational material, however, assumes, perhaps falsely, that members of these communities are literate.

These AIDS prevention efforts have been predominantly ethnic specific. For instance, educational materials have been targeted at different ethnic communities. AIDS presentations given at the Asian AIDS Project, AIDS Project Los Angeles, and Asian Health Services in Oakland are all language and culture specific. At the Asian AIDS Project, educational activities have also targeted specific occupational groups, such as Asian attorneys, social workers, and substance abuse rehabilitation staff.

The third feature of current Asian AIDS education programs is that they deemphasize issues of sex and homosexuality. Most of the educational materials address but do not focus on specific unsafe sexual practices and homosexuality. The cultural inhibition around such topics may also be the reason printed materials are popular: Brochures and leaflets can be read in the privacy of one's home. It is not surprising, then, that public presentations at the Asian AIDS Project are not usually well attended unless organized for captive audiences such as schools, summer youth programs, and church congregations. Furthermore, many requests for presentations have been for single-sex audiences.

Fourth, except for the Stop AIDS Project of the Asian AIDS Project, the prevention programs are aimed primarily at the heterosexual Asian communities. It is likely that this is a result of the involvement of Asian health agencies, who have not historically provided services directly to the gay and lesbian community. At the same time, mainstream Asian agencies with services for the gay community have not initiated programs for Asian gays.

Finally, community organizing has been a key element in the development of the more comprehensive AIDS prevention programs targeting Asians. For example, the Asian communities in San Francisco and Los Angeles either have coalitions organized around the issue of AIDS or are active in advocating for services. In San Francisco, community coalitions include the Asian AIDS Task Force, the Gay Asian Pacific Alliance, the Pilipino AIDS Advisory Task Force, and the Japanese Community Youth Council AIDS Advisory Committee. The two coalitions active in Los Angeles are the Asian Pacific Planning Council and the Asian Pacific Lesbians and Gays. These community coalitions are seen as critical components of an effective prevention strategy that is beginning to change community and cultural norms about sexuality and homosexuality as well as increasing visible support for an individual's adoption of risk-reduction practices.

Conclusions

Health behavior change models can potentially assist us in developing AIDS education programs that are effective. However, the applicability of the three models discussed above to the Asian community differs due to the impact of the social and subjective norms of that community. In addition, the social and subjective norms are complicated by the diversity within the Asian community. The Asian community is not only ethnically diverse, but also includes different generations and varying psychological adaptations among heterosexual and gay members.

Of the three models, the health belief model probably has the most utility for the Asian community. In the context of this model, the dissemination of information that serves to raise the awareness that Asians are susceptible to AIDS is important. However, the model suggests that the intensity of this message should not be at such a level that it would cause hysteria. Overreaction to an AIDS prevention message is a real concern among Asian-Americans, given notions regarding etiology of contagious disease.

AIDS prevention brings into the forefront four topics that are difficult if not taboo for Asians to discuss in public: illness, death, sexuality, and homosexuality. Illness and death are taboo subjects because they are considered bad luck and, in societies where the self-fulfilling prophesy is a norm, there is a prevalent belief that discussion may bring on the condition or some other kind of misfortune.

Sexuality is not considered an appropriate topic for normal discussion, except in the company of married, same-sex individuals. Homosexuality is a highly charged topic because it involves both child and parents in a negative situation of unfulfilled duties and responsibilities. By implication, the homosexual child who does not have progeny is unfilial, and the parents have somehow failed in their role.

Recommendations

(1) Preventive interventions have to be framed in such a way that information can be disseminated without intensifying the discomfort around taboo issues. Otherwise, the discomfort may interfere with the comprehension of the critical messages. Consistent with this, written material, audiovisual presentations, and small, same-sex group discussion may be more effective than large group presentations.

(2) Ethnic-specific media may be a cost-effective vehicle for communication of AIDS education messages to a large audience in a nonthreatening manner.

(3) Delivering the message that Asians are susceptible to AIDS is an effective approach to engaging this population in responding to AIDS. How-

ever, this message should be at a level that elicits personal concern but not hysteria.

(4) Community organizing and education of local leadership are necessary to develop positive subjective norms within the various communities. This positive reinforcement may include an increased openness in discussing AIDS and the impact of AIDS on the community, the development of social support for people with AIDS and their families, increased individual responsibility for AIDS education and prevention, and reduced discrimination against gays, lesbians, or people with AIDS.

References

Abramson, P. R. (1986). The cultural context of Japanese sexuality. *Psychologia, 21*(1), 1–9.

Bandura, A. (1982). Self-efficacy mechanism in human agency. *American Psychologist, 37*, 122–147.

Bartholomew, C., Charles, W., Saxinger, C., Blattner, W., Robert-Guroff, M., Raju, C., Ratan, T., Ince, W., Quamina, D., Basbeo-Maharaj, K., & Gallo, R. C. (1985). Racial and other characteristics of human T-cell leukemia/lymphoma (HTLV-I) and AIDS (HTLV-III) in Trinidad. *British Medical Journal: Clinical Research, 290*, 1243–1246.

Becker, M. (Ed.). (1974). *The health belief model and personal health behavior.* Thorofare, NJ: Charles B. Slack.

Centers for Disease Control. (1989). *AIDS weekly surveillance report, United States AIDS Activity.* Atlanta: Author.

Coleman, S. (1983). *Family planning in Japanese society.* Princeton, NJ: Princeton University Press.

DeVos, G., & Wagatsuma, H. (1966). *Japan's invisible race: Caste in culture and personality.* Berkeley: University of California Press.

Hart, D. V. (1968) Homosexuality and transvestism in the Philippines: The Cebuan Pilipino Bayot and Likin-on. *Behavior Science Notes, HRAFO Bulletin, 3*, 211–248.

Iguchi, M. Y., Aoki, B., Ngin, P., & Ja, D. (1988). *AIDS prevalence in U.S. Asian and Pacific Islander populations.* Manuscript submitted for publication.

Jacobs, R. (1987). A model for AIDS prevention. *Focus: A Guide to AIDS Research, 2*, 2–3.

Jue, S. (1987). Identifying and meeting the needs of minority clients with AIDS. In National Association of Social Workers, *Responding to AIDS: Psychosocial initiatives.* Silver Springs, MD: National Association of Social Workers, Inc.

Kalish, R., & Reynolds, D. K. (1981). *Death and ethnicity: A psychological study.* Farmington, NY: Baywood.

Kitano, K. J. (1988). *Correlates of AIDS-associated high-risk behavior among Chinese and Pilipino gay men.* Unpublished master's thesis, University of California, Berkeley.

Koo, L. C. (1982). *Nourishment of life: Health in Chinese society.* Hong Kong: Commercial Press.

Ohnuki-Tierney, E. (1984). *Illness and culture in contemporary Japan.* Cambridge: Cambridge University Press.

San Francisco Department of Public Health. (1988, March 15). *AIDS in San Francisco: Status report for fiscal year 1987–88 and projections of service needs and costs for 1988–93.* San Francisco: Author.

San Francisco Department of Public Health. (1989). *AIDS monthly surveillance report: Summary of cases meeting the CDC surveillance definition in San Francisco* (cases reported through 1/2/89). San Francisco: Author.

Sechrest, L. (1969). Philippine culture, stress and psychopathology. In W. Caudill & T. Lin (Eds.), *Mental health research in Asia and the Pacific.* Honolulu: East-West Center Press.

Sechrest, L., & Flores, L. (1969). Homosexuality in the Philippines and in the United States: The handwriting on the wall. *Journal of Social Psychiatry, 79,* 3–12.

Sue, S. (1977) Psychological theory and implications for Asian Americans. *Personnel and Guidance Journal, 55,* 381–389.

Winkelstein, W., & Samuel, M. (1987). Prevalence of human immunodeficiency virus infection in ethnic minority homosexual/bisexual men. *Journal of the American Medical Association, 257,* 1901.

Yim, M., Hayashi, T., Yanagihara, E., Kardin, M., & Nakamura, J. (1986). HTLV-I-associated T-cell leukemia in Hawaii. *American Journal of Medical Science, 292,* 325–327.

18

Women and HIV Infection: Issues in Prevention and Behavior Change

Susan D. Cochran

The prevention of human immunodeficiency viral infection in women, and, by extension, the prevention of AIDS and AIDS-related disease in women and their offspring, present psychologists with a difficult challenge. Although HIV is a biological, and not a social, entity, its transmission from one person to another, for the most part, occurs within the social context of interpersonal relationships. For women at risk of contracting HIV, these relationships are most likely to be with men, whether the men are sexual partners or fellow IV drug users (Friedland & Klein, 1987; Guinan & Hardy, 1987). For HIV-infected women at risk for transmitting the virus, these relationships are again with men and also with their own unborn children. In order to understand the intimate behavioral choices of women related to HIV prevention, we need to be cognizant of the complicated social context in which their decisions for behavior change are made.

This chapter focuses on two very disparate populations of women: those currently most at risk for HIV (poor, urban, Black and Hispanic/Latina women) and those who are potentially at risk for HIV infection should the virus become more prevalent throughout the population (sexually active young adult women from the middle class). In doing so, the chapter limits itself primarily to issues of sexual transmission.

Author's Note: This work was supported in part by an award from the National Institute of Mental Health (Grant 1 R01 MH 42584–01) and a California State University, Northridge, Foundation Grant. Correspondence should be addressed to Dr. Susan Cochran, Department of Psychology, California State University, Northridge, CA 91330.

Patterns of HIV Infection in Women

A first step in understanding women and HIV infection is an examination of the epidemiologic patterns of current AIDS cases. To date, nearly 91% of reported AIDS cases have occurred in males and only 9.2% in females (Centers for Disease Control, 1989). The proportion of female to male cases has stayed fairly stable over time, hovering around 7% of total AIDS cases (Guinan & Hardy, 1987), although more recent statistics suggest that an increasingly higher percentage of AIDS cases reported involve women. In 1988, women accounted for nearly 11% of newly reported cases (Centers for Disease Control, 1989).

AIDS in women presents a markedly different picture from that observed epidemiologically in men (Centers for Disease Control, 1987). Among men, the major transmission vector involves same-sex sexual behaviors, or homosexual contact. Of reported cases in men over the age of 13 years, 76% are classified by the CDC as occurring in homosexual or bisexual men. A second major route of transmission involves the sharing of drug paraphernalia in conjunction with intravenous drug use, acting as a primary or secondary risk factor in 25% of adult male cases. Only 24% of total adult male cases involve exclusively heterosexual men. Heterosexual sexual contact as a transmission vector accounts for merely 2% of reported cases.

In contrast, for women, AIDS is almost exclusively a disease of heterosexuals. To date, only one possible case of female-to-female sexual transmission in the United States has been documented (Marmor et al., 1986). Of the first 2,200 U.S. AIDS cases in women diagnosed since 1981, only 46 women (less than 1%) acknowledged sexual contact with other women (Kahn, 1987); 78% of these lesbian and bisexual women were IV drug users.

It appears that the major incursion of HIV into the female population has occurred within a subpopulation of individuals directly or indirectly involved with IV drug use (Guinan & Hardy, 1987). Nearly half of the women with AIDS are present or former IV drug users. In addition, between 1981 and 1986, two-thirds of women who contracted AIDS through heterosexual intercourse did so by having sex with an IV drug user (Guinan & Hardy, 1987).

Women can infect others with HIV through similar routes of sharing IV drug paraphernalia or sexual contact, although for the latter, the relative transmission efficacy between men and women during heterosexual intercourse is still being debated (Curran et al., 1988). Additionally, HIV can be transmitted from mother to child during pregnancy, possibly at childbirth, and immediately postpartum through breast milk (Curran et al., 1988).

The well-noted overrepresentation of Blacks and Hispanics among AIDS cases is even more pronounced for women than it is for men (Bakeman, McCray, Lumb, Jackson, & Whitley, 1987; Cochran, Mays, & Roberts, 1988; Mays & Cochran, 1987, 1988). The reasons for this reflect both behavioral differences among ethnic groups and the differential prevalence of HIV within some poor, urban, Black and Hispanic populations (Cochran & Mays, 1988; Mays & Cochran, 1987, 1988, 1989b; Worth & Rodriguez, 1987).

When we think about primary prevention, ethnic differences in patterns of infection have another important implication. White women are more likely than ethnic women to have contracted HIV through blood transfusions, a medical procedure occurring more typically among older women who are beyond their prime childbearing years. As a result of this, 34% of White women with AIDS are over 39 years old, in contrast to 17% of Black women and 16% of Hispanic women. Thus HIV seropositive ethnic minority women are more likely than similarly infected White women to risk transmitting HIV to their offspring. Reflecting this, most infants with AIDS are born to Black (57%) or Hispanic (23%) women.

Friedland and Klein (1987) have underscored the point that HIV is not an efficient virus. In most instances it takes frequent and sufficient contact with HIV for infection to occur. In certain subpopulations, such as hemophiliacs, high rates of infection happened quickly because of repeated and substantial contact with HIV in contaminated blood products (Mason, Olson, & Parish, 1988).

For women from the lower socioeconomic strata of the Black community and certain segments of the Hispanic community, there are behaviors that also facilitate a relatively more efficient transmission of the virus. Some of these are quite proximal to transmission, for example, high levels of intravenous drug use with sharing of drug paraphernalia. Some are more distal and socioculturally based. These include engaging in behaviors where HIV is more likely to be present, instability of relationships, little or no prenatal care, health problems, unemployment and underemployment, and poverty (Amaro, 1989; Mays & Cochran, 1988, 1989b; Richardson, 1988). Given the inefficient nature of the virus, these sociocultural factors assume more importance as mediators of HIV transmission.

With this as a backdrop, we can now turn to some of the issues that arise when developing HIV primary prevention strategies for higher-risk women. These issues include women's perceptions of HIV risk, cultural differences in the meanings of sexual behavior, the role of sexual behavior in women's lives, and economic barriers to prevention efforts.

Prevention Issues in Black Women

One focus is on the specific issues that affect Black women from the lower socioeconomic strata. These women occupy a behavioral location within society that places them in particularly close proximity to HIV infection. Studies of IV drug use show significantly higher prevalence of IV drug addiction within the Black community when compared to the White community (Gary & Berry, 1985). As a result, Black women may be more likely than White women to be IV drug users and, even if not users themselves, more likely to be sexually involved with individuals who are. In addition, 9% of Black women with AIDS in the United States were born in areas of central, eastern, or southern Africa or specific Caribbean countries, geographic regions where HIV infection is thought to be primarily transmitted through heterosexual contact (Centers for Disease Control, 1989). Virtually none of the White or Hispanic women with AIDS was born in these regions.

Perceptions of AIDS Risk

In assessing AIDS-related risk-reduction behaviors, it is important to examine perceived risk as a context for understanding behavior change (Mays & Cochran, 1989b). Without the perception of risk, women may not be motivated to alter sexual practices, and even with the perception of risk, should this risk perception be inaccurate, they may change their behavior, but not effectively. Unsafe sexual behavior will not be perceived as risky if (a) women are unaware of the relation between behavior and level of risk, (b) women are aware but devalue the risk to the group (e.g., Black women as opposed to White women), or (c) women are aware of risk to the group but devalue the extent of personal risk (Weinstein, 1987).

With the onset of the AIDS epidemic, Blacks initially perceived the problem, as did many in this country, as primarily a concern of White gay men (Mays & Cochran, 1987). Indeed, in 1986–87, when Blacks were already overrepresented among reported AIDS cases, a survey of Black women attending college revealed that they inaccurately perceived Whites as significantly more at risk for AIDS than Blacks (Mays & Cochran, 1989c). Sampling from this same Black population one year later showed a significant change in their perceptions of risk, so that they now more accurately perceived the risk of AIDS to Blacks, but still only 6% always insisted that their sexual partners use condoms during sexual intercourse (Mays & Cochran, 1989c). These young Black women represent one of the most highly educated segments of the Black population, and we do not know if similar changes in risk perception have occurred among other Black women.

Understanding poor Black women's responses to AIDS entails both knowledge of their perceptions of its relative riskiness in comparison to more immediate day-to-day threats and the existence of resources available for them to behave differently. Pressing survival needs, family demands, and sheer fatigue from the burden of economic pressures plague many poor individuals and compete for some of these women's attention. Life circumstances may also lead them to view risks differently from middle-class or White women. For example, in the case of possible perinatal transmission by HIV-positive women, advice to avoid pregnancy or seek abortion in the event pregnancy occurs may seem straightforward, but it overlooks other realities in these women's lives. Children and motherhood are highly valued in the Black community, giving some women a path by which to achieve or a way to hold onto a tenuous relationship (Mays & Cochran, 1988). Also, Black women are 2.25 times more likely than White women to have prenatal care only in the third trimester or not at all (U.S. Department of Health and Human Services, 1986), thereby negating abortion as an option.

Cultural Differences in the Meaning of Sexual Behavior

As scientists, we know very little empirically about the inner processes of sexual behavior among poor Black Americans. Many of our data on the sexual behavior of Black women focus on specific sexual behavior outcomes, such as pregnancy rates or incidence and prevalence of sexually transmitted diseases, or markers of sexual activity, such as age at first sexual intercourse or choice of contraceptive method. These data show clearly that differences between Blacks and other ethnic groups, including Whites, do exist (Wyatt, Peters, & Guthrie, in press).

Black adults are more likely than Whites to be unmarried and therefore presumably experience greater instability in their love relationships (Mays & Cochran, 1988, 1989b). Also, Black adolescents are more likely than Whites to begin sexual intercourse at an earlier age, although in adolescence they may have less frequent sexual intercourse and fewer partners than White adolescents (Farley & Allen, 1987; Flick, 1986; Gibbs, 1986; Hofferth, Kahn, & Baldwin, 1987; Wyatt, in press). Inner-city Black adolescent females have more negative attitudes toward contraception, make less effective use of contraceptives, and more positively value fertility than White females (Gibbs, 1986). Black women are less likely than White women to have their partners use condoms for contraceptive purposes (Farley & Allen, 1987). In 1982, less than 8% of married Black women between the ages of 15 and 44 relied on condoms for contraceptive purposes (Farley & Allen, 1987).

Overall, in the poorer Black community there may be a greater likelihood of sexual activities for survival or in exchange or barter for needed resources (Mays & Cochran, 1988, 1989b). These behavioral differences in Black women result from sociocultural and economic differences between the Black community and White America. Interventions aimed at altering patterns of sexual behavior among Black women will not be effective if they ignore these differences. Effective HIV prevention programs may require long-term interventions aimed at solving many of the ills of poverty, illiteracy, and inadequate or ineffective government assistance programs that fail in achieving their goals.

Weinstein (1987) describes three possible functions of sexual behavior: procreation, recreation, and an expression of emotional connectedness. However, there are other possible components to sexuality that may assume greater importance in economically deprived communities. One additional component to sexuality is the notion of sexual behavior as survival. Women who work in the sex industry understand this function of sexual behavior (Alexander, 1987). But women do not need to be paid for sex directly to reap economic or social status benefits from sexual involvements with men. In an economically impoverished community, sexual attractiveness is an important resource for Black women, 65% of whom over the age of 15 years are not married (compared to 43% of White women) (U.S. Bureau of the Census, 1983). Sexual involvement may significantly improve a woman's economic position (Mays & Cochran, 1989a, 1989b). For a woman to insist that her sexual partner use condoms when other readily available partners may not could destroy her hold on a developing relationship. Indeed, an insistence on premarital celibacy may seriously undermine a poor woman's ability to transform a new dating relationship into a serious, committed one, as sexuality may be an important component in generating attachment to her partner.

Other functions of sexual behavior are sex as power or as an expression of oneself in the world, or self-procreation. For some living in impoverished segments of the Black community, feelings of powerlessness and efforts to overcome the negative effects of lower status are intimately woven into the ways in which men and women express their sexuality (Harrison, 1977; Wilkeson, Poussaint, Small, & Shapiro, 1983). For example, among young Black adolescent females, sexual activity is sometimes a method for achieving a desired traditional female adult role (Gibbs, 1986). Underemployed or unemployed teenagers and adults who are coping with the inequalities of society while seeking a sense of belonging, creativity, or achievement may find sexuality to be a way to demonstrate womanhood and independence through having children and being sexually experienced (Wilson, 1986).

Viewing sexual behavior as a statement of self-identity is not new in the fight against AIDS. Many risk-reduction interventions directed at the gay male community seek to meld individuals' needs for self-expression with the practice of safer sex (Shilts, 1987). There are similar issues for Black women. In developing prevention strategies, psychologists can use these issues to reach Black women more effectively. Risk-reduction interventions that help adolescent Black females to develop achievable life plans first and then fit the issues of sexuality and risk reduction into that schema may be more effective than interventions that focus simply on sexual behavior (Gibbs, 1986). Research suggests that adolescent females who are better contraceptors and, one might assume, would be quicker to change their behavior to reduce HIV risk are those who view unwanted pregnancy from sexual activity as interfering with life plans and who feel more confident and responsible in handling contraceptive tasks (Flick, 1986; Levinson, 1986). Programs aimed at preventing unplanned adolescent pregnancies recognize that sexual activity occurs within a social context and that interventions need to be more broadly focused than simply providing sex education (Quinn, 1986).

Male-Female Relationships

Although it appears that Blacks hold the same ideals for marriage and family relationships as Whites, in practice the sex-ratio imbalance among Black heterosexuals has influenced the development of alternative forms of male-female relationships (Tucker & Mitchell-Kernan, in press). *Sex-ratio imbalance* refers to differences between the genders in number of eligible partners with whom to establish a relationship. Among Blacks, there are far fewer eligible males than available females. The effect of this is greater instability of relationships and higher rates of sexual activity outside of marriage (Tucker & Mitchell-Kernan, in press). At a psychological level, the overrepresented gender, in this case women, experiences options in choosing mates as limited and may be more likely to tolerate objectionable behavior. The underrepresented gender, men, may view options as limitless, resulting in less pressure to develop commitments, greater power within relationships, and fewer behavioral controls (Tucker & Mitchell-Kernan, in press). Sex-ratio imbalance, coupled with the economic realities of poverty that encourage individuals to seek relationship partners who can provide financial support (Scott, 1980), creates an environment in which friendship-based models of close relationships may not work (Mays & Cochran, 1989b).

This has important implications for development of preventive intervention models with Black women. Interventions that emphasize egalitarian negotiation, as among best friends, will fail to address the often divergent goals of relationship partners. Let me give you an example of this:

> A working-class Black woman in her late 30s whom I was seeing in treatment began a dating relationship with a Black man in his early 50s. As a single mother with many pressing financial debts, she currently views her relationships with men as falling into one of two camps. The first is a romantic, idealized relationship where she is sexually and emotionally attracted to the man and seeks permanency of the relationship for these emotional reasons. The second type of relationship, more commonly experienced by her, is simply pragmatic. In the latter relationship, she generally is not especially attracted to the man himself but feels that he will spend money on her, perhaps give her money to spend on herself, or provide assistance in raising her young daughter. Her desires for financial support include help in paying for extensive car repairs, long-standing charge card debts, and the monthly rent on her apartment. These are in addition to expenses associated with dating, such as dinners out and movies.
>
> Over the last 8 months she has had several brief relationships of mostly the pragmatic kind and is grateful when her partner suggests using a condom, although often he will do so in a way that makes her feel accused of being diseased or someone he does not care about very much. Her interests in condom use are more for contraception than HIV prevention, although she acknowledges that it is probably good to prevent catching something she doesn't need to be bothered with. But she does not insist on condom use for two reasons: She feels it is the man's responsibility, and she is concerned that he may have a negative reaction if she suggests using condoms. From her perspective, there is

no possibility that she is HIV infected; her only concern is that the romantically exciting men she dates are infected.

Her relationship with this new man fell into the second category of pragmatic dating. She very quickly reassured herself that he was not HIV infected by bringing up the general topic of homosexuality and watching his reaction to it. He passed; he displayed no interest either way, saying whatever those people do is their own business. His strategy with her was also indirect, though more awkward. Soon after they began going out he handed her a letter. In the letter, he brought up the issue of AIDS and sexual histories, and closed by citing C. E. Koop's advice that it never hurts to ask. The letter itself was fairly inarticulate and angered her because it demonstrated his ineptitude in dating. She told him if he wanted to use a condom then he should, much to his apparent relief.

The story, however, does not end there. After a couple of months of getting to know her better as a person, he decided that she was safe and asked to have unprotected intercourse. At the time, she was coming to see that his financial help was going to be more tenuous than she had hoped for, while his demands on her for emotional support were more than she wanted to give. She refused in punishment for his earlier letter. Thus, for the time being, at least, these two individuals continue to practice safer sex, although not for reasons motivated by prevention concerns.

This situation illustrates very clearly the difficulties of primary prevention for some Black women. First, the woman in this situation does not perceive herself to be at great risk for HIV. She views AIDS as a result of immorality rather than sexual behavior and as a problem for certain isolated segments of the community—a not uncommon view of sexually transmitted diseases (Brandt, 1987). Second, her decisions surrounding behavioral choices are primarily motivated by the immediacy of her current life concerns. For some individuals, prevention behaviors can be a luxury to be afforded only if they do not conflict with other primary needs. Third, some may not have the behavioral repertoires to "negotiate" safer sex with words, written or spoken. Social norms, however, that dictate safer sex could spare individuals from such difficulties, something that is becoming more apparent from research on gay male sexual behavior change (Becker & Joseph, 1988). Fourth, prevention behaviors can serve many utilities within interpersonal relationships, including in this instance an expression of her dissatisfaction with her dating partner. And fifth, actions in one situation may influence future inclinations to engage in primary prevention. Behavioral principles predict that punishing a behavior decreases the likelihood that it will recur. In this example, one is left to contemplate what this man will do with his next sexual partner. The odds are slim that he will write another letter and face the wrath of his partner. He may also choose not to talk about safer sex to avoid committing himself to perpetual condom use if he changes his mind later in the dating relationship. Prevention efforts that are driven by an understanding of the inner motivations and decision-making trees of individuals are likely to be the most effective in predicting, in the short term, HIV risk-reduction behaviors.

Prevention Issues in Hispanic/Latina Women

Shifting focus now to poor, urban Hispanic/Latina women in inner cities, we find that there is even less known about their sexual lives and concerns about AIDS. An especially important issue in developing prevention programs is the diversity of this ethnic minority group. Although in the epidemiology of AIDS, all Hispanics are treated alike, in reality, several distinct subpopulations exist, including those with ties to Mexico, other Central and South American countries, Puerto Rico, and Cuba (Amaro, 1989). Parenthetically, this is also true for women from other ethnic minority groups classified by the Centers for Disease Control. Differences among the various Hispanic subpopulations exist, particularly for expressions of intimate sexual behaviors. This makes the process of developing AIDS prevention programs that are culturally appropriate much more complicated than simply the translation of an English-language intervention directly into the Spanish language. Ideally, multiple indigenously generated strategies will be developed, since no one approach can be expected to transcend the cultural diversity of the Hispanic population.

In addition, when we think in terms of behavioral locations of individuals in relationship to HIV, some Latina women, such as poor Puerto Rican women in New York City, are closer behaviorally to HIV (Worth & Rodriguez, 1987) than women from some other Hispanic subpopulations. Values and attitudes toward sexual behavior and the ability to enact risk-reduction activities may be influenced by recency of immigration and economic resources. For example, when there is little privacy due to a high density of individuals within a household, preplanning safe sexual behavior may be difficult. Instead, sexual activity may be more likely to occur spontaneously, when privacy unexpectedly develops.

The next sections very briefly discuss some relevant issues for Hispanic/Latina women. In doing so, differences among subcultures are not addressed. Instead the focus is at the level of general cultural values. For any individual, some of these issues may be more or less important and subtly influenced by her specific cultural background.

Cultural Differences in the Meaning of Sexual Behavior

Traditionally, sexual behavior in Hispanic culture has occurred within a system of *machismo* for men and *marianismo* (Burgos & Perez, 1986; Pavich, 1986; Wilkeson et al., 1983). Men were expected to be sexually experienced. In contrast, women were to be naive and virginal until marriage. Single women were to be sexually attractive, but chaste. As an example, in Mexico this emphasis on chastity before marriage has resulted in possibly higher rates of heterosexual anal intercourse in order to preserve vaginal virginity and homosexual behavior in heterosexual males (Carrier, 1985, 1989). It is unknown to what extent this also occurs in the United States. For women, also, there may be little training in body knowledge. Indications that this lack of emphasis on sex education possibly still continues emerge from several studies drawn from samples in diverse geographic locations (Davis & Harris, 1982; Moore & Erickson, 1985; Padilla & Grady, 1987).

In this cultural context, where traditionally women are not educated about sexuality, public, detailed AIDS education can clash with community values. Other issues are also problematic, including advocating the use of condoms, which conflicts with both the teachings of the Catholic church and cultural reticence in discussing openly such intimate matters. Indeed, three San Francisco studies that directly assessed knowledge of HIV transmission found important misconceptions among some Hispanic participants (DiClemente, Boyer, & Morales, 1988; Fairbank, Bregman, & Maullin, Inc., 1987; Marin, Marin, & Juarez, 1987).

Male-Female Relationships

The organization of male-female relationships may also complicate preventive approaches. For women, *respeto*, or respect for authority including one's husband or boyfriend, and sexual modesty mean adopting a role in which fulfilling male needs is paramount (Burgos & Perez, 1986; Poma, 1987; Wilkeson et al., 1983). Asking a partner to use condoms, when women are expected to be sexually inexperienced and obedient to male desires, may stigmatize a woman as "loose" (Mantell, Schinke, & Akabas, 1988). Within some traditional Latin cultures, authorization for use of contraceptives lies with the husband, of whom approximately 25% oppose any form of birth control (Poma, 1987). Similarly, public health messages requesting women to discuss sexual practices with their sexual partners do so in ignorance of cultural norms governing sexual behavior.

From this perspective, expecting some segments of Hispanic women to carry the burden of encouraging men to practice safer sex may be somewhat unrealistic. Our prevention strategies must work within existing cultural, sex-role, and class norms.

Prevention Issues in Young Adult Women

At present, young, sexually active single women from the middle class do not appear to be at high risk for HIV infection, although the history of sexually transmitted diseases (STDs) suggests that when there is no means of secondary prevention (i.e., curative treatments), as is the current situation with AIDS, lifetime prevalence rates of STDs can reach very high levels in the absence of effective primary prevention (Brandt, 1987). There are several reasons to concern ourselves with this population.

First, teenagers and young adults represent a segment of the population already involved in high rates of sexual behavior outside of long-term monogamous relationships (Chilman, 1979; Holmes, 1981) and are more likely to be experimenting with drug use. Although at present the onset of AIDS is most common between the ages of 25 and 40 years, incidence rates of other STDs indicate that young adults under the age of 25 already practice behaviors that will increase their risk for contracting HIV should the virus become widely distributed within the population.

Second, prevention of HIV infection in this population of young women will dramatically prevent high rates of perinatal transmission because these women are in their prime childbearing years.

And third, young, middle-class, sexually active adults are fairly easy to study. The development of effective HIV prevention methodology is going to require a multitude of studies. Using relatively inexpensive and readily accessible populations will facilitate these research efforts. However, in doing so, we need to be cognizant that the most common research population, college students, may not represent the highest-risk individuals even within their own age cohort.

What are the prevention issues for young sexually active women? This chapter will focus on three: Do young sexually active women know about AIDS and perceive themselves to be at risk for HIV?

Have this knowledge and perceived risk been translated into behavior change? Is this behavior change likely to be effective in reducing their HIV risk?

Recent research has documented deficiencies in adolescents' knowledge and beliefs about AIDS (Baldwin & Baldwin, 1988; Carroll, 1988; DiClemente, Zorn, & Temoshok, 1986; DiClemente et al., 1988; Price, Desmond, & Kukulka, 1985). In our own work in Southern California, we have found that most women students know that sexual activity is one means of getting AIDS and that using condoms reduces risk (Cochran, 1988; Mays & Cochran, 1989c). However, 9% of approximately 350 college women polled in 1987 believed that one can get AIDS from toilet seats; 16% believed that one can get AIDS by sharing food, drink, or eating utensils with an HIV-infected individual.

In the winter of 1986 and the fall of 1987, my students and I collected questionnaires covering sexual behavior and AIDS-related concerns from large samples of undergraduates. By a frequency matching procedure, we then generated samples from both time points matched for gender, age, ethnicity, and religion (Cochran, Keidan, & Kalechstein, 1989). At both time points, subjects were asked how much they worry about getting AIDS. Men and women did not differ in their levels of worry, but worry about AIDS has increased significantly over time. Subjects were also asked what was the probability that they would contract an HIV infection during their lifetimes. At both points in time, women rated their odds of getting AIDS as significantly higher than the odds that men gave themselves. There were also significant differences across time, with subjects rating themselves as more vulnerable in fall 1987 as opposed to 20 months earlier. These findings underscore the changing face of AIDS. Today, college undergraduates are probably much more concerned about AIDS than they were even three years ago.

The next question, however, is, Do these cognitive factors of worry and perceived risk translate into behavior change? I attempted to address that question in a study exploring both rational and irrational predictors of behavior change (Cochran & Peplau, 1989). From the health belief model (Becker & Maiman, 1975), it was postulated that perceptions of being at risk for STDs, including AIDS and herpes, and sexual behavior experiences, such as number of lifetime partners, sexual practices, and previous treatment for an STD, cause individuals to practice safer sex if they are cued to action through worry about contracting an STD. Recognizing, also, that AIDS, in the minds of many, is intimately linked to homosexuality (Langone, 1985; Pleck,

322   Susan D. Cochran

O'Donnell, O'Donnell, & Snarey, 1986), a stigmatized social status, it was predicted that homophobia might cause individuals heightened worry about contracting AIDS, thus leading to risk reduction.

Using structural equation modeling, this model was fit for male and female subjects, separately, predicting that perceptions of being at risk, sexual experiences, and homophobia "cause" levels of worry about contracting STDs, which then "cause" risk reduction. Since the data were correlational, assumptions of causality are for heuristic purposes only. Results of this analysis indicated that, for both men and women, worry does predict number of risk-reduction behaviors enacted. However, predictors of worry differ somewhat between the two genders. For men, sexual behavior experiences are unrelated to worry; only perceptions of being at risk and homophobia predict worry. For women, in contrast, sexual behavior significantly predicts worry and perception of being at risk shows a trend to predict worry, but homophobia is unrelated to levels of worry. These results suggest that different factors may facilitate risk reduction for men and women. This has clear implications for designing preventive interventions: We will need to tailor these interventions to the separate concerns of young men and women. For women, highlighting relationships between behavioral experiences and risk may prove to be effective in producing behavior change.

This study, however, does not address the question of what it is that young women are doing to reduce their risk of getting AIDS. Using data from matched samples, my students and I compared risk-reduction strategies used by women in 1986 with those strategies used in 1987 (Cochran et al., 1989). Women were asked whether or not they were using seven different strategies for reducing their AIDS risk: waiting longer to have sex, limiting number of partners, avoiding anal sex, talking to new partners about risk factors, insisting on condom use, avoiding oral sex, and practicing celibacy. The two most preferred strategies at both points in time were waiting longer and limiting their number of sexual partners. These were endorsed by 36% to 47% of the women, depending on the question and when we asked it. In 1987, women were significantly more likely to use three additional strategies (avoiding anal sex, talking to new partners, and insisting on condoms) to reduce their AIDS risk. Even though the insistence on condom use jumped dramatically from 10% to 25% of women polled, clearly many women have yet to adopt this risk-reduction strategy.

The final issue is whether or not these risk-reduction strategies are likely to be effective. One of the most interpersonal of strategies that women are increasingly more likely to use is talking to their partners about risk factors for AIDS. For this strategy to be effective, one has to make two very interesting assumptions. The first is that people do not lie. And, since obviously that is not correct, the second is that one will know when one is being lied to.

In the 1987 questionnaire, this issue of lying in the negotiation of safer sex was directly addressed (Cochran, 1988; Cochran & Mays, 1989a). We first asked our sample to what extent they thought that men and women will lie when asked about their risk factors for AIDS. There was remarkable agreement between men and women. Both agreed that men will lie significantly more than women will. But this may simply reflect stereotypes that people have of men's and women's behavior.

We next asked subjects if they had ever lied to someone in order to have sex. Men were significantly more likely than women to admit to having told a lie (35% versus 10%); 38% of men reported that they had lied about having ejaculatory control when they did not, and 14% of women admitted that they had lied when asked by their partners about contraception and the likelihood of pregnancy. In addition, men were significantly more likely than women to report that (a) they had told a potential partner that they cared more for her than they really did, (b) they had been sexually involved with more than one person at a time, and (c) they had used a dating tactic of cutting dates short and acting hurt, disappointed, or disinterested when a potential partner was reluctant to have sex. When we asked subjects about their dating experiences of being lied to by partners, we found, again, that the experience of partner dishonesty was quite prevalent.

Finally, we gave subjects several scenarios in which they were asked to tell us what they would do in a hypothetical situation. In all of the scenarios, honesty threatened the opportunity either to have sex or to maintain a desired relationship. For example, in one scenario, subjects, in this case men, were told that they had "met a girl who is really hot. But she is worried about AIDS. You're pretty certain that you haven't been exposed to AIDS . . . because all of your previous partners seem okay and you're healthy. She asks you if you have had the AIDS test. You know if you say no she won't have sex with you unless you wear a condom and you don't have one with you." A total of 20% of the men said that they would lie and say that they had had the test and tested negative. Only 4% of women reported that they would tell this lie. In general, a sizable percentage of both genders indicated that they would not be honest, although men tended to be less willing to be honest than women.

This study demonstrates very clearly that the strategy of asking one's

324   Susan D. Cochran

partner about AIDS risk factors is itself a risky technique, particularly for women, since it appears that men will more frequently be dishonest. But this is a strategy that is often suggested in risk-reduction advice and is increasingly being used by young women. Obviously, in our preventive interventions we need to distinguish between the goal of increasing communication between sex partners to facilitate implementation of safer sex practices and using information gained during this process to circumvent the consistent practice of safer sex.

Conclusions

The history of society's response to the problem of sexually transmitted diseases is colored by our social construction of these diseases (Brandt, 1987). So, for example, we see individuals as acquiring STDs through volitional behavior of somewhat immoral motivation. It is also fairly easy, given women's traditional role in society, to view the issue of women and AIDS as primarily a problem of women as potential "infection vectors" of men and children, rather than as individuals who themselves are affected by this disease (Mays & Cochran, 1989a).

In these few pages, I have tried to highlight the social context for AIDS within the lives of two disparate populations of women: those at highest risk and those who will be at risk should HIV's prevalence increase throughout the population. In developing prevention strategies for women, we need to be sensitive to the influence of sexual dynamics, class and economic factors, the interpersonal nature of AIDS-related transactions, and the potential interpersonal costs for women in sexual risk reduction. Unlike contraception, where women can act independently of men to some extent, women-generated AIDS sexual risk reduction frequently requires women to influence the behaviors of men.

References

Alexander, P. (1987). Prostitutes are being scapegoated for heterosexual AIDS. In F. Delacoste & P. Alexander (Eds.), *Sex work: Writings by women in the sex industry* (pp. 248–263). Pittsburgh, PA: Cleis.
Amaro, H. (1989). Considerations for prevention of HIV infection among Hispanic women. *Psychology of Women Quarterly, 12,* 429–444.
Bakeman, R., McCray, E., Lumb, J. R., Jackson, R. E., & Whitley, P. N. (1987). The incidence of AIDS among Blacks and Hispanics. *Journal of the National Medical Association, 79,* 921–928.

Baldwin, J. D., & Baldwin, J. I. (1988). Factors affecting AIDS-related sexual risk-taking behavior among college students. *Journal of Sex Research, 25,* 181–196.

Becker, M. H., & Joseph, J. G. (1988). AIDS and behavioral change to reduce risk: A review. *American Journal of Public Health, 78,* 394–410.

Becker, M. H., & Maiman, L. A. (1975). Sociobehavioral determinants of compliance with health and medical care recommendations. *Medical Care, 13,* 10–24.

Brandt, A. M. (1987). *No magic bullet: A social history of venereal disease in the United States since 1880.* New York: Oxford University Press.

Burgos, N. M., & Perez, Y.I.D. (1986). An exploration of human sexuality in the Puerto Rican culture. *Journal of Social Work and Human Sexuality, 4,* 135–150.

Carrier, J. M. (1985). Mexican male bisexuality. In F. Klein & T. Wolf (Eds.), *Bisexualities: Theory and research* (pp. 75–85). New York: Haworth.

Carrier, J. M. (1989). Sexual behavior and the spread of AIDS in Mexico. *Medical Anthropology, 10,* 129–142.

Carroll, L. (1988). Concern with AIDS and the sexual behavior of college students. *Journal of Marriage and the Family, 50,* 405–411.

Centers for Disease Control. (1987). Human immunodeficiency virus infection in the United States: A review of current knowledge. *Morbidity and Mortality Weekly Report, 36*(Suppl. S-6), 1–48.

Centers for Disease Control. (1989, January 2). *Acquired immunodeficiency syndrome (AIDS) weekly surveillance report, United States AIDS activity.* Atlanta: Author.

Chilman, C. S. (1979). *Adolescent sexuality in a changing American society* (DHEW Publication No. NIH 79–1426). Washington, DC: Government Printing Office.

Cochran, S. D. (1988, August). *Risky behavior and disclosure: Is it safe if you ask?* Paper presented at the annual meetings of the American Psychological Association, Atlanta.

Cochran, S. D., Keidan, J., & Kalechstein, A. (1989). *Changes in AIDS-related beliefs and behaviors among young adults.* Manuscript submitted for publication.

Cochran, S. D., & Mays, V. M. (1988) Epidemiologic and sociocultural factors in the transmission of HIV infection in Black gay and bisexual men. In M. Shernoff & W. A. Scott (Eds.), *A sourcebook of gay/lesbian health care* (2nd ed., pp. 202–211). Washington, DC: National Gay and Lesbian Health Foundation.

Cochran, S. D., & Mays, V. M. (1989a). *AIDS-related sexual behavior and disclosure: Is it safe if you ask?* Unpublished manuscript.

Cochran, S. D., & Mays, V. M. (1989b). Women and AIDS-related concerns: Roles for psychologists in helping the worried well. *American Psychologist, 44,* 529–535.

Cochran, S. D., Mays, V. M., & Roberts, V. (1988). Ethnic minorities and AIDS. In A. Lewis (Ed.), *Nursing care of the person with AIDS/ARC* (pp. 17–24). Rockville, MD: Aspen.

Cochran, S. D., & Peplau, L. A. (1989). *Sexual risk reduction behaviors in sexually active heterosexual young adults.* Manuscript submitted for publication.

Curran, J. W., Jaffe, H. W., Hardy, A. M., Morgan, W. M., Selik, R. M., & Dondero, T. J. (1988). Epidemiology of HIV infection and AIDS in the United States. *Science, 239,* 610–616.

Davis, S. M., & Harris, M. B. (1982). Sexual knowledge, sexual interests, and sources of sexual information of rural and urban adolescents from three cultures. *Adolescence, 17,* 471–492.

DiClemente, R. J., Boyer, C. B., & Morales, E. S. (1988). Minorities and AIDS: Knowledge, attitudes, and misconceptions among Black and Latino adolescents. *American Journal of Public Health, 78,* 55–57.

DiClemente, R. J., Zorn, J., & Temoshok, L. (1986). Adolescents and AIDS: A survey of knowledge, beliefs, and attitudes about AIDS in San Francisco. *American Journal of Public Health, 76,* 1443–1445.

Fairbank, Bregman, & Maullin, Inc. (1987). *Report on a baseline survey of AIDS risk behaviors and attitudes in San Francisco's Latino communities* (Conducted for the San Francisco Health Department AIDS Activity Office). Unpublished manuscript.

Farley, R., & Allen, W. R. (1987). *The color line and the quality of life in America.* New York: Russell Sage Foundation.

Flick, L. H. (1986). Paths to adolescent parenthood: Implications for prevention. *Public Health Reports, 101,* 132–147.

Friedland, G. H., & Klein, R. S. (1987). Transmission of the human immunodeficiency virus. *New England Journal of Medicine, 317,* 1125–1135.

Gary, L. E., & Berry, G. L. (1985). Predicting attitudes toward substance use in a Black community: Implications for prevention. *Community Mental Health Journal, 21,* 112–118.

Gibbs, J. T. (1986). Psychosocial correlates of sexual attitudes and behaviors in urban early adolescent females: Implications for intervention. *Journal of Social Work and Human Sexuality, 5,* 81–97.

Guinan, M. E., & Hardy, A. (1987). Epidemiology of AIDS in women in the United States. *Journal of the American Medical Association, 257,* 2039–2042.

Harrison, A. O. (1977). Family planning attitudes among Black females. *Journal of Social and Behavioral Sciences, 23,* 136–145.

Hofferth, S. L., Kahn, J. R., & Baldwin, W. (1987). Premarital sexual activity among U.S. teenage women over the past three decades. *Family Planning Perspectives, 19,* 46–53.

Holmes, K. K. (1981). Sexually transmitted disease: An overview and perspectives on the next decade. In U.S. Department of Health and Human Services, *Sexually transmitted diseases: 1980 status report* (DHHS Publication No. NIH 81–2213). Washington, DC: Government Printing Office.

Kahn, E. (1987). Lesbians and AIDS: Everything you need to know about AIDS prevention. *On Our Backs,* pp. 13–15.

Langone, J. (1985, December). AIDS. *Discover,* pp. 28–53.

Levinson, R. A. (1986). Contraceptive self-efficacy: A perspective on teenage girls' contraceptive behavior. *Journal of Sex Research, 22,* 347–369.

Mantell, J. E., Schinke, S. P., & Akabas, S. H. (1988). Women and AIDS prevention. *Journal of Primary Prevention, 9*(1–2), 18–40.

Marin, B. V., Marin, G., & Juarez, R. (1987, August). *Attitudes, expectancies and norms regarding AIDS among Hispanics.* Paper presented at the annual meetings of the American Psychological Association, New York.

Marmor, M. J., Weiss, L. R., Lyden, M., Weiss, S. H., Saxinger, W. C., Spira, T. J., & Feorino, P. M. (1986). Possible female to female transmission of human immunodeficiency virus. *Annals of Internal Medicine, 105,* 969.

Mason, P. J., Olson, R. A., & Parish, K. L. (1988). AIDS, hemophilia, and prevention efforts within a comprehensive care program. *American Psychologist, 43,* 971–976.

Mays, V. M., & Cochran, S. D. (1987). Acquired Immunodeficiency Syndrome and Black Americans: Special psychosocial issues. *Public Health Reports, 102,* 224–231.

Mays, V. M., & Cochran, S. D. (1988). Interpretation of AIDS risk and risk reduction activities by Black and Hispanic women. *American Psychologist, 43,* 949–957.

Mays, V. M., & Cochran, S. D. (1989a). *Acquired Immunodeficiency Syndrome and women.* Manuscript submitted for publication.

Mays, V. M., & Cochran, S. D. (1989b). Methodological issues in the assessment and prediction of AIDS risk-related sexual behavior among Black Americans. In B. Voeller, M. Gottlieb, & J. Reinisch (Eds.), *AIDS and sex: An integrated biomedical and biobehavioral approach.* New York: Oxford University Press.

Mays, V. M., & Cochran, S. D. (1989c). [Sexual risk reduction among young ethnic minority heterosexuals]. Unpublished raw data.

Moore, D. S., & Erickson, P. I. (1985). Age, gender, and ethnic differences in sexual and contraceptive knowledge, attitudes, and behaviors. *Family & Community Health, 8,* 38–51.

Padilla, E. R., & Grady, K. E. (1987). Sexuality among Mexican Americans: A case of sexual stereotyping. *Journal of Personality and Social Psychology, 52,* 5–10.

Pavich, E. G. (1986). A Chicana perspective on Mexican culture and sexuality. *Journal of Social Work and Human Sexuality, 4,* 4765.

Pleck, J. H., O'Donnell, L., O'Donnell, C., & Snarey, J. (1986, August). *AIDS-phobia, contact with AIDS, and AIDS-related job stress in hospital workers.* Paper presented at the annual meetings of the American Psychological Association, Washington, DC.

Poma, P. O. (1987). Pregnancy in Hispanic women. *Journal of the National Medical Association, 79,* 929–935.

Price, J. H., Desmond, S., & Kukulka, G. (1985). High school students' perceptions and misperceptions of AIDS. *Journal of School Health, 55,* 107–109.

Quinn, J. (1986). Rooted in research: Effective adolescent pregnancy prevention programs. *Journal of Social Work and Human Sexuality, 5,* 99–111.

Richardson, D. (1988). *Women and AIDS.* New York: Methuen.

Scott, J. W. (1980). Black polygamous family formation: Case studies of legal wives and consensual "wives." *Alternative Lifestyles, 3,* 41–64.

Shilts, R. (1987). *And the band played on: Politics, people and the AIDS epidemic.* New York: St. Martin's.

Tucker, M. B., & Mitchell-Kernan, C. (in press). Sex ratio imbalance among Afro-Americans: Conceptual and methodological issues. In R. Jones (Ed.), *Black adult development and aging.* Berkeley, CA: Cobb & Henry.

U.S. Bureau of the Census. (1983). *General population characteristics, 1980.* Washington, DC: Government Printing Office.

U.S. Department of Health and Human Services. (1986). *Health status of the disadvantaged: Chartbook 1986* (DHHS Publication No. [HRSA] HRS-P-DV86–2). Washington, DC: Government Printing Office.

Weinstein, N. (1987, October). *Perceptions of risk.* Paper presented at the Centers for Disease Control Conference on Behavioral Aspects of High Risk Sexual Behavior, Atlanta.

Wilkeson, A. G., Poussaint, A. F., Small, E. C., & Shapiro, E. (1983). Human sexuality and the American minority experience. In C. Nadelson (Ed.), *Treatment interventions in human sexuality* (pp. 279–324). New York: Plenum.

Wilson, P. (1986). Black culture and sexuality. *Journal of Social Work and Human Sexuality, 4,* 29–46.

Worth, D., & Rodriguez, R. (1987). Latina women and AIDS. *Radical America, 20*(6), 63–67.

Wyatt, G. E. (in press). Why we know so little about Afro-American sexuality. In R. Jones (Ed.), *Black adult development and aging.* Berkeley, CA: Cobb & Henry.

Wyatt, G. E., Peters, S. D., & Guthrie, D. (in press). Kinsey revisited part II: Comparisons of the sexual socializations and sexual behavior of Black women over 33 years. *Archives of Sexual Behavior.*

Commentary

Juan Ramos

The authors in this section do an excellent job in defining the situation of AIDS and ethnic minority men and women both in general and in specifics. They cite the flaws in the assumptions underlying ongoing prevention efforts, and suggest promising approaches based on alternative assumptions. They point to the critical need to redirect efforts incorporating relevant assumptions and knowledge about minorities. They also describe in some depth the complex systemic and societal issues that impinge on ethnic minorities. The richness of sociocultural, religious, generational, language, class, and acculturation factors may either facilitate and clarify or impede and distort the efforts to develop effective AIDS prevention interventions. While community-based values and perspectives and data-based results support interventions directed at individuals, the more difficult, but probably more promising, preventive interventions must be directed at groups, families, and communities. These must affect norms, heighten a sense of urgency, and set a social movement in motion.

The section does a credible job in covering a wide range of critical subjects, including those mentioned above. The chapters raise the level of awareness, and make an appeal for the substantial work that lies ahead if reduction of HIV infection is to become a reality.

The section provides information that can facilitate evaluation of the ongoing efforts and lead to the development of relevant and new preventive interventions. Both majority and ethnic minority men and women will benefit by reading the whole section as well as the chapters most pertinent to their concerns. All must work together to reduce the likelihood of a situation in 1993 that finds ethnic minority men and women being the groups most affected by HIV/AIDS because of the failure of current preventive interventions so well-described in the section.

19

Mexican-American Intravenous Drug Users' Needle-Sharing Practices: Implications for AIDS Prevention

Alberto G. Mata, Jr.
Jaime S. Jorquez

We were asked to provide a review of Mexican-American[1] intravenous drug use and needle-sharing behaviors, to identify potential influences promoting or deterring these practices, and to discuss how these practices have been affected by the growing attention and concern with acquired immunodeficiency syndrome. Thus we began our efforts by focusing on these general topics:

(1) reviewing the literature (Chaisson, Moss, & Onishi, 1987; Cohen et al., 1985; DiClemente & Boyer, 1987; Feldman, 1985; Watters, Newmeyer, & Cheng, 1986) and exploring with a handful of experts their knowledge and understanding of Mexican-American IV drug use practices, particularly as they concern needle sharing;

(2) given the rising concern over AIDS, exploring and discussing with these experts their knowledge about changes in IV drug use practices and related health risk behaviors; and

(3) exploring and examining factors that contribute to the practice of needle sharing and potential measures to attenuate IV drug use among Hispanics.

The importance of examining this subpopulation is underscored by the fact that IV drug use constitutes a major health risk behavior among Mexican-American IV drug users. IV drug use and needle-sharing practices have been implicated in the spread of AIDS not only among IV drug users (Des Jarlais, Friedman, & Hopkins, 1985) but also among their sexual partners and, perinatally, their children (Bakeman, Lumb, & Smith, 1986; Centers for Disease Control, 1986; Rogers & Williams, 1987; Winkelstein & Samuel, 1987; Worth & Rodriguez, 1987, pp. 5–7). It is also important to examine Mexican-American IV drug use because it is prevalent in many low-income Mexican-American communities. Another reason to examine this subpopulation is the widely held belief that *tecatos* (Mexican-American addicts), their networks, and social world are resistant, if not unresponsive, to societal and community pressures and campaigns to eradicate, if not lessen, their influence.

Background and Historical Context

Since World War II, racial and ethnic minority substance abusers have drawn the attention and concern of many, not only from within the barrio, but also from without. By the 1950s, policymakers, practitioners, and service providers began to draw attention to the problem of marijuana and heroin addiction among Mexican-American youth and young adults in the Southwest (Casavantes, 1977; Moore & Mata, 1982; Morales, 1984).

Within a relatively short period of time, in most major southwestern inner-city and port-of-entry barrios, the social world of the *pelados* (youth and young adults who tend to hang around on street corners) had not only gained a strong foothold but had also spread to other communities in the Southwest. The social world of the pelado soon began to be typified by the emergence of three distinct social types in the barrio: the *vato loco* ("crazy dude"—not bound by street or societal norms), the *pinto* (ex-prisoner), and the tecato. These important new character types began to compose a social hierarchy that action-oriented barrio youth would emulate.

Gradual involvements in local barrio street scenes served as initiating experiences and practicing grounds for a career with heroin. The move from the world of the pelado to the world of the tecato entailed an apprenticeship. The move from the role of observer to that of participant required knowing someone who already had knowledge of how to "turn on," to "hustle," and to "cop." If one were "lucky," it would be a *veterano* (a tecato who has been around and knows the ropes). While each IV drug use scene would bear some localized traits, those into *la vida loca* (literally, the crazy life—the addict life-style) soon came to share a common language and subculture that would serve them well across town, in prison, and throughout their spiral of addiction. By the 1950s, a full-blown tecato subculture could be observed in almost all major cities in the Southwest, with an argot and a life-style distinct from others in the barrio (Casavantes, 1976).

By the late 1950s, attention began to focus on the spread of heroin use among adolescent Mexican-Americans, particularly those involved with gangs. While there was great concern, societal reactions were mostly punitive and resulted in large numbers of Chicanos being arrested and incarcerated in jails, forestry camps, or prisons. The incarceration of large numbers of Hispanics from diverse regions of the nation had the unintended consequences of reinforcing and homogenizing both the pinto and the tecato subcultures (Casavantes, 1976; Davidson, 1970; Irwin, 1970; Moore, 1978; Moore & Long, 1981). As novice Hispanic drug users entered these correctional settings, they encountered racially segmented and antagonistic drug user networks. Thus the novice tecato became enmeshed with others who had shared in similar socializing experiences. In this milieu, individuals from many different localities began to exchange mutually reinforcing pinto/tecato perspectives, codes of conduct, conventions, and crime and drug use "technologies," and also reinforced shared norms in such areas as food, clothing, jobs, information, and even drugs and sex (Bullington, 1977; Davidson, 1970; Irwin, 1970).

Coinciding with the civil rights and mental health movements of the mid-1960s, societal responses to the drug problem began to be less coercive, less punitive, and more treatment oriented (Inciardi, 1986). In this era, Mexican-American IV drug users' reliance on barrio-born and -maintained personal and social networks lessened in some ways. For example, Mexican-Americans in institutional and community drug abuse treatment programs commonly met nonbarrio drug users from diverse social, economic, racial, and ethnic backgrounds. These social experiences, in part, contributed materially to breaking the insularity of the tecato subculture and to the opening of the barrio drug scene to nonbarrio outsiders and vice versa.

To those who could read the signs, throughout the late 1960s and into the 1970s, the tecato subculture remained visible, secure, and firmly entrenched. Concurrently, a variety of distinct and competing drug scenes in the barrio were also flourishing. For example, *chavalos* (youth) were into the "sniffing thing" (inhalants); teens and young adults were into "pills" and "barbs" (amphetamines and barbiturates); and some *safados* (especially prone to risk taking) were using LSD, PCP, and amyl nitrite. For the truly innovative and trendy users, there was always a new "drug" to experience and take to the limit, such as cocaine, crack, smoking opium, and designer drugs (Crider, Gfroerer,

& Blanken, 1986). It bears mention that alcohol and marijuana remained universal staples of each of the drug scenes (Mata, 1984,
1986).

One could argue that, by the 1970s, both gangs and barrio drug use
scenes were quasi-institutionalized (Bullington, 1977; Moore, 1978).

The Problem in Perspective

Official national, state, and local reports continually indicate that
Mexican-Americans are overrepresented in narcotics arrests
(Aumann, Hernandez, Medina, Stewart, & Wherley, 1972; Moore &
Mata, 1982; Morales, 1984), narcotics-related offenses (Irwin, 1970),
drug treatment rolls (National Institute on Drug Abuse, 1982, 1986),
and medical examiners' statistics (U.S. Department of Justice, 1980).
These reports have a number of serious limitations (Desmond &
Maddux, 1984). In most instances, ethnic identifiers remain key problems. In some reports and studies, the focus is on broad categories
such as "Hispanics." Arrest, conviction, and imprisonment reports
combine opiate use with cocaine use. Other reports fail to clearly
differentiate users from nonusers who have been convicted for
narcotics-related offenses or from convicted felons whose convictions
are narcotics related.

Treatment data involving the five southwestern states do not provide data about all narcotics users in treatment. In fact, most reports
generally reflect only those using publicly funded services and not
private ones (Scott, Orzen, Musillo, & Cole, 1973). Last, but more
important, while these data do provide some sense of the incidence
and prevalence of drug use and occasionally information about mode
of drug administration and age and year of drug abuse onset (Ball &
Chambers, 1970), there is little that can be gleaned from them about
needle-sharing practices and related topics.

Taking their lead from Chein et al.'s (1964) study *The Road to H:
Narcotics, Delinquency and Social Policy,* several studies focused on
Mexican-American heroin and other drug use in the late 1960s and
early 1970s. One example is Redlinger's (1970) qualitative case study
focused on drug marketing and distribution patterns in San Antonio,
Texas. The work of Bullington, Munns, and Geis (1969) focused on
heroin use and its consequences, particularly as it concerned treatment. This work was soon followed by Moore's (1978) examination of
continuities and discontinuities in the drug use careers of barrio youth
and young adults. These studies provide important firsthand ac-

counts about major dimensions and themes of Mexican-American drug use, such as barrio contexts, careers in drugs, and barrio perspectives.

While these studies generated important data on and better understanding of heroin use in the barrio, they did not provide data focused on specific drug-using behaviors such as learning to use and share injection equipment ("works," or *fierros*) or dealing with *malias* (opiate withdrawal syndrome) (Howard & Borger, 1974). Studies of heroin relapse (Jorquez, 1983, 1984; Schasre, 1966) and women and heroin in the barrio (Moore & Mata, 1982) provided data and insights about IV-drug-using behaviors in the barrio. While these later studies did focus some attention on the problem of IV drug use ("turning on" and "getting down"), on tecatos' and their significant others' attitudes about the health consequences of IV drug use, and on the process of extrication from la vida loca, they provided few data about needle sharing and factors associated with health risks.

It is at this point that we saw the need to develop our own data sources. Although we began with knowledge and familiarity gained from our earlier studies, the need for additional data sources became readily apparent.

Our initial probes consisted of discussions and on-site visits with both IV drug users and service providers with whom we had preexisting relationships. Responses to our original research questions concerning IV-drug-using behaviors and needle-sharing practices suggested that drug- and works-sharing practices of most Mexican-American IV drug users were not extensive, pervasive, or entrenched. For example, a Chicano former IV drug user with numerous contacts with the San Antonio, Austin, and Chicago IV-drug-using scenes held that almost all self-respecting and aware IV drug users now possess their own works. Another knowledgeable contact, in Phoenix, strongly argued that, while needle sharing occurred, it was not as serious a problem as it is in the East, in the Midwest, and on the West Coast (as needles were relatively easy and cheap to obtain). If any needle sharing was going on, it would be among young, *mocoso* (wet-nosed) tecatos.

A Chicano former IV drug user, now working as a paraprofessional counselor, noted that needles were readily available in drug stores and that *aguajes* (shooting galleries) were a part of the past—more of a problem elsewhere than in the border communities of Texas and Arizona.

Our initial probes were developed from long-term users' information. It was soon clear that we were obtaining valid and relevant observations and insights about a segment of Mexican-American IV drug users, but not one that extended to a wide range of actors and settings. From other sources, we soon became aware of, and interested in following leads about, the problem that new Chicano IV drug users were presenting at treatment programs. We found it was easier to obtain needles and syringes in some southwestern states than in others. We also found that many Mexican-American IV drug users were still sharing their works or stashing their used fierros and *algodones* (cottons) for "a rainy day" when they might find themselves short on luck. There seemed to be conflicting and puzzling aspects to what we were learning about current IV drug use scenes among Chicanos. It is here that we began to develop separate and distinct information sources.

Methodology

When we asked our respondents about their past and current IV-drug-using experiences, they could not relate to the queries about needle sharing and works sharing as we had anticipated. However, when we explored their own drug use experiences, particularly in relation to the first time they "turned on" or their "sharing of drugs," we found that we struck a responsive chord. In exploring their initial IV drug use experiences, they related that they had been "turned on" by others and had seen others "get off" from the same "stuff" (heroin) and possibly the same *erres* or works.

Our initial exploratory efforts extended only to key experts and informants in major cities. As professionals and practitioners, they were knowledgeable of the Chicano heroin addict scenes in their respective cities. The cities included Wilmington, San Pedro, East Los Angeles, and Oakland (California); Denver (Colorado); Albuquerque (New Mexico); Phoenix and Tucson (Arizona); and El Paso, Houston, San Antonio, Harlingen, and Austin (Texas). In these inquiries, we learned of the pervasiveness of Mexican-American IV drug use. To supplement these data, we also conducted ad hoc telephone interviews with our Mexican-American drug abuse treatment personnel contacts in the communities mentioned above and with others.

Given our limited research resources, we focused our efforts on three major urban regions in Texas and two in Arizona. We did this because we saw an opportunity to gather data where syringes are relatively easy to obtain legally rather than in states where this is not the case (such as California and Colorado), and, also, because these are regions where heroin use among Chicanos is well established.

Since there was some indication that drug users were no longer primarily tied to barrio-born and -maintained social networks and that some IV drug users were involved in other drug scenes, we focused some attention on the nature of IV-drug-using networks outside the barrio. We looked for a range of experiences common to addicts in our respondents' drug-using social networks. We also wanted to explore the continuities and discontinuities (i.e., starting and ending drug use "runs") in their drug use patterns and explore factors that promote or deter barrio IV drug users' needle- or works-sharing practices. The salience and representativeness of the data were cross-checked with other data sources.

We chose to develop four distinct data sources and frames of reference focusing on a major IV drug use scene in each of the five cities. The first data source involved key medical, counseling, and substance abuse treatment personnel who had been identified as being most knowledgeable about IV drug use in their respective target areas or communities. A second source of data involved individual and group discussions with IV drug users who were in treatment or a related institutional setting. The third source of data involved interviews and discussions with police narcotics officers who were identified as being the most knowledgeable about the IV drug use scene in the barrio(s). The final source of data involved individual interviews with active IV drug users at large in the community and not in treatment.

An ethnographic interview guide was used to gather data from respondents known to have information relevant to IV drug use. Some respondents were interviewed singly and others, in groups. The interview settings included such places as job sites, youth programs, drug abuse treatment programs, jails, barrio streets, barrio porches, and parks. While some interviews were conducted in English, many respondents were interviewed in a mixture of Spanish and English, and sometimes Mexican-American street argot (*calo*) was used.

IV Drug Use in the Barrio

One of the first observations that we would like to make is that Mexican-American IV drug use scenes are currently flourishing throughout the Southwest. We discovered that IV heroin use is found not only in the expected Mexican-U.S. border towns and larger inner-city barrios of such places as East Los Angeles, Phoenix, Albuquerque, El Paso, and San Antonio, but also in many smaller cities, towns, and rural villages where barrios exist. For the last 10 to 20 years, there have been growing indications that tecatos were becoming a part of most barrios, regardless of their size. While heroin use is widespread, our information suggests that southwestern Mexican-Americans are using it at levels that are relatively affordable and not likely to require extremes of crime to maintain the habit ($10- to $20-a-day habits). A common observation was that Mexican heroin is available and cheap, especially for Mexican-Americans with Mexican connections.

A second observation is that in many southwestern barrios, various drug use scenes exist. In large part, they tend to remain age-graded phenomena, but generally evolve and coexist with each other. Eventually, they may come to draw upon distinct segments of the larger community. Each of these scenes requires different identities, attachments, skills, commitments, and personal/social investments.

The important distinction to be drawn here concerns the varying degree of insularity that these different drug use scenes exhibit with respect to racial and ethnic composition. Mexican-American drug users' social networks range from being barrio oriented, completely insular, localized, and virtually impermeable to outsiders (as in "gangs") to being open to interethnic and intercommunity drug use networks. For the most part, we found that Mexican-American IV drug use scenes located in well-defined, insular barrios were more localized and more socially cohesive. By contrast, we also found drug user networks (especially on city fringes where there is racial and ethnic mixing) where Mexican-Americans were highly involved but were less influential concerning such things as dress codes, life-styles, and drug use preferences and patterns. As one drug abuse counselor reported, there are tecatos who "hang around" with Anglos and Blacks. Their concern is not with whom they associate but that they "score and get well."

A third observation from our study is that polydrug use is more typical than it once was. While drug users may have a particular preference for a given drug, it is not uncommon for them to switch from drug to drug depending on circumstances and opportunities. In most southwestern locales, it was suggested that cocaine, alcohol, and marijuana were regarded as barrio staples. Most respondents mentioned that cocaine for snorting and injecting and for "speedballing" with heroin is currently very popular among barrio Mexican-Americans and undocumented Mexicans. Among youth and young adults, PCP, crack, LSD, and inhalants were sometimes mentioned as being problematic in some, but not all, barrio communities. The more important suggestion here is that Mexican-Americans' IV drug use is extending to substances other than heroin, yet IV drug use still remains heroin dominant.

A fourth observation concerns the role of personal social support networks for both barrio and nonbarrio drug users. While recognizing that different drug use scenes now exist and different barrio orientations also exist, we discovered that, among drug users, there was a continuing reliance on personal social support networks for learning to use drugs, obtaining drugs, and avoiding arrest; for information and resource exchanges; and for coping with the exigencies of illicit drug use. This particular observation has important implications for understanding factors that promote the sharing of drugs, works, information, and resources. These personal social support systems or networks could be utilized, once better understood, to introduce new behavioral norms conducive to dealing with communicable diseases.

A fifth observation concerns the difference between controlled and less controlled users. We found that controlled IV drug users tended to be older and more experienced. They tended to use various precautions, such as less frequent drug use and less drugs used, and they were more careful about whom they shared their drugs and IV injection works with. They also were more likely to be involved with other users of a similar cautious orientation, to know each other more intimately and for some period of time, and to be less prone to high-risk escapades. By contrast, novices, "hardheads," "gutter types" (*cucarachas*), and "burnouts" were drug users who were reported to be careless (regarding police surveillance, using "dirty" works, or being "burnt" and "ripped off") and more concerned with getting loaded. The key implication we would like to draw attention to concerns the need to explore and understand the process by which users move from being less controlled to more controlled.

The sixth major observation in our study involves IV drug users' awareness of health risk factors. It appears that controlled users have grasped the potential for contracting illnesses such as hepatitis and, more recently, AIDS. Learning what factors or experiences lend themselves to the internalization of this health awareness is beyond the scope of our preliminary research efforts. We found evidence that controlled users are concerned and are taking some measures to reduce their health risks. Among less controlled users, we found that there was also an awareness of the many serious consequences of shooting up drugs, but there was little evidence to suggest that they had internalized the seriousness of communicable diseases related to IV drug use.

In discussing with Chicano addicts their knowledge of AIDS, we found that almost all had some level of awareness. However, among most novice heroin users and "hardheads," we found strong tendencies to deny or minimize the AIDS threat. Within this group, there were expressions that AIDS was a White, gay male disease affecting areas of the country far away from their backyards. For both controlled and less controlled users, the topic of safer sexual practices was much more difficult to raise and fully discuss. Most clinicians and more "open-minded" tecatos suggested that initial efforts and contacts with high-risk individuals be on a one-to-one basis; at the same time, both saw a great need for community outreach efforts that are culturally relevant and sensitive.

With respect to awareness of health risks, we were warned that the current AIDS situation is an opportunity for harmful myths and ineffective or dangerous behavioral adjustments to enter the IV-drug-using world. For example, our attention was drawn to the fact that tecatos commonly treat opiate overdoses by placing the victim in cold water, packing ice around the genitals, and injecting substances like salt, coffee, or milk into the victim's veins. It was also suggested to us that immediate measures to introduce legitimate medical information could arrest the institutionalization of dangerous myths and practices concerning IV drug use and AIDS.

A seventh observation concerns IV drug use and alternative sexual preferences. We found that Mexican-American gay and lesbian worlds have existed for some time. While Chicano homosexual worlds exist in larger urban communities, such as Los Angeles, Houston, and Phoenix, and even in the larger border communities, in virtually all these places homosexuality remains a strong taboo, a denigrated and deprecated life-style. Unlike the tecato subculture, Chicano gay and lesbian social scenes were usually outside the view and influence of their barrios. Most of our contacts (IV drug users and experts knowledgeable about both scenes) remarked on how distant the IV drug use and gay worlds remained from each other. This is not to say that, for some Chicano gays and lesbians, drug use is not a part of their social worlds.

What may be a more fruitful line to explore with both Chicano IV drug users and gay Mexican-Americans is an assessment concerning their health risk behaviors and unsafe sexual practices. It is imperative that such an assessment be made and that the results lead to the development of curricula, materials, and services designed to address these health risk issues. These products must then be delivered to four specific populations. We suggest beginning with (a) the sexual partners of IV drug users; (b) IV-drug-using men and women, their families, and their children; (c) institutionalized persons in settings such as jails, detention centers, and prisons; and (d) high-risk youth (school dropouts, homeless/runaway youth, and adjudicated delinquents).

Comments

The personal social networks of barrio IV drug users serve to meet their need to belong, to meet expressive social and psychological needs, and also to address utilitarian needs and wants, such as learning to use drugs, to cop, to fix, to hustle, and to maintain a habit. These personal social networks are even applied to an addict's attempts to end a run or to quit using drugs altogether. This is facilitated by calling on barrio *carnales* (acquaintances and friends) who have "connections" (entrée to treatment programs) or know how to "kick" at home.

Efforts to curb IV drug use and needle sharing must begin with the understanding that these practices are embedded and maintained by a set of ongoing personal relations and exchanges in IV drug users' personal social networks. Needle sharing must be seen as part of the larger picture of drug-sharing practices. Drug sharing is at once a means to socialize, to belong, and to provide some measure of protection from the exigencies of la vida loca. More immediately, it is a means of coping with one's craving for drugs. Thus in southwestern states with strict laws and enforcement patterns focusing on needles and related paraphernalia, needle sharing is expedient, economical, and, of course, "gratifying."

With few exceptions, among Mexican-American IV drug users, needle-sharing practices associated with shooting galleries are rare, yet needle sharing as a drug use practice in this group is quite common. Among more controlled users, the frequency of drug use and whom they use with is more routinized and restricted. Among less controlled users, the factors promoting drug use, frequency, and needle sharing are more variable and problematic. For these users, caution, care, and attention to legal and health issues are overridden by the pressing need to *alivianarse* (get well/straight). It is common for less controlled users to inject within walking distance of their connection (motel, park, house/apartment, or the dealer's car).

For many drug abuse treatment, criminal justice, and other professionals, the Mexican-American IV drug user remains hard to reach and unresponsive to treatment. Our observations suggest that both less controlled and controlled IV drug users are open to various strategies and modes of intervention and treatment. The two key dimensions that we suggest can break the spiral of addiction are identifying the stage of drug involvement and linking it to the appropriate treatment interventions, and developing and maintaining entrée to Mexican-American IV drug user networks.

In comparison to AIDS among IV drug users in the Northeast, AIDS among IV drug users in the Southwest, particularly among Mexican-Americans, may be characterized as being in the first stages of the epidemic.

We noted that AIDS awareness was found among most users and also among their IV-drug-using acquaintances and their families, yet the internalization of the serious consequences of this disease was not evident. As Mexican-American addicts continue to engage in needle-sharing practices, they remain important vectors of AIDS virus transmission to nonusers, that is, their sexual partners and their children. Therefore, it is imperative that we undertake projects that help these IV drug users to internalize the seriousness of this disease and the consequences of continuing to engage in high-risk behaviors—specifically, IV drug use, sharing of injection equipment, and unsafe sexual practices. Contrary to the contention that addicts do not care enough or are unable to respond, we suggest that *some* have learned from their "bottoming out" experiences and their familiarity with the many problems associated with the spiral of addiction. Whether it be a severe bout with hepatitis or their "just being sick and tired of being sick and tired," there are natural points of intervention that we can draw on to access them. Successful intervention will require aggressive case finding and concrete information and assistance (Friedman, Des Jarlais, & Goldsmith, in press).

Recommendations

Prevention Efforts

It is recommended that a series of well-coordinated community efforts be instituted and adequately supported to prevent Mexican-American youth from starting drug- and alcohol-using careers. Existing programs should be encouraged to coordinate their efforts and also should be provided necessary support: money, human resources, and technical assistance (Friedman, Des Jarlais, & Sotheran, 1986). To prevent IV drug use among Mexican-Americans at risk for entering the spiral of addiction, we recommend the following:

(1) the development of culturally sensitive educational programs designed to inform all at risk—Mexican-Americans and others who reside in barrios—about the negative consequences of using drugs and to encourage positive alternatives (programs should involve a broad spectrum of Mexican-Americans working closely with agencies and people who are sensitive to the Mexican-American culture);

(2) the development of local councils of barrio people (including undocumented Mexicans and Central Americans) to facilitate and improve community efforts in drug abuse and health risk prevention; and

(3) the development of culturally sensitive, trained professionals and indigenous barrio people, including ex-addicts who are respected by drug users, to work in the barrio and provide educational/prevention services to the general population and to special at-risk subpopulations (Beschner & Friedman, 1979).

Active IV Drug Users in Treatment

The population of Mexican-American IV drug users in treatment at any time depends greatly on available treatment services, their attractiveness to Mexican-American IV drug users, the obstacles (money, hassles, and so on) in accessing such programs, and other factors. Drug abuse treatment provides the opportunity to help addicts internalize the seriousness of their health risk behaviors to themselves, their sexual partners, and their children. In treatment, addicts can be exposed to information, educational aids, and resources to help them not only to cope with their addiction but also to internalize behaviors that minimize their risk for exposure to AIDS and other communicable diseases, such as hepatitis. Since relapse to drug abuse is common following treatment, programs should make risk-reduction efforts a priority. Also, these addicts in treatment can, in turn, influence other addicts in their personal social networks to begin to consider their health risks.

Active IV Drug Users Out of Treatment

For active Mexican-American IV drug users out of treatment and at large in the community, we recommend three basic but well-integrated elements for dealing with the transmission of AIDS and other communicable diseases through needle-sharing and unsafe sexual practices:

(1) Efforts must be made by trained individuals with high credibility and respect among Mexican-American addicts to locate and make appropriate entrée into addicts' barrio social networks. Such individuals could come from the ranks of ex-addicts and other "street-wise" individuals.

(2) Once meaningfully engaged with active addicts' social networks, these trained community health education workers would provide information on AIDS and its transmission, instructions on safer sexual practices, and information on how to reduce risk during drug use. These workers could also gather epidemiological data that would be useful in planning and evaluating risk-reduction programs (Akins & Beschner, 1980).

(3) The community health education workers must not simply inform addicts but must encourage and reinforce behavior change. Addicts who are ready for treatment would be assisted in this process. The mission is to attempt, carefully, to induce active IV drug users to develop incentives to stop or curtail IV drug use and unsafe sexual practices. Here, great care must be taken to ensure that workers do not gain the reputation of "lame do-gooders." Community health education workers must have official legitimacy so that they can gain the cooperation of barrio people, drug users, treatment program personnel, the police, probation and parole officers, and medical personnel.

Sexual Partners, Families, and Children

Efforts are needed to reach the sexual partners and families of IV drug users to alert them to the AIDS risk faced by addicts, to alert them regarding the risk of sexual and perinatal transmission of AIDS, and to inform sexual partners of specific steps to reduce their risk as well as that of future offspring. These risk-reduction efforts should include media campaigns to sensitize barrio communities to health risks; educational workshops to be offered through churches, schools, and other community organizations; and individualized educational strategies to be provided at health clinics and by indigenous outreach workers. Prostitutes would constitute an important target group.

Note

1. The terms *Mexican-American* and *Chicano* are recognized as having different meanings, but for purposes of this chapter they are used interchangeably.

References

Akins, C., & Beschner, G. (Eds.). (1980). *Ethnography: A research tool for policymakers in the drug and alcohol fields* (National Institute on Drug Abuse, DHHS Publication No. [ADM]80–946). Washington, DC: Government Printing Office.

Aumann, J., Hernandez, M., Medina, M., Stewart, C., & Wherley, N. (1972). *The Chicano addict: An analysis of factors influencing rehabilitation in a treatment and prevention program.* Phoenix, AZ: Valle del Sol.

Bakeman, R., Lumb, J. R., & Smith, W. S. (1986). AIDS statistics and the risk for minorities. *AIDS Research, 2*(3), 249–252.

Ball, J. C., & Chambers, C. D. (1970). *The epidemiology of opiate addiction in the United States.* Springfield, IL: Charles C. Thomas.

Beschner, G. M., & Friedman, A. S. (1979). *Youth drug abuse: Problems, issues and treatment.* Lexington, MA: Lexington.

Bullington, B. (1977). *Heroin use in the barrio,* Lexington, MA: Lexington.

Bullington, B., Munns, J. G., & Geis, G. (1969). Purchase of conformity: Ex-narcotic addicts among the bourgeoisie. *Social Problems, 16*(4), 456–463.

Casavantes, E. J. (1976). *El tecato: Cultural and sociologic factors affecting drug use among Chicanos* (2nd ed.). Washington, DC: National Coalition of Spanish Speaking Mental Health Organizations.

Centers for Disease Control. (1986). Acquired Immunodeficiency Syndrome (AIDS) among Blacks and Hispanics—United States. *Morbidity and Mortality Weekly Report, 36,* 655–666.

Chaisson, R. E., Moss, A. R., & Onishi, R. (1987). Human immunodeficiency virus infection in heterosexual intravenous drug users in San Francisco. *American Journal of Public Health, 77,* 169–172.

Chein, I., et al. (1964). *The road to H: Narcotics, delinquency and social policy.* New York: Basic Books.

Cohen, H., et al. (1985, April). *Risk factors for HTLV III/LAV seropositivity among intravenous drug users.* Paper presented at the First International Conference on AIDS, Atlanta.

Crider, R. A., Gfroerer, J. C., & Blanken, A. J. (1986). Black tar heroin field investigation. In *Drug abuse trends and research issues: Proceedings of the Community Epidemiology Work Group, December 1986* (National Institute on Drug Abuse Administrative Report), pp. III11-III34.

Davidson, T. (1970). *Chicano prisoners.* San Francisco: Holt, Rinehart & Winston.

Des Jarlais, D. C., Friedman, S. R., & Hopkins, W. (1985). Risk reduction for the Acquired Immunodeficiency Syndrome among intravenous drug users. *Annals of Internal Medicine, 103,* 755–759.

Desmond, D. P., & Maddux, J. F. (1984). Mexican American heroin addicts. *American Journal of Drug and Alcohol Abuse, 10*(3), 317–346.

Feldman, D. A. (1985). AIDS and social change. *Human Organization, 44*(4), 343–348.

Friedman, S. R., Des Jarlais, D. C., & Goldsmith, D. S. (in press). An overview of current AIDS prevention efforts aimed at intravenous drug users. *Journal of Drug Issues.*

Friedman, S. R., Des Jarlais, D. C., & Sotheran, J. L. (1986). AIDS health education for intravenous drug users. *Health Education Quarterly, 13*(4), 383–393.

Howard, J., & Borger, P. (1974). Needle sharing in the Haight: Some social and psychological functions. In D. Smith & G. R. Gay (Eds.), *It's so good don't even try it once: Heroin in perspective.* Englewood Cliffs, NJ: Spectrum.

344   Mata and Jorquez

Inciardi, I. J. (1986). *The war on drugs.* Englewood Cliffs, NJ: Prentice-Hall.

Irwin, J. (1970). *The felon.* Englewood Cliffs, NJ: Prentice-Hall.

Jorquez, J. S. (1983). The retirement phase of heroin using careers. *Journal of Drug Issues, 13*(3), 343–365.

Jorquez, J. S. (1984). Heroin use in the barrio: Solving the problem of relapse or keeping the tecato gusano asleep. *American Journal of Drug and Alcohol Abuse, 10*(1), 63–75.

Mata, A. G. (1984). *Inhalant use in small rural south Texas communities.* Paper presented to Governor M. White's Commission on Inhalant Abuse, San Antonio, TX.

Mata, A. G., Jr. (1986). Marijuana use in a small rural community. In *Drug abuse trends and research issues: Proceedings of the Community Epidemiology Work Group, December 1986* (National Institute on Drug Abuse administrative report), pp. III, 119-III, 148.

Moore, J. W. (1978). *Homeboys: Gangs, drugs, and prison in the barrios of Los Angeles.* Philadelphia: Temple University Press.

Moore, J. W., & Long, J. (1981). *Barrio impact of high incarceration rates.* Los Angeles: Chicano Pinto Research Project.

Moore, J. W., & Mata, A. G. (1982). *Women and heroin in a Chicano community: A final report.* Los Angeles: Chicano Pinto Research Project.

Morales, A. (1984). Substance abuse and Mexican American youth: An overview. *Journal of Drug Issues, 14*(2), 297–311.

National Institute on Drug Abuse. (1982). *The 1982 National Drug and Alcohol Treatment Utilization Survey.* Washington, DC: Alcohol, Drug Abuse, and Mental Health Administration.

National Institute on Drug Abuse. (1986). *Drug abuse trends and research issues: Proceedings of the Community Epidemiology Work Group, June 1986.* Washington, DC: Author.

Redlinger, L. D. (1970). *Dealing in dope.* Unpublished doctoral dissertation, Northwestern University.

Rogers, M. F., & Williams, W. W. (1987). AIDS in Blacks and Hispanics: Implications for prevention. *Issues in Science and Technology, 3*(3), 89–94.

Schasre, R. (1966). Cessation patterns among neophyte heroin users. *International Journal of the Addictions, 1*(2), 23–32.

Scott, N. R., Orzen, W., Musillo, C., & Cole, P. T. (1973). Methadone in the Southwest: A three-year follow-up of Chicano heroin addicts. *American Journal of Orthopsychiatry, 43*(3), 355–361.

U.S. Department of Justice. (1980). *Project DAWN annual report* (Drug Enforcement Agency/Department of Health and Human Services). Washington, DC: Government Printing Office.

Watters, J. K., Newmeyer, J. A., & Cheng, Y.-T. (1986, October). *Human immunodeficiency virus infection and risk factors among intravenous drug users in San Francisco.* Paper presented at the annual meeting of the American Public Health Association, Las Vegas.

Winkelstein, W., & Samuel, M. (1987). Prevalence of human immunodeficiency virus infection in ethnic minority homosexual/bisexual men. *Journal of the American Medical Association, 257,* 1901.

Worth, D., & Rodriguez, R. (1987). *Latina women and AIDS.* New York: SIECUS.

Commentary

Edward S. Morales

The importance of the subcultures within cultural and ethnic communities is central to understanding the AIDS epidemic within groups with a high prevalence of high-risk behaviors. The life-styles of Mexican-American intravenous drug users differ from those IV users from other ethnic and racial groups, which has implications for AIDS prevention interventions. Mata and Jorquez provide a fundamental ethnographic description of the IV drug user and the variations in life-styles within the Mexican-American community, suggesting subgroups within the IV-drug-using population that center on generational differences, class, geographical residence, acculturation, and experience in drug use. Epidemiological data concerning needle sharing and sexual practices among Mexican-Americans are sorely needed if we are to understand the magnitude of the AIDS transmission problem as well as identify specific ways in which Mexican-Americans continue to be at risk for AIDS.

Although needle sharing is one of several vectors for transmitting HIV efficiently, little information was derived from the study concerning sexual practices among IV users. Mata and Jorquez note that the topic of safer sexual practices among IV users is difficult to raise and fully discuss. The role of HIV transmission through high-risk sexual practice affects the sexual partners of IV users and those who tend to be sexually active, especially adolescents and young adults. Generational differences in drug use among Mexican-Americans seem to have differential risks for the transmission of HIV. Among these same adolescents and young adults Mata and Jorquez note that the choice of drugs is different, and they report the frequent use of PCP, crack, LSD, and inhalants as well as the "barrio staples," specifically, alcohol, cocaine, and marijuana. It may be expected that these adolescents and young adults may use these drugs to enhance their sexual experience, which in turn impairs their judgment in the use of safer sex guidelines.

Many of the barriers to AIDS information and drug abuse prevention for Mexican-Americans seem common to other ethnic and racial communities. These barriers include (a) the lack of drug treatment

345

services, (b) lack of credibility of the delivery of the health message, (c) suspicion of medical and health professionals, (d) negative perception of those at risk for AIDS, (e) poverty and the life-style in the barrio or ghetto, (f) poor health practices among drug users, and (g) the lack of formal involvement of adolescents and young adults in the community structure, function, and decision-making process. For most communities those in the targeted groups, particularly gay and bisexual men and IV drug users, live different life-styles, have different support groups, and face different challenges due to their life-styles. Additionally, the personality and temperament of controlled versus less controlled drug users appear to relate to the psychological concept of adequate and poor impulse control, a concept that is applicable across populations. What seem unique to Mexican-American drug users are (a) acculturation to the United States and the drug use world, (b) availability of less expensive drugs through connections in Mexico, and (c) the socialization process in the drug-using world, such as language and customs.

The role of personal social support networks for both barrio and nonbarrio drug users can be central to an effective AIDS prevention strategy. In applying the health belief model (Beck & Frankel, 1981) to AIDS prevention a key factor in changing behavior has been noted to be a change in social norms and expectancies. As the norms for needle sharing and sexual practices change by adopting the AIDS risk-reduction guidelines within the community, there is increased peer pressure and expectation to comply with the new social norms. The use of safer sex educational workshops in the form of "safe sex socials" at the homes of those at risk has been shown to be popular and successful through programs such as the Stop AIDS Project in San Francisco and other cities and the AIDS educational program for IV drug users in San Francisco's outreach efforts. These latter programs teach addicts to clean their works with bleach and about AIDS prevention. They have reported an increased use of bleach and a reduction in needle sharing among their clients. Interventions to teach addicts how to develop their skills in AIDS risk reduction, including changing sexual practices, are currently being researched; the preliminary results have revealed increases in skill attainment and changes in AIDS risk-taking behavior.

The recommendations for AIDS prevention efforts outlined by Mata and Jorquez are based on the principle of community involvement at every level with target groups identified, combined with plans and commitments from the community to adopt the AIDS risk-reduction guidelines, thereby reducing transmission of HIV. The uniqueness of the AIDS epidemic forces all communities to confront a variety of barriers simultaneously, some of which have been chronic and long-standing. A barrier in the Mexican-American community may lie in limited or overcommitted community and leadership resources, affecting its ability to address AIDS prevention adequately. Community involvement at every level also means that the community—every man, woman, and child—must recognize AIDS as a community problem. The community must agree to reject treating persons at risk as outcasts or as responsible for AIDS prevention efforts. For the Mexican-American community, using the strength of its culture, its sense of community responsibility, and its strong need for participation is essential for AIDS prevention.

References

Beck, A., & Frankel, A. (1981). A conceptualization of threat communications and protective health behavior. *Social Psychological Quarterly, 44*, 204–217.

Rogers, R. W. (1975). A protection motivation theory of fear appeals and attitude change. *Journal of Psychology, 92*, 93–114.

Rosenstock, I. M. (1974). The health belief model in preventive behavior. *Health Education Monographs, 2*, 355–385.

PART V

An Agenda for Psychological Training and Research

This section of the book groups three disparate but not completely unrelated chapters. Flora and Thoresen present a compelling argument for an integrated approach to AIDS prevention, utilizing the synergistic and additive effects of several levels of intervention extending from the individual to the community and media levels, all based upon cognitive social learning theory. They urge the use of social marketing strategies to tailor messages to particular groups. As background, they review several interventions with adolescents, assessing their successes and failures. They are clearly aiming for the most powerful combination of weapons intended for application to ethnic minority teenagers. Flora and Thoresen provide concrete examples of the possibilities inherent in a well-thought-out, theoretically based, and competently evaluated intervention program aimed at priority populations and behavior.

Sheridan reviews a program that supports AIDS education of mental health professionals. She is hardly reticent about the possibility of contributions from the behavioral sciences and exhorts mental health professionals to use this knowledge across the spectrum of AIDS-related activities, to become the leaders in the fight against the disease. The chapter is full of challenging questions, situations, anecdotes, and observations that inform us about why leadership has been slow to develop and suggestions about how we might facilitate the process. The emphasis is on the provision of care and the multiple contributions of which professionals are capable before the disease starts and throughout its course. Impediments to the success of leadership are also examined.

Clearly, Flora and Thoresen have given us examples of excellent intervention research by behavioral scientists, and Sheridan makes a strong case for the leadership potential of mental health professionals based on knowledge from the behavioral sciences. Schneider suggests a research and training agenda for psychologists, emphasizing that many kinds of psychologists can make contributions in the battle to understand and eradicate AIDS. He reviews the content of several new announcements requesting applications that are remarkable for the breadth of their content and the diversity of their sponsorship, since many of them are cosponsored by NIMH and several other federal agencies. The resources are at hand to do the kinds of things suggested by Flora and Thoresen and by Sheridan. It remains for our currently uninvolved colleagues to take up the challenge.

The final three chapters in this section discuss programs at specific agencies: the National Institute on Alcohol and Alcohol Abuse, the National Institute on Drug Abuse, and the National Institute of Mental Health.

20

An AIDS Research and Training Agenda for Psychology

Stanley F. Schneider

AIDS[1] is a behaviorally transmitted disease. AIDS is an immune system disease. AIDS is a social disease. AIDS is a disease affecting the neurovirological functions. AIDS is a disease of the brain. AIDS is a disease the prevention and transmission of which is affected by culture. All of these are true. AIDS is an excellent example of a biopsychosocial phenomenon, since it probably involves mutual interactions of the neural, immune, and endocrine systems, and of all of these with behavior, in a sociocultural context. If one were asked to invent a disease that was more fascinating, more perplexing, more challenging scientifically, socially, ethically, and legally than AIDS, one would be hard put to do so.

AIDS is also a preventable disease, although it involves behaviors that are powerfully motivated and resistant to change. There is hardly an area of psychology that cannot make some contribution to our knowledge about AIDS. Primary prevention activities concern themselves with forestalling the further spread of the disease. There is a need to understand the major behaviors involved in transmission, sexual behavior and intravenous drug use, to develop strategies to change these behaviors if they involve risk, and to maintain such changes. We know very little about sexual behaviors and about the behaviors associated with intravenous drug use; there is critical need for a sophisticated, culturally sensitive knowledge base in these areas. The development of various kinds of interventions at various levels is required. These may affect individuals, groups of various sizes, institutions, and communities, utilizing methods as disparate as cognitive behavioral therapy, educational materials, and mass media approaches. In addition, it is absolutely essential that interventions be subject to planned variation, that they be suited to target populations, and, above all, that they be rigorously evaluated. There is sufficient work in the areas briefly described above to involve social, community, cognitive, clinical, and health psychologists as well as evaluation researchers and others.

These areas are reflected in one of several announcements that will be issued by the time the proceedings of this conference appear. The particular announcement in question is called Research on Behavior Change and Prevention Strategies to Reduce Transmission of HIV, and it represents the interests of all Alcohol, Drug Abuse, and Mental Health Administration (ADAMHA) institutes, several National Institutes of Health (NIH) components, and the Centers for Disease Control (CDC). It is the announcement that may be of greatest interest to this audience, since a major focus is prevention. Research topics are presented under four broad headings: (a) Determinants, Development, and Distribution of Risk Behaviors; (b) Research on Behavioral Interventions to Prevent AIDS; (c) Research on the Diffusion/ Implementation of AIDS Prevention Programs; and (d) Methodological Research. Since HIV and AIDS also affect children, adolescents, and the elderly, all periods of the life span must be studied. Developmentalists, personality researchers, and those interested in the aged will find that their research skills are needed. So will counseling psychologists, for the entire relationship of serotesting and counseling is fraught with questions. The need for ethnic minority researchers and the devastating impact of AIDS upon ethnic minority populations are priority concerns. There is also considerable agreement that, from the perspective of primary prevention, children and adolescents are important populations to reach. Preventive intervention programs should be mounted in schools, workplaces, the community at large, and among informal support groups. Basic research from such areas as attitude change, persuasion, communication, and use of mass media can be of enormous importance in AIDS research. School psychologists, organizational psychologists, and media psychologists can contribute to the effort.

There are vehicles for the participation of biopsychologists, and two of the forthcoming announcements deal with (a) Brain, Immune System, Behavioral, and Neurological Aspects of HIV Infection; and (b) Central Nervous System Effects of HIV Infection: Neurobiological, Neurovirological, and Neurobehavioral Studies. The first of these covers the entire domain of what has come to be called psychoneuroimmunology, which brings together neuroscientists, immunologists, cognitive psychologists, and neuropsychologists. The second announcement emphasizes the fields of molecular biology, neurobiology, and neurovirology more directly, but several sections of the announcement deal with neuropsychological deficits and AIDS dementia, including their behavioral outcomes. Both of these announcements are cosponsored by NIMH, the National Institute of Child Health and Human Development (NICHD), and the National Institute of Neurological Diseases and Stroke (NINDS). The substantive areas of research interest in these announcements should provoke considerable thought about the training of psychologists for research in AIDS.

A fourth announcement will be concerned with the measurement, course, and treatment of HIV-related mental disorders and will interest clinical psychologists and psychopharmacologists particularly, but by no means exclusively. Psychosocial, neuropsychological, and psychiatric measures need to be adapted to the course of HIV disease and to the populations affected by it, and clinical treatment and secondary prevention are important areas of emphasis. The fifth announcement focuses on the problem of HIV infection in the severely mentally ill and on risk reduction in this population. In addition, it provides support for research on the service needs and models of service delivery for HIV-infected mentally ill, including work on the financing of services, the impact of laws and regulations on service delivery, and various measures to facilitate research with this neglected class of subjects.

These announcements cover a research agenda of incredible breadth and richness. The involvement of several NIH institutes (NINDS, NICHD, the National Institute on Aging [NIA], the National Heart, Lung, and Blood Institute [NHLBI], and the National Center for Nursing Research), the three ADAMHA institutes, and the CDC in one or another of the announcements attests to the interest and support of a wider array of federal agencies than ever before. The NIMH has taken the lead role in each of these announcements, but the others were eager to participate. Revisions in other mechanisms of support are also pertinent. The Research Scientist Development Award (Level 1), the Physician Scientist Award, and the Clinical Investigator Award are to be replaced by a Scientist Development Award (SDA) and a Scientist Development Award for Clinicians (SDAC). The SDA and SDAC are principally intended for developing scientists, persons who have never held a research grant (small grants are an exception). However, the SDA allows up to two years of support for established investigators seeking to make a significant change of research field. Investigators requiring supervised research experience to make a change to AIDS research could qualify for support under this program. In addition, the Small Grants Program is to be revised, with research support of up to $50,000 per year for two years. Again, the program has a major purpose to support newer, less experienced investigators, or those at institutions without well-developed research resources, but small grants are also available to more experienced investigators for exploratory studies that represent a significant change in research direction, or for pilot studies for the development/ testing of new methods or techniques. This is another program that should be utilized for AIDS-related research.

A great deal of the work that has been done up to this point by psychologists is concentrated in two major areas: (a) studies of psychosocial factors and determinants of risk-taking behavior, mainly in gay, White populations and to some extent in intravenous drug users; and (b) studies that may be broadly classified under the rubric of psychoimmunology, with much less involvement until now of the neural aspects. This is not surprising, since these are heavily affected target populations for the disease, and the various psychological-immune system interactions represent a natural interest fallout of AIDS. Much of the work on interventions is derived from clinical or counseling cognitive-behavioral models, conducted at the individual or small group level. More attention needs to be paid to ethnic minority populations and to adolescents as an age group (and to women and the older adult population, both comparatively neglected); to larger-scale interventions, including those based on mass media, very carefully varied and evaluated; to research on sexual behavior, including contexts of such behavior and communication about it, which has virtually disappeared from the psychologists' palettes; to the developmental course of the disease in infected children; to the real integration of psychological, immunological, and neural factors in disease progression; to the social impact of the disease, including its effects upon institutions and upon such things as stigma; to the ever-mounting chronic disease population, their well-being and the well-being of those close to them, and to the impact of this population on health care professionals and on the health care system; to the broad mass of heterosexuals for whom the disease, now gone from the front pages, has again become somebody else's concern and a matter for denial; and to carefully conducted neuropsychological assessments with added performance measures that will inform about functioning on the job. This is only a partial menu, but it is enough to occupy us for a while.

Two additional announcements will be issued, one for institutional research training grants and one for individual research training fellowships in HIV infection. The substantive areas covered by these announcements will be similar to those included in the research announcements reviewed previously. One characteristic of the research announcements, reflected as well in the breadth of their sponsorship, is their interdisciplinary and multidisciplinary nature. If I emphasize nothing else in these comments, it is essential to make one point, that psychology must give up its insularity in order to deal with AIDS. Psychologists of all kinds can make important contributions to the understanding and eventual amelioration of this dreadful disease, but they must inform themselves about its epidemiology, molecular neurobiology, virology, immunology, and treatment prospects in order to have the knowledge base necessary to appreciate its current status. We are dealing with a remarkably variable and complicated virus, one that not only affects different people differently but affects the same person in different ways at different times. Indeed, the genetic expression of the virus is so unreliable that it is likely that an individual at a given time has "enormous numbers of slightly different viruses" (Marx, 1988, p. 1039). This in turn is probably related to the variable lag period from asymptomatic seropositivity to full-blown AIDS, a problem that complicates prediction of the course of the disease.

Psychologists should avail themselves of opportunities to participate in multidisciplinary training programs, such as those already supported by NIMH, that tend to provide a firm foundation in other areas for persons whose original training was in the behavioral sciences, neurosciences, or immunology. At the very least, an introduction to these important substantive areas must be provided. At the predoctoral level, it is unlikely that cross-training and real interdisciplinary training will occur because most research graduate education programs in psychology do not venture outside the discipline, or even to remoter areas inside the discipline. In clinical psychology and other programs that prepare for research and applications of psychology, accreditation requirements limit the possibilities even more. But some exposure to these nonpsychological areas and to actual research on AIDS-related problems can do a good deal to overcome some of these barriers. Students will find themselves engaged in one way or another with those who speak other research languages, and this can benefit them if their supervisors are open to the prospect. By all means, a reality unduplicated elsewhere will be found by exposure to persons with AIDS, who ideally should be seen and worked with throughout the course of the illness. It would be appropriate, and fitting, to see some health psychology training programs lead the way in this effort to incorporate AIDS-related material into graduate training. At the postdoctoral level, a much more concentrated exposure to the intensity and breadth of AIDS research issues is possible, and the goals should include an increased ease and sophistication in handling ideas and concepts across the spectrum of AIDS research in order to mesh psychological hypotheses and measures sensibly with other aspects important in the disease process. Not long ago, I heard a remarkable presentation of a research project at one of our AIDS research centers. The project was conducted by a health psychologist and an immunologist. The psychologist presented the immunologic aspects of the research, and the immunologist the psychological aspects, each of them rendered in exquisite and knowledgeable detail. These investigators had truly learned to understand and speak the language of the other, and the quality and originality of their research showed the fruits of such understanding.

Training programs will require a good deal of experimentation, and we should be open to several models. This is especially so because people are working together on AIDS who have not collaborated previously, and the nature of the epidemic itself is such that it will continue to surprise us and to demand adaptations. Beyond any of the more or less formal aspects of training, however, there needs to be the conviction that AIDS is an important problem, something worth the devotion of one's time and energy, for, make no mistake about it, AIDS will consume these resources. Most people prefer to go about their daily work and lives as though the disease did not exist, and it has not been easy to recruit psychologists to work on AIDS. They would prefer not to be bothered by it. One of the sad signs of the insularity I spoke of can be seen in the attendance at the conference that produced this book. Usually, these conferences attract substantial numbers of community psychologists, since many of them are absolutely dedicated to primary prevention. They also have the capability to create, test, and evaluate many of the kinds of interventions that would be invaluable in fighting this disease. Yet almost none of the Division 27, the Division of Community Psychology, regulars was there. What we had was mainly the circle of AIDS researchers and advocates, people who are tireless and totally committed, but who need the help of others. There are opportunities, there are resources, there is a catastrophic problem, and psychologists have something to contribute to its solution. I conclude as I have previously to my colleagues: The world is waiting.

Note

1. In this chapter, the term *AIDS* is used to include HIV infection and the entire course of the disease.

Reference

Marx, J. L. (1988). The AIDS virus can take on many guises. *Science, 241*, 1039–1040.

21

Mental Health Practitioners and Their Roles in the AIDS Crisis

Kathleen Sheridan

Framework

AIDS has often been called a behavioral disease as well as an infectious disease. That behavioral scientists should play a vital role in this health care crisis may seem self-evident, yet we continue to face some obstacles in making a convincing case for our presence. While most observers seem to agree that education and prevention are our only available strategies against transmission of the human immunodeficiency virus, this acknowledgment is quite conditional. That is, once a vaccine against HIV and cures for AIDS are discovered, needs for education and prevention will diminish. Parallel reasoning suggests that only so far as education and prevention go, so go the contributions of behavioral scientists. Beyond education and prevention, opportunities for mental health professionals have been neither vigorously pursued nor eagerly welcomed with any consistency.

The 1988 Vermont Conference on Psychological Approaches to the Prevention of the Acquired Immune Deficiency Syndrome (AIDS) highlighted many avenues for involvement by mental health professionals. This discussion attempts both to broaden our perspectives regarding these opportunities and to concretize some education and training strategies necessary to meet them.

At the outset, it is important to acknowledge my several frames of reference so that readers have a fair opportunity to evaluate this offering in light of their own perspectives. First, my comments about mental health professionals include all of us as a collective group. For instance, I combine clinical and health psychologists, psychiatrists,

Author's Note: This chapter reports work funded in part by NIMH Contract 278–87–004 (ES).

and social workers into that group. Further, I tend to use the phrases *mental health professionals* and *behavioral scientists* interchangeably, although I am exquisitely aware of the tension and debate that arise when someone dares such a global fit. Typically, we devote more energy to distinctions: whether one who interacts with persons can also be at ease with concepts, not to mention numbers and technology; whether clinical observations (with or without counting), program evaluations, and applied and field research are real research; and whether, within the smaller realm of psychology, the scientist-practitioner actually exists.

Second, I am convinced that nothing we do—as scientists, practitioners, or teachers—is value-free (see also Howard, 1985). As one of my first graduate school professors often claimed, "As soon as you're born, at the latest, you've got a point of view." I have in fact never thought it necessary or efficient to claim that what we do is value-free. The influence of values on any endeavor seems ultimately enriching and, "speaking scientifically," at least ought to be recognized for what it contributes to the variance.

The third issue is an applied extension of my second point. Within any context where a mental health professional encounters consumer/client/patient/subject/student/colleague/audience/the public, that professional brings a unique constellation to the situation. Whether one dubs that countertransference (heaven forbid!), habit, or the more colloquial "baggage" is again a value choice. My point is simply that such a constellation needs to be acknowledged and its influences figured into the process and outcome of the encounter.

My fourth point has very practical consequences for me, but that I operate within its framework is not accidental. And it is a point that deserves special attention. As the reader is aware, federal monies for the support of AIDS education for health professionals emanate from at least three sources, the Centers for Disease Control (CDC), Health Resources and Service Administration (HRSA), and the National Institute of Mental Health (NIMH). Some CDC contracts are aimed at blood bank staff and those who work in sexually transmitted disease clinics; CDC has for a long while been the major source of continuing education in AIDS for these line staff. HRSA has aimed its efforts at establishing some nine regional centers to provide a degree of oversight and coordination in AIDS health practitioner education efforts.

NIMH funds 21 practitioner education projects across the country. NIMH emphasizes two focal issues that, while important in the CDC and HRSA initiatives, are not treated with commensurate clarity and weight by them. A major focus of the NIMH efforts is that all education must consider the potentially formidable influences of attitudes, fears, prejudices, and other psychological variables that might affect the rendering of quality professional services. The second major focus is that all AIDS education programs for practitioners contain an evaluative component to assess their effectiveness. Notwithstanding the enormous difficulties inherent in achieving each of these prominent ingredients, the fact of their existence significantly shapes our initiatives.

Behavioral scientists have the potential for critical involvement in every aspect of the AIDS challenge. Further, it is my belief that behavioral scientists should continue to assume leadership aggressively in the many spectra of AIDS. Not only must we concentrate on prevention strategies and their evaluation, we are particularly suited to develop education for the public, for those who are at risk, and, uniquely, for those in health care professions. We have the capacity to create and study health service models. And we must lend our expertise and leadership to understanding the psychosocial factors affecting, and providing psychological interventions for, those who are HIV infected or have AIDS, and their loved ones.

Professional Education and Training Issues in AIDS

Over the past two years, the first nine centers funded by NIMH to provide health practitioner AIDS education set innovative and challenging goals, and undertook an enormous amount of work. Not incidentally, none of this work at Northwestern (and I venture to suggest the same is true for other centers) could occur without NIMH funding. At Northwestern University Medical School, for example, curricular and extracurricular programs were developed and implemented for dental, law, medical, nursing, and graduate clinical psychology students, and for medical, psychology and psychiatry residents.

In addition to the groups traditionally included in the definition of health care practitioners, we deliberately expanded our charge in order to reach key persons in the community whose involvement we considered vital if one of our major goals was to provide quality services. Thus we initially targeted hospital and insurance executives and administrators, police, and the largest religious group in our area, the Archdiocese of Chicago. Our rationale was that to widen access to health resources for those communities where services are not easily available, we needed to enlist the cooperation of police, pastors, and religious school principals to assist us.

Lyons, Sheridan, and Larson (1988–89) developed and described a four-component model for education upon which our practitioner programs have been based. Once target audiences are identified, the content domains are tailored to their respective needs and expectations. Educational modes ideally combine didactic, dialogue, and modeling formats enhanced by audiovisual emphases, print materials, and opportunities for small group discussion and time to process the information. While the programs are all based on in-person presentations, we offer one additional educational service. Often, as a result of or as part of contracting for an AIDS education program, an organization will develop an AIDS policy for its staff and toward the constituents it serves. We have agreed to assist groups in developing such policies.

Essential to this education is the understanding that the factual information is not being presented in a vacuum. The epidemiological, virological, diagnostic, and HIV transmission material, for instance, is highly emotionally laden. A program should incorporate methods for allowing participants to deal with their feelings about the material. Often participants are reluctant to ask questions or to raise their concerns in a large audience. If time and facilities allow, opportunities for small group discussion of the material and feelings might be included. Or paper and pencils might be provided to allow people to write out questions for the presenters rather than ask them aloud.

Since the information is so often difficult to hear, emotionally, repetition of the content is indicated. This repetition can be arranged in a variety of ways. For instance, if the program is incorporated into a series of weekly in-service training seminars, each session can begin with a summary of what was discussed the prior week. Or if the program is incorporated into a graduate curriculum, say, for medical students, the first presentation can be a section in introductory clinical medicine (first year), reviewed as part of blood-drawing techniques (second year), and expanded in the behavioral science sequences (third and fourth years). In many institutional settings, annual or semiannual programs on AIDS can easily incorporate repetition and updating of information.

The outcomes of the program are both short and longer term. The aims are to communicate new knowledge, correct misinformation, and improve accuracy of perceptions of risk. Simple pre- and postprogram questionnaires can provide reasonably accurate evidence that these short-term goals are being met (Sheridan, Phair, McCarthy, Fitzgibbon, & Sheridan, 1988; Sheridan, Sheridan, McCarthy, & Fitzgibbon, 1988). Meeting longer-term goals—retention of knowledge and utilization of that knowledge in helping prevent risk

of HIV infection and in quality service delivery—is much more difficult from an evaluative perspective.

Some generalizations about our short-term outcome evaluations
seem appropriate at this point. Factual information is best communi-
cated when it is relevant and specific to daily situations encountered
by the audience. Much of the correcting of misinformation occurs
around how HIV virus is transmitted and how it is not. Fewer health
care practitioners than expected were as attentive to infection precaution procedures as perhaps they should be (Moretti, Ayer, &
Derefinko, 1988). Short-term education effects also included a higher
degree of certainty about what audiences knew and felt about AIDS in
their workplaces (Sheridan, Lyons, Fitzgibbon, Sheridan, & Mc-
Carthy, 1988).

Currently, follow-up questionnaires are being administered to
groups who attended programs 6–12 months ago. Strategies to evaluate the impact of health practitioner education on actual service delivery to AIDS patients or HIV-infected persons present complex research design questions. However, such evaluation is an essential next
step to which we are committed.

Finally, given our growing experience with AIDS practitioner education, we offer the following observations. First, when a program is
designed for a staff of a discrete organization, such a program will
have its best chance of success if administrative and supervisory personnel also attend. Relatedly, in instances where a longer-term goal
includes development of an organization's policy with regard to HIV-
infected staff or clients, participation by staff in developing such policy and in communicating that policy is very enhancing.

Second, we are aware that audiences who attend most AIDS education programs are self-selected. We have not conducted many mandatory programs; in fact, we advise those with whom we work not to
mandate attendance. Given our limited resources, we have made a
deliberate decision to concentrate on those persons who choose to
attend. Even with our extensive police education program, while police administration requires officers to fill out attendance cards for all
in-service training, we have encouraged the administration not to follow up on those who missed their scheduled AIDS education sessions.
It is, however, interesting to note that nonattendance among police
has been rare.

Third, we have discovered a shared shortcoming with regard to the
various health professional groups with whom we have worked. In
practically every profession in which we might have expected more
expertise—for instance, medicine, nursing, psychiatry, psychology, so-

cial work—there is a glaring inability among practitioners to conduct a thorough sexual history of patients or clients, even when clearly indicated. While this inability is especially vivid in the case of homosexual histories, it is remarkably evident with regard to heterosexual history taking as well (Sheridan & Phair, 1988a).

Fourth, we want to emphasize an important distinction between AIDS education and more specialized clinical training in HIV infection and AIDS. For the most part, I have discussed only AIDS education, basic and preliminary to what needs to be incorporated into professional curricula and continuing education as greater knowledge becomes available and more specialization is necessary.

Finally, practitioner education programs must be knowledgeable about and pay attention to the ethical and legal responsibilities within which audiences operate. Programs must also be cognizant of federal and state legislation affecting persons who are HIV infected or who have AIDS. Particularly important are questions regarding confidentiality and discrimination in medical settings, in employment and educational settings, and with regard to insurance coverage and housing.

Mental Health Leadership Roles in AIDS

The mental health professional can define his or her role as simply or as complexly as seems agreeable or fitting. He or she can lend expertise as scientist, clinician, educator singly or in combination. The universe of potential impact in AIDS can be viewed along two continua. The first ranges from macrolevels to microlevels of influence, extending from wide medico-social-political contexts to the health care delivery level and to the actual clinical encounter. Clearly, at any level(s) within which he or she chooses to exert influence, the professional can again exercise one or any combination of roles.

Medico-Social-Political Contexts

Since AIDS was defined and HIV identified in the early 1980s, many sociopolitical influences have affected timely, sufficient responses to the subsequent health care crisis. Issues within mental health itself have contributed to our somewhat reticent and late involvement in AIDS. These issues deserve recognition and require rectification for our contributions to be more effective. Historically, behavioral scientists and mental health professionals have had relatively little impact within the groups of individuals whom we have identified as being at risk for HIV infection, namely, the gay and bisexual communities, IV drug users (and chemically dependent populations generally), and Blacks and Hispanics. Of course, respective reasons for this inactivity differ.

First, an ambivalent dance continues between the gay and bisexual communities and mental health. Notwithstanding the elimination of homosexuality from diagnostic manuals as a disorder category about ten years ago, questionable attitudes and suspicions persist from the provider side.

Professionals trained, say, prior to the 1970s, particularly in the psychoanalytic mode, still formulate theories of early developmental conflict causing psychosexual fixation at pregenital stages. Thus they seem, at least implicitly, to view homosexuality as a lesser developmental achievement than heterosexuality.

More recent generations of practitioners consider pantheoretical explanations for homosexuality, ranging from biochemical bases (Ellis & Ames, 1987) to political imperatives—nonetheless, they often convey pejorative perspectives. Putting aside what individual professionals or scientists really do think about homosexuality, their attitudes are perceived by many in the gay community as negative or merely tolerant at best. To be sure, resistances to mental health also originate from within the homosexual community itself. However, our focus here is on the provider side of the equation.

Second, intravenous drug abusers have long been identified as a clinical population. Drug abuse, its impact on children, adolescents, and the disadvantaged, and its relationship to crime and violence are prominent subjects for public health initiatives, government commissions, and funded research projects. Nevertheless, IV drug abusers remain one of the groups with whom mental health has had very little success in prevention, treatment, and cure.

Third, the problems of access to health care for Black and Hispanic communities are well documented (Lyons, Hammer, Larson, Visotsky, & Burns, 1987). Access to mental health resources, not to mention relevant mental health resources, appears even more scarce. Our professions, by and large, are not meeting critical needs for these minority communities; nor, importantly, do we attract Blacks and Hispanics to enter our professions as scientists/practitioners. At local levels of influence, the results of our poor performance with these groups have been several. First, in the absence of professionally based resources (perceived or real), the psychosocial aspects of HIV infection and AIDS have been primarily handled by grass-roots, mostly volunteer movements. Early prototypes include the Shanti Project in Berkeley,

the Gay Men's Health Crisis in New York, and the Howard Brown
Memorial Clinic in Chicago. These community-based groups strug-
gled mightily early, but have emerged into quite complex, successful
organizational entities.

Some sad conflicts remain. For instance, in some communities
volunteer-based psychological services are perceived as good, caring,
and supportive, while professionally based services are viewed as
"negative," majoritarian, and institutional, and thus bad. One particularly tragic effect of this rift is the apparent high rate of suicide attempts and successes among seropositive persons or those with AIDS
that have gone unpredicted, undetected, and underreported.

Second, in part due to our lack of success with or absence in potentially high-prevalence communities, public health officials have had
difficulty obtaining hard data regarding rates of HIV infection
among IV drug users (including prostitutes, high percentages of
whom are estimated to be drug users) and Black and Hispanic adults.
We have begun to gather data on IV-drug-abusing pregnant women
who are seropositive and who are minority members (Rich, 1986). We
also know that HIV prevalence is overrepresented in drug-user and
minority communities in New York, New Jersey, Florida, Southern
California, and coastal areas of Texas (Deucher, 1984; Morgan &
Curran, 1986). Nevertheless, behavioral scientists must lead in developing methodologies to determine the extent of the problem, the
needs for services, and their availability in minority and underserved
communities (R. S. Boruch, personal communication, February 2,
1988).

Health Care Delivery Systems

Two of many AIDS issues that require data-based analyses are models of care and costs of care. Only recently have health care providers
considered the possibility that AIDS demands service delivery systems
of a different nature from what is currently available. The working
assumption (probably well founded in economic reality) has been that
existing resources should be reallocated to accommodate AIDS.

Although several studies are in process, only two models have been
examined in any consistent way—the San Francisco General Hospital
model and the New York City hospitals model, the latter really reflecting traditional inpatient care. For a time, Houston, Texas had an
AIDS hospital, a project probably not very thoughtfully conceived,
that was forced to close because of uncompensated costs of care for

indigent patients ("AIDS Hospital," 1987). Both coastal models were developed under siege of the crisis as it hit San Francisco and New York. Thus services emerged out of need, not out of planning.

In the past three years, the hospice case management philosophy has been touted as the model alternative to inpatient care for persons with AIDS. Yet, little empirical evidence exists to support the hospice philosophy as a preferred model (Brooks, 1983; Haid, Fowley, Nicklin, & Letourneau, 1984; Lyons et al., 1987; Lyons, Von Roenn, Sheridan, & Anderson, 1988). A critical need, then, is evaluation of service delivery for HIV and AIDS, ranging from antibody test sites to ambulatory treatment centers, hospice and home-based care, extended care—skilled and custodial—and inpatient resources, including integrated and segregated systems.

Cost-benefit analyses must include at least four questions. Who are the consumers and what are their needs? What services work best for what kinds of consumers, using a complexity of outcome measures (resource utilization, economic and psychological costs, quality of care, quality of life, quality of death)? Who pays (or who should pay) for such services—the patient, private insurers, employers, state or federal resources, or some combination of all resources? How ought health care resources be newly designed or reallocated in light of projections of health care needs in the next five to ten years?

Thorough cost analyses by Hardy, Rauch, Echenberg, Morgan, and Curran (1986) and Scitovsky and Rice (1987) projected $8 billion to $16 billion in health care costs by 1992 for approximately 175,000 AIDS cases. These projections, however, reflect 1984 dollars and are based on the coastal care models. Long-term, prospective service delivery analyses are vital now if we are to prepare adequately for the numbers of expected AIDS patients in the 1990s. Cost analyses that factor in the effects of treatment such as zidovudine (not available during the earlier studies) on prolonging patient life, of better and earlier diagnoses of clinical manifestations of AIDS, and of growing reliance on ambulatory and other alternative care models must be continuing enterprises.

Biopsychosocial multidisciplinary approaches. Any delivery system that would attempt to confront AIDS from a purely infectious disease perspective or a solely medical perspective is very inefficient and unresponsive. (At this point in our experience, it is difficult to believe that the adjective *biopsychosocial* was not coined exclusively in response to AIDS.) Any quality response must be comprehensive, integrated, and multidisciplinary. Development and evaluation of innovative models of care are enterprises waiting for our participation.

Sheridan and Phair (1988b) describe a model AIDS biopsychosocial program as a confluence of services, basic and applied research, education, and clinical training. Jointly directed by psychology and infectious diseases, the ambulatory services program includes antibody testing and counseling, zidovudine clinics, psychological services (group psychotherapy; stress management; psychological and neuropsychological assessment; couple, individual, and family therapies; and support groups for health practitioners), and legal and dental services or referrals. Closely relating to ambulatory care are hospice and nonsegregated inpatient programs.

Disciplines represented include clinical and health psychology, infectious diseases, internal medicine, oncology, psychiatry, virology, law, dentistry, pediatrics, neurology, hematology, immunology, nursing, and social work. Opportunities for direct services, research, and clinical training at the practicum, clerkship, residency, and postdoctoral levels can be available for all specialties.

The Consumer-Provider Encounter

The second continuum from which to view the various ways mental health professionals can be involved takes place at the micro level, the encounter, suggested by the first continuum. At this level a variety of person-to-person encounters can occur between, say, the psychologist and group therapy members, researcher and subject, educator and audience, or colleague and colleague.

This second continuum views the disease process longitudinally, at a point before HIV infection, during the life of HIV infection through progression to AIDS, and to the outcome stage. Sheridan and Sheridan (1988) have described the potential roles of psychologists as consultants to persons who are HIV positive and who have AIDS. The present discussion will focus on more general issues at each point along the continuum.

Prevention and education. With regard to prevention efforts, Joseph et al. (1987) and Ekstrand and Coates (1988) have shown sturdy positive changes in risk-related behaviors among homosexual males in Chicago and San Francisco. Prevention and its evaluation, to repeat the obvious, are crucial. Serious challenges remain, however, in prevention strategies and evaluation methods with regard to others presumed to be at high risk for HIV infection, including IV drug users and minority members, particularly the young and the underserved.

Behavioral scientists have rich backgrounds to apply to the area of public education about AIDS. Mass media endeavors, from polished

368   Kathleen Sheridan

products to public service announcements, can benefit from our understanding of marketing techniques for intended audiences and evaluation of the effectiveness of the messages. With a more selected segment, behavioral scientists should be more appreciative than any other professional group about the complex dynamics that depict the groups we have categorized as the "worried well."

Process of infection. When working with persons who are HIV infected, we need to proceed with considerable flexibility and juggle some assumptions we may have applied to other populations we encounter in mental health. First, we cannot assume that a generalized psychological profile fits all HIV-infected individuals. Nor can we assume that membership in a group at risk—for example, homosexuals or pregnant teenagers—implies a group psychological profile applicable to each member of that group. Second, we cannot assume that an HIV-infected person has a preinfection history of psychological conflicts or, indeed, of psychiatric diagnoses.

On the other hand, we may err just as readily by borrowing too much from another arena, that of the medical patient. Unquestionably, work with psychosocial components in nonpsychiatric illness contains a wealth of valuable information relevant for infected persons or those with AIDS. But some specific differences may be important.

The first HIV-infected persons and AIDS patients generally came from the homosexual community. Relative to the typical medical patient, members of this group appear more informed about and more assertive and collaborative in planning their treatment, and may or may not enjoy quality, supportive persons to help them cope with infection or AIDS. Hemophiliac seropositive patients, even though they bring long histories of familiarity with medical care, present some unique and complex motivational problems. As part of adapting to an illness, hemophilia, which potentially shortens their lives, these men often marry at young ages, with specific intent to have children. Many hemophiliacs acknowledge that having children is a way to prolong their lives symbolically. Seropositivity presents these patients with a serious impediment; proceeding with the important goal of procreation may jeopardize the health of spouses and offspring.

If we accept any psychodynamic explanations about chemical dependency, we can suggest that IV drug users engage in behaviors that have both self-soothing (perceived) and self-destructive (real) qualities. If that suggestion is accurate, expecting that these patients will be responsible, compliant health care consumers when seropositivity is diagnosed seems very unrealistic.

The body of knowledge about AIDS is rapidly growing and changing. Keeping current with relevant developments may be an unmeetable challenge. For instance, a serious mental health problem that illustrates this knowledge explosion concerns differential diagnosis of functional and neuropsychological concomitants to infection and AIDS. Early reports based on autopsy (Navia & Price, 1987) suggested serious organic involvement in AIDS, and led to a syndrome named AIDS dementia complex (Price, Sidtis, & Rosenblum, 1988). Next came the suspicion that symptoms of this complex were detectable early on in the disease process, perhaps appearing prior to any other clinical manifestation of AIDS. Most of us began to estimate the incidence of neurological complications in persons infected or those with AIDS with guesses ranging from 10% to 65%, often basing our estimates on studies using very small samples (e.g., Grant et al., 1987).

Recent data from the Multicenter AIDS Cohort Study based on comparisons between 819 seropositive and 836 seronegative homosexual men (Selnes et al., 1988) do not demonstrate statistically significant prevalence of neuropsychological abnormalities in *healthy* HIV-infected men over seronegative subjects. These new data clearly add important information based on many more subjects that temper, refine, and raise additional areas of inquiry about the neuropsychological implications of HIV infection and of AIDS. These new data have certainly reinforced the wisdom of large sample studies, replication, and the value of longitudinal investigations of the disease process.

We strongly suspect that psychological interventions are important resources for infected persons and those with AIDS and that such interventions can be best provided by mental health professionals or with consultation and support from us. We are very aware, as discussed earlier, that this assertion runs counter to the opinions of some interest groups, who suggest that psychosocial care can and should be handled primarily by families, friends, and religious and community groups. Psychosocial care does not need the professional or scientific presence that medical care requires. Other interest groups suggest that professional involvement is patronizing, formalistic, stereotyping, and, thus, not genuinely *caring*.

Nevertheless, valuable interventions exist that need expertise to implement and empirically verify. Depending on the personality and environmental resources available to a person who is infected or who has AIDS, a variety of interventions are possible. Some people may not need or want assistance at all. Some may derive maximal benefit from support groups. Others can learn many valuable coping strategies via stress management. Still others can be best served by referral to established chemical dependency programs, if abuse issues are prominent.

Working with this medical population requires therapeutic flexibility and a willingness to consider a variety of interventions, in which patients often wish to participate concurrently. It is common for patients to attend group therapy, stress management, acupuncture, imaging, and relaxation programs simultaneously. Working with persons who have AIDS, particularly those who are nearing end stages of the disease, requires that the mental health professional maintain a sensitive balance as both therapist and educator/advocate. In the latter role, the therapist may play a more directive, advice-giving part than he or she is accustomed to, or would play with other persons. For instance, direct advice to consider living wills, or to establish durable powers of attorney, or initiation of discussion of do-not-resuscitate orders may be indicated with some patients. Therapists may, at the suggestion or with the consent of the patient, meet with lovers, friends, and family—practices less often considered with other populations.

Outcomes. Clinical outcomes for infected persons or those with AIDS are varied. A determination that a person is HIV positive typically means a lifetime of concern and monitoring of that individual's health status. Such a process inherently suggests tension, stress, anxiety, depression, and interpersonal difficulties. Progressive deterioration of cognitive and other physical functions requires other dramatic life adjustments, including educational goals, employment, financial planning, and quality-of-life issues. Awareness of and preparation for death are poignant periods that test the compassionate capacity of the caregiver. Death requires special attention to the bereavement period, surely by the mental health professional, and likely involves other caregivers and family and friends of the deceased.

Importantly, mental health professionals are not immune from the effects of working with dying persons. Even if all other countertransference issues (e.g., homophobia, prejudice) are acknowledged or resolved, the prospect of death and our helplessness to prevent its occurrence are issues that profoundly affect us and our relationships with AIDS patients.

No matter the point at which the behavioral scientist encounters AIDS, and no matter what combination of roles that person chooses to exercise, the professional must appreciate that interdisciplinary collaboration is essential. The mental health professional vis-á-vis his or her peer in oncology, or infectious diseases, or epidemiology, or nursing is a collaborator, a student, and a teacher. He or she is particularly poised to be a source of emotional support. This contribution is a singular benefit that mental health can provide. Understanding human motivation, the interplay of attitudes, feelings, and interpersonal behavior is the essential strength of any health care system.

For instance, the mental health professional can be a valuable member of the team that interviews prospective staff and helps weigh, on a case-by-case basis, which applicants would be successful. Sensitive motivational issues are involved. Should a health care professional whose lover, spouse, brother, or sister is HIV positive or who has AIDS or who has died be hired? Are the motivations of the professional who is a member of a risk group—say, a homosexual, a hemophiliac, an ex-addict—potentially constructive or detrimental? What about the psychological, not physical, strengths of the staff member who is seropositive or who has AIDS? The mental health team member can be particularly alert to issues of overidentification between staff and patients, and can prepare staff for potential difficulties in dealing with some patients. For instance, some staff find it very difficult to deal empathically with a drug-using pregnant woman who is seropositive and already has an infant who is seropositive or who has AIDS.

Presentation of these two continua and discussion of some of their points are necessarily incomplete in explication and inclusiveness. It is my hope that each issue raised will catalyze more questions for behavioral scientists to answer and more areas on which they can have an impact. The opportunities for creative, collegial influence are limitless and crucial—both before and after vaccines and cures for HIV and AIDS are discovered.

Recommendations and Conclusions

The messages in this discussion are simple, straightforward challenges. The universe of human issues surrounding AIDS calls for strong leadership to provide solutions. This leadership is available in the behavioral sciences. Consequently, we are obligated to educate ourselves, our colleagues, and the public, and to work with those at risk, who are infected, and who are ill. We are obligated to generate health delivery systems capable of rendering quality care to all persons affected by AIDS, and, through education and its empirical test, eliminate social, political, and economic barriers to such care. We are obligated to bring to person-to-person encounters informed diagnostic skills, selected therapeutic strategies, willing collaboration, genuine self-knowledge and reflection, and respect for people in life and in death.

References

AIDS hospital a failure. (1987, November). *Register Report, 14*, 14.

Brooks, C. H. (1983). The potential cost savings of hospice care: A review of the literature. *Health Matrix, 1*, 49–55.

Deucher, N. (1984). AIDS in New York City with particular reference to the psychosocial aspects. *British Journal of Psychiatry, 145*, 612–619.

Ekstrand, M. L., & Coates, T. J. (1988). Prevalence and change in AIDS high risk behavior among gay and bisexual men [Abstract]. *Proceedings of the IVth International Conference on AIDS*, Book 1, 466.

Ellis, L., & Ames, M. A. (1987). Neurohormonal functioning and sexual orientation: A theory of homosexuality-heterosexuality. *Psychological Bulletin, 101*, 233–258.

Grant, I., Atkinson, J. H., Hesselink, J. R., Kennedy, C. J., Richman, D. D., Spector, S. S., & McCutchan, J. A. (1987). Evidence for early central nervous system involvement in acquired immune deficiency syndrome (AIDS) and other human immunodeficiency virus (HIV) infections: Studies with neurophysiologic testing and magnetic resonance imagery. *Annals of Internal Medicine, 107*, 828–836.

Haid, M., Fowley, M., Nicklin, O., & Letourneau, E. (1984). People and dollars: The experience of one hospice. *Southern Journal of Medicine, 77*, 470–472.

Hardy, A. M., Rauch, K., Echenberg, D., Morgan, W. M., & Curran, J. W. (1986). The economic impact of the first 10,000 cases of acquired immune deficiency syndrome in the United States. *Journal of the American Medical Association, 255*, 209–215.

Howard, G. S. (1985). The role of values in the science of psychology. *American Psychologist, 40*, 255–265.

Joseph, J. G., Montgomery, S. B., Emmons, C., Kessler, R. C., Ostrow, D. G., Wortman, C. B., O'Brien, K., Eller, M., & Eshleman, S. (1987). Magnitude and determinants of behavioral risk reduction: Longitudinal analysis of a cohort at risk for AIDS. *Psychology and Health, 1*, 73–95.

Lyons, J. S., Hammer, J. S., Larson, D. B., Visotsky, H. M., & Burns, B. (1987). Impact of prospective payment on psychosocial services in the general hospital. *Medical Care, 25*, 140–147.

Lyons, J. S., Sheridan, K., & Larson, D. (1988–89). An AIDS educational model for health care professionals. *Journal of Health Education, 19*, 12–15.

Lyons, J. S., Von Roenn, J., Sheridan, E. P., & Anderson, B. A. (1988). *Comparing hospital and hospice charges for persons with AIDS: A pilot study.* Unpublished manuscript.

Moretti, R. J., Ayer, W. A., & Derefinko, A. J. (1988). *Dentists' attitudes and practices regarding HIV patients.* Manuscript submitted for publication.

Morgan, W. M., & Curran, J. W. (1986). Acquired Immunodeficiency Syndrome: Current and future trends. *Public Health Reports, 101*, 459–465.

Navia, B. A., & Price, R. W. (1987). The Acquired Immune Deficiency Syndrome dementia complex as the presenting or sole manifestation of human immunodeficiency virus infection. *Archives of Neurology, 44*, 65–69.

Price, R. W., Sidtis, J. J., & Rosenblum, M. (1988). The AIDS dementia complex: Some current questions. *Annals of Neurology, 23*(Suppl.), S27-S33.

Rich, K. C. (1986). Immunologic function and AIDS in drug exposed infants. In I. J. Chasnoff (Ed.), *Drug use in pregnancy*. Lancaster, England: MTP.

Scitovsky, A. A., & Rice, D. P. (1987). AIDS: The cost in dollars. *Internist, 28*, 9–15.

Selnes, O. A., Miller, E. N., Becker, J. T., Cohen, B. A., McArthur, J. C., Visscher, B., Gordon, B., Satz, P., Ginzburg, H. M., & Polk, B. F. (1988). Normal neuropsychological performance in healthy HIV-1 infected homosexual men: The Multicenter AIDS Cohort Study (MACS) [Abstract]. *Proceedings of the IVth International Conference on AIDS*, Book 2, 399.

Sheridan, K., Lyons, J. S., Fitzgibbon, M., Sheridan, E. P., & McCarthy, M. (1988). *Effects of an AIDS education program on police knowledge and perceptions of risk*. Manuscript submitted for publication.

Sheridan, K., & Phair, J. P. (1988a). *AIDS: A paradigm for the doctor-patient relationship*. Manuscript submitted for publication.

Sheridan, K., & Phair, J. P. (1988b). AIDS biopsychosocial services: A comprehensive health care delivery model [Abstract]. *Proceedings of the IVth International Conference on AIDS*, Book 1, 484.

Sheridan, K., Phair, J. P., McCarthy, M., Fitzgibbon, M., & Sheridan, E. P. (1988). AIDS education: A midwestern U.S. city's response [Abstract]. *Proceedings of the IVth International Conference on AIDS*, Book 1, 362.

Sheridan, K., & Sheridan, E. P. (1988). Psychological consultation to persons with AIDS. *Professional Psychology: Research and Practice, 19*, 532–535.

Sheridan, K., Sheridan, E. P., McCarthy, M., & Fitzgibbon, M. (1988). Effect of AIDS education on police knowledge and attitudes [Abstract]. *Proceedings of the IVth International Conference on AIDS*, Book 1, 365.

22

Components of a Comprehensive Strategy for Reducing the Risk of AIDS in Adolescents

June A. Flora
Carl E. Thoresen

The threat of an AIDS epidemic among America's youth is an ever increasing public health concern (Institute of Medicine, 1986). While the number of adolescents with AIDS is relatively small and the presence of the human immunodeficiency virus among teens is unknown, the risks are considerable (Centers for Disease Control, 1988b). Ways to prevent HIV transmission as well as AIDS can be viewed from many different theoretical and intervention perspectives, such as psychosocial, communication, or public health viewpoints. Given various perspectives, the unclear theoretical bases of most current efforts to prevent HIV transmission, and the range of groups at risk (e.g., Black females, Hispanic males, runaways), we argue that a comprehensive intervention concerning AIDS-related issues and youth is urgently needed.

This comprehensive strategy is derived from the following assumptions: (a) that effective intervention must be derived from theory, particularly theory that explains human behavior as the ongoing interaction of cognitive, behavioral, physiological, and sociocultural (contextual) influences; (b) that to reach multiple audiences and to sustain programs over time, strategies for prevention of AIDS should include multiple levels of intervention, varying from individuals, social net-

Authors' Note: We wish to thank Susan Blake, Ph.D., at the American Red Cross in Washington, D.C., and Joel Killen, Ph.D., at the Stanford Center for Research in Disease Prevention, for their comments on earlier drafts of this chapter. Reprint requests should be addressed to June A. Flora, Ph.D., Institute for Communication Research, McClatchy Hall, Stanford University, Stanford, CA 94305.

works (e.g., family, peer group), and local organizations (e.g., schools, religious organizations, social organizations and clubs) to whole communities (e.g., mass media, political and governmental organizations); (c) that interventions must be integrated in such a way as to capitalize on the unique features both within and between levels, so that additive and synergistic effects are obtained; and (d) that methods for tailoring messages/programs to the special needs of population subgroups (e.g., high-risk youth, Black teens, females) are required.

We will discuss the problems of AIDS relevant to adolescents, identifying high-risk behaviors and population subgroups. Because of the current lack of carefully evaluated behavior-change-oriented AIDS prevention efforts with adolescents, we will review relevant facets of other prevention efforts, such as teenage pregnancy prevention, smoking prevention, and cardiovascular disease (CVD) risk reduction. Finally, we review components of a comprehensive AIDS prevention strategy (Flora & Thoresen, 1988).

The Problem

The risks of AIDS in adolescents emerge from epidemiologic data on HIV infection, contraceptive use, sexual behavior, sexually transmitted diseases (STDs), and substance use. First we will examine risks for adolescents and then review how these risks prevail in particular adolescent subgroups.

The implications of risk for HIV in adolescents include the following:

(1) While few cases of AIDS exist in adolescents, a large proportion (21%) of the current AIDS cases are found in young adults in their 20s. Given the long incubation period between HIV infection and an AIDS diagnosis (estimated to be an average of seven years) these young adults were probably infected while teenagers (Centers for Disease Control, 1988b). Thus some of the current cases of AIDS may have been contracted while the individuals were adolescents.

(2) Unprotected sexual intercourse increases the risk of becoming infected with HIV (Centers for Disease Control, 1988a). While there are gender and race variations, recent surveys of the age of first intercourse in females find that by age 15 approximately 18% have had intercourse. This rate increases by about 10% a year, until at age 19, 66% have engaged in sexual intercourse (Hayes, 1987; Hofferth, Kahn, & Baldwin, 1987; Smith, Nenney, & McGill, 1986; Zelnik & Kanter, 1980). Approximately 10–20% (varying somewhat by popula-

tion and year) more males than females are engaging in sexual intercourse every year until age 20 (Hayes, 1987). Black males and females are engaging in sexual activity earlier and attain higher rates of nonvirginity by age 16 (Furstenberg, Morgan, Moore, & Peterson, 1987). Of unmarried, sexually active women aged 15–19, 27% have never used any method of birth control and 39% have used a method but not every time (compiled by the Center for Population Options, cited in Hersch, 1988). In a recent study of teens attending a clinic, 27% of female and 41% of male middle-class teens reported using condoms at least once, but only 2% of females and 8% of males used condoms regularly (Kegeles, Adler, & Irwin, 1988). In general, most studies of teen contraceptive use find that the earlier the age of onset of sexual activity, the greater the likelihood that no contraceptive will be used at time of first intercourse.

Little is known about the sexual behavior of teens, such as how many have intercourse only once, frequency of intercourse, number of partners, and the nature of the relationship with the first partner (Brooks-Gunn, Boyer, & Hein, 1988). However, in one study focused on teens 15 years of age or older, at least one-third report having sex once a week or more (Hofferth & Hayes, 1987). In another study, of those who are sexually active, over 50% report having had two or more partners (Zelnik, 1983).

There are few data on the numbers of adolescents who identify themselves as homosexual or have had some homosexual experience, but those data that are available indicate that a significant proportion of teenage men (5–8%) may have had some homosexual experience and that their partners were several years older (average 7 years) than they, providing a bridge to potentially infected adults (Brooks-Gunn et al., 1988; Remafedi, 1987; Sorensen, 1973).

(3) Another indicator of high-risk behavior in teens is the rate of contraction of sexually transmitted diseases. The incidence of these diseases has been increasing sharply; approximately 2.5 million teenagers are infected with an STD each year (Centers for Disease Control, 1988b). In fact, 10–24-year-olds accounted for 62.5% of gonorrhea cases and 40% of syphilis cases in 1985 (Center for Population Options, cited in Hersch, 1988). Overall, sexually active adolescents have the highest rates of STDs of all age groups.

(4) Intravenous drug use is also a risk factor for HIV infection. Currently, 25% of all adult and adolescent cases of acquired immunodeficiency syndrome in the United States are IV drug users. The percentage of AIDS among heterosexual IV drug users is growing. These cases are heavily concentrated along the East Coast, and

have been reported in 50 states, the District of Columbia, and Puerto Rico. Blacks and Hispanics are overrepresented among heterosexual IV drug users with AIDS; Blacks account for 51% of cases (Blacks constitute 12% of the U.S. population) and 30% are Hispanic/Latino (6% of the population) (Schuster, 1988).

While reliable data are often lacking, the potential risk for teenagers clearly exists. A small number of high school students in a nationally representative sample recently reported IV drug use, but 57% reported having tried illicit drugs, with a third having tried drugs other than marijuana (Johnston, Bachman, & O'Malley, 1987). Longitudinal studies of cohorts of adolescents implicate tobacco and alcohol as gateway substances to marijuana and harder drugs (Schuster, 1988). While the number of adolescents using IV drugs is currently small, there is greater risk for teens who use tobacco and alcohol. Further, nearly 30% of all students will drop out before high school graduation. Youths who have dropped out have higher rates of intravenous drug use than those in school (Center for Population Options, cited in Hersch, 1988). The concern about IV drug use is not only for infection among users but also for potential spread of the virus to their sexual partners and their children.

High-Risk Populations

While risk of HIV infection exists for many teens, it is particularly great in some subgroups: runaway youth, Black and Hispanic adolescents, and youth who live in economically deprived communities. Consider runaway teens, disenfranchised youth who occupy the streets of most large urban centers in this country. Over a million adolescents run away each year; more than half of these run away at least three times. More than 180,000 runaways are involved in illegal activities such as drug use, prostitution, and drug trafficking. Shelters serve less than half of this population. It is estimated that there are from 20,000 to 40,000 homeless youth in New York City alone, and 1.2 million nationwide (Hersch, 1988). These disenfranchised youth are at risk for HIV from drugs and unsafe sexual activity and are likely to pose risks for their sexual partners (both those on the streets and those with whom they come in contact as they reenter the community).

Being Black or Hispanic/Latino and living in urban and economically deprived areas constitute considerable increased risk for HIV (Centers for Disease Control, 1986). Blacks and Hispanics/Latinos suffer a dramatically higher prevalence of AIDS: 25% and 24%, respectively, of all reported cases. As mentioned earlier, Blacks and Hispanics are more likely to have acquired AIDS from IV drug use or from being partners of IV drug users (Centers for Disease Control, 1986). Black teens in particular are at high risk, because they engage in sexual intercourse at a younger age and at higher rates than do Whites or Hispanics until age 20. Early onset of intercourse is associated with longer periods of unprotected sex (Zelnik & Kanter, 1980).

Education and economic factors are related to adolescents' sexual behaviors (as well as their attitudes, values, and knowledge) (Hayes, 1987). Mothers' educational attainment and age of onset of sexual activity are related. In addition, sexual activity has been shown to vary with high school dropout rate (especially for Black females) (Hayes, 1987). Finally, Black and Hispanic teens in San Francisco are roughly twice as likely to misunderstand how HIV is transmitted than White teenagers (DiClemente, Boyer, & Morales, 1988). These race-, ethnic-, socioeconomic status-, and gender-specific factors point out the critical need to understand the "consumers" of AIDS prevention programs and to tailor programs to meet the needs of these groups.

Overall, adolescents remain ignorant or confused about the causes and the preventive behaviors relevant to AIDS (DiClemente et al., 1988; DiClemente, Zorn, & Temoshok, 1986). Further, youth have distorted views of their own vulnerability. For example, after exposure to intensive media coverage of AIDS in Northern California, adolescents did not report changing their sexual behavior (Kegeles et al., 1988). Indeed, their use of condoms actually diminished over time following exposure to AIDS information. In a study of youth living in Boston, of those who changed their behavior, only one in five changed it in effective ways (Strunin & Hingson, 1987).

These data indicate that teens are at risk for HIV infection, and some population subgroups are at even greater risk. Further, there are many barriers to reaching youth to teach them about safe behavior (e.g., runaways) and to inducing and maintaining behavior change (e.g., social and cultural mores, skill in relationships, addiction, perceived risk). Youth who live outside of the structure of the home and school, engage in high-risk behaviors (i.e., having multiple partners, unprotected sex, and IV drug use), and have limited access to information and health services are at increased risk of being exposed to HIV, of transmitting the virus to their children, and of exposing their sexual partners to increased risk.

Levels of Intervention

Much of public health practice is predicated on the belief that health behavior is the result of influences at many levels of analysis. Interventions can and should be conducted at each of these levels. Most intervention research in the health area targets individual-level changes and employs individual-level change strategies (Abrams, Elder, Carlton, Lasater, & Artz, 1986; Thoresen, 1984). Higher-level change strategies involving groups, organizations, and communities are much rarer. While more research is needed for a better understanding of the reciprocal nature of micro- and macro-level factors, much can be learned by examining the elements that enhance or accelerate social change processes within each level (e.g., school-based smoking prevention, classroom sex education, and community-based reduction of teenage pregnancy).

In a recent report from the Office of Technology Assessment of the U.S. Congress (1988), it was recommended that AIDS prevention programs for youth should be integrated into more comprehensive communitywide programs, including school, parents, media, and youth and family agencies. While many prevention efforts are currently under way, few are well evaluated and fewer still examine the effects of education on behavior (U.S. Congress, 1988). Because of the lack of data on current efforts and urgent need to understand behavior change related to AIDS prevention, we examine three areas of behavior change: prevention of teenage pregnancy, substance abuse prevention, and cardiovascular disease prevention.

Sex Education and Pregnancy Prevention Programs

Three main streams of research and treatment can be identified in the sex education and pregnancy prevention literature: individual or classroom instruction, school-based health clinics (SBCs), and school- or community wide programs. Even though interventions take place at different levels, all are aimed at changing the behavior of adolescents. For example, sex education typically focuses on individual students, attempting to alter sex-related behavior via social, cognitive, and sometimes emotional changes.

Classroom and Group Approaches

The most commonly used strategy to change adolescent sexual behavior is a classroom-based approach. While well-controlled empirical studies of sex education are scarce and the findings are often contradictory, most researchers agree that sex education seems to influence some interim objectives (e.g., knowledge) but does not change others (e.g., beliefs about one's own sexual behavior or attitudes about premarital sex or birth control); more important, sex education does not appear to change sexual behavior significantly (either to increase or decrease sexual activity) (Kirby, 1984, 1985). There is some limited evidence suggesting that certain subgroups who receive sex education are more likely to use contraceptives at first intercourse and less likely to experience unintended pregnancy (Zelnik & Kim, 1982).

Classroom- or school-based efforts have not proven as effective as generally hoped. Several researchers have noted that such programs typically focus on providing sex-related information and, less frequently, on increasing access to birth control (Kirby, 1985). Most classroom- or school-based efforts do not include behavioral skills training, inoculation against peer and other pressures to have sex, problem solving, or behavioral rehearsal.

The efforts of Schinke and Gilchrist and their colleagues offer a promising exception to the traditional information-based classroom strategy (see, for example, Gilchrist & Schinke, 1983; Schinke, 1984; Schinke, Blythe, & Gilchrist, 1981). In one study, ten 50-minute classroom sessions were provided to 15–16-year-old students in a sex education program that highlighted the integration of information, understanding, and skills training in targeted problem-solving situations. Compared to students in the control condition, those participating in the special program increased knowledge about sex and contraception, improved attitudes about safer sex practices, and actually behaved more effectively in videotaped simulations focused on selected situations, such as talking with possible partners about sex and use of contraceptives. Noteworthy of this work is the use of a well-grounded theoretical rationale—cognitive behavioral theory—with the consequence that students were explicitly instructed in how to alter their behaviors through skills training in such areas as how to discuss sex with a partner, how to make agreements (contracts), and how to resist having sex under certain conditions. While major outcomes of these programs remain unknown (e.g., actual use of contraceptives, reduced frequency of multiple sex partners, changes in pregnancy rates), the results provide a useful example of how to use a well-conceived theoretical framework focused on change processes (not just the acquisition of information) and how such a framework provides guidance in what should be the ingredients of a prevention program.

Individually Oriented Programs in School-Based Clinics

SBCs represent a different model for change, but also attempt to modify contraceptive and sexual behavior. The focus or level of treatment in SBCs remains at the individual level. Parents, school district trustees, and other community groups are usually involved, but they are not considered major targets of the intervention. Studies of the effectiveness of SBCs are to date limited. However, two studies offer promising results. Edwards, Steinman, Arnold, and Hakanson (1980) report a notable decrease in adolescent pregnancy rates in an SBC in Minneapolis—a reduction of over 60% (79/1,000 to 26/1,000) during a decade (1973–1983). In the second study, a school-related clinic program in Baltimore achieved increases in knowledge and use of contraceptives, and after 28 months a 30% decrease in pregnancy rates in treatment schools, compared to a 58% increase in control schools (Zabin, Hirsch, Smith, Street, & Hardy, 1986). Particularly impressive in this study was the result that adolescents attending the SBC delayed their onset of sexual intercourse by an average of seven months. Thus the fear that sex-related education programs or services would increase sexual activities in adolescents has not been supported (Dryfoos & Klerman, 1988; Zabin et al., 1986).

Community-Based Prevention

Community wide interventions combine individuals, classrooms, schools, and other community groups and institutions. To date only one community-based program to prevent adolescent pregnancy has been reported. This innovative and successful example involves students, parents, teachers, ministers and other church representatives, community leaders, and local health officials (Vincent, Clearie, & Schlucheter, 1987). Over a period of 2 to 3 years there was a 36% decline in average estimated pregnancy rates in the treated portion of a county in South Carolina, a 14% decline in a comparison portion of the target county, and 6–16% increase in three comparison counties. Although the relative contributions of each intervention component are not reported, it is significant that an integrated preventive social and education effort across several community institutions was associated with reducing rates of pregnancy.

The successes and failures of pregnancy prevention programs at the individual, group, and community levels have several implications for AIDS prevention programs. The results of the research reviewed indicate that (a) programs based on knowledge alone are not effective in inducing behavior change; (b) efforts that incorporate skills training (e.g., developing resistance skills, behavioral rehearsal, social modeling with performance feedback) are likely to improve the chances of obtaining behavior change; (c) approaches that integrate individual and school, family, and institutional efforts are likely to achieve greater behavior change; (d) current research contributes little to our understanding of how to tailor messages or to utilize appropriate channels of communication to reach different audience subgroups; and (e) with rare exception, current research is not clearly based on a theoretical rationale focused on altering behavior and contexts.

School-Based Smoking Prevention Programs

School-based smoking (and substance abuse) prevention offers some important lessons for AIDS prevention in adolescents. After a period of little success in prevention, researchers began in the 1970s to focus on the social influences associated with the onset of smoking in adolescents. These influences included peers, family, and the media. In the first study of its kind, Evans and colleagues (1974) used social inoculation theory (McGuire, 1964) to teach adolescents how to counter the persuasive social pressures to smoke. Principles of social and participant modeling, focused feedback, and guided behavioral rehearsal derived from Bandura's (1977) social learning theory were combined with inoculation theory to create a comprehensive theoretical framework to guide the design of smoking prevention programs. Through the use of older trained peers as group leaders to deliver part of the program that includes active role playing and social reinforcement of counterarguing techniques to resist pressures to smoke, this line of research has demonstrated that young adolescents can learn how to reduce the risk of starting to smoke (Evans et al., 1974; Telch, Killen, McAlister, Perry, & Maccoby, 1982). Studies have demonstrated a delay of onset of smoking of 30%-70%, over periods of up to 5 years. These results have been reported in several regions of the United States and in several other countries (e.g., Norway, Australia, and Finland).

Smoking prevention programs offer a viable framework for designing school- or classroom-based AIDS prevention programs. As in pregnancy prevention research, less has been learned about how to tailor programs to subgroups of the intended clientele. For example, Hansen, Marotte, and Fielding (1988) reported overall success in preventing smoking in adolescents, but the rate of success differed considerably for different populations and for different schools. The program was more effective for females than for males and was most effective with White students. In fact, at the 4-year follow-up only White students showed a significantly lower rate of smoking. For Asian, Native American, and Black students, there were no differences between treatment schools and the control schools. Further, some schools showed treatment effects while others failed to demonstrate changes.

The experience in smoking prevention studies can provide valuable theoretical, programmatic, and methodological guidance for future AIDS prevention studies with adolescents. Specifically, smoking studies suggest that (a) social psychological theories, such as cognitive social learning theory (Bandura, 1986) and social inoculation theory (McGuire, 1964), can serve as effective guides for program development; (b) the classroom and the school can be effective channels for influencing the behavior of adolescents; (c) high-status peers are often effective in delivering much of a prevention program to students; and (d) different programs may need to be designed for various audiences (e.g., based on gender, race, and ethnicity).

Community-Based Approaches to Reducing Cardiovascular Disease

Recently, Perry, Klepp, and Shultz (1988) advocated community wide approaches for primary prevention of CVD in adolescents. The benefits of a community approach include (a) the capability of reaching a broad spectrum of adolescents and families, (b) the ability to target adolescents at all levels of risk, and (c) the flexibility of allowing for the possibility of other changes in the community (structural and normative) that may, in turn, alleviate and change risk. To date, there have been few population wide community-based prevention programs that have been specifically designed for youth. However, each of the three national CVD prevention community studies have youth components (Blackburn et al., 1984; Farquhar et al., 1985; Lasater et al., 1984). Each of these programs has integrated youth programs into overall efforts to bring about positive changes in individuals, families, health professions, and community institutions. The following discussion will consider some examples from one of these programs.

The Stanford Five City Project (FCP) is a 14-year field trial investigating the efficacy of community wide health education to reduce the risk of cardiovascular disease through the use of mass media and face-to-face education. The FCP is an outgrowth of the earlier Stanford

384   Flora and Thoresen

Three Community Study (TCS). The TCS demonstrated a 25% reduction in a composite CVD risk score using a 2-year mass media campaign in one community. In a second community receiving mass media and intensive face-to-face instruction, there was a 30% reduction in the CVD risk score. CVD risk reduction was due to reductions in cholesterol, smoking rates, and blood pressure. Both treatment communities showed reductions in risk significantly different from a control community, which increased in risk (Farquhar et al., 1977).

Several theoretical perspectives were incorporated into the design of TCS and FCP educational materials and programs, including cognitive social learning theory (Bandura, 1986), the communication-persuasion model (McGuire, 1981), the hierarchy of effects model (Ray, 1983), and social network diffusion theory (Rogers, 1983). These perspectives have been integrated into a paradigm called the communication-behavior change (CBC) model. This model is based on the contention that cognitive and behavioral outcomes (i.e., awareness, knowledge, motivation, action, skills, and behavior maintenance) are achieved by providing a combination of information, incentives, and skills training.

Social marketing principles were used to tailor programs to audience needs, to select channels of communication (media, group, or institutional), and to pretest materials with audience members. Social marketing principles (Kotler & Zaltman, 1971) can lead program planners through a process of understanding consumers' health information needs and designing a mix of health products (programs) targeted to specific audience subgroups. Social marketing uses considerations of products, promotion, pricing, and placement to guide implementation of theoretically derived messages (Lefebvre & Flora, in press). Using social marketing principles, the Stanford FCP developed a combination of broadcast television materials, mass mail health tip sheets, and newspaper stories and columns coupled with booklets, self-help kits, correspondence courses, and prevention programs for youth and children. Programs were also developed for families, workplaces, and physicians' offices.

While the final results of the FCP are not yet complete, small field studies of the effectiveness of specific programs have demonstrated (a) significant improvements in adolescents' nutrition knowledge and self-reported diet from a school-based program (King et al., 1988), (b) a 13% quit rate at 2 months and a 11% rate at 6 months for participants using self-help quit-smoking kits (Sallis et al., 1986), (c) a 22% reduction in smoking in a community-smoking cessation contest (King, Flora, Fortmann, & Taylor, 1987), and (d) significant increase in sales of healthy foods in some restaurants participating in a labeling program (Albright, Flora, & Fortmann, 1988). These field studies demonstrate that behavior can be modified using interventions at several levels of audience organization (self-help print media, schools, community wide events, and restaurants). These field study results coupled with the overall success of the TCS highlight the potential of community wide efforts for AIDS prevention.

Several important lessons can be gleaned from these comprehensive community-based programs. First, community-based programs utilize multiple channels of communication; often these channels reflect different levels of intervention (e.g., media versus schools). For AIDS prevention, appropriate channels would include schools, community services, family and household networks, social groups, and the media. Second, community-based programs allow for and attempt to facilitate the synergistic interaction of interventions in multiple channels. For example, in AIDS prevention, school-based programs could build skills to negotiate safe sex or delay of sex with partners, to resist pressures to engage in sex (or unprotected sex), while the media can heighten awareness that youth are at risk, and that families need to discuss sex and AIDS and to support the efforts in school and community services. Third, social marketing is an essential component of a strategy that aims to reach multiple audiences who have varying levels of understanding, motivation, and skills concerning the targeted behavior. Social marketing can guide program planners through a process of planning that includes audience needs analysis, audience segmentation, program and materials pretesting with groups of the target audience, identification of channels of communication, and feedback about the process of the intervention. This understanding of the consumer will not only allow program planners to reach segments of the population that have to date been difficult to reach but will also provide guidance in how to improve the effectiveness of those communications.

Summary

A review of three relevant areas of intervention research illustrates that behavior change can be achieved by employing multiple levels of intervention. Individual-, school-, and community-level efforts have proved successful in prevention of teenage pregnancy. School-based programs derived from a strong theoretical base have demonstrated that smoking can be prevented in adolescents for several years. Community studies in prevention of cardiovascular disease have illustrated the need to target audience subgroups, to select program planning perspectives that help tailor messages to specific groups, and to include the media in a comprehensive strategy. Finally, messages/programs can be integrated to support one another both within and between levels of intervention.

A comprehensive strategy that is well integrated is needed for AIDS prevention (Flora & Thoresen, 1988). This strategy should include (a) integration of cognitive social learning theory into the design and implementation of programs, (b) development of interventions at multiple levels of analysis (e.g., individual, family, school, community, and media), (c) selection of specific target audiences, (d) use of social marketing principles to tailor messages to specific audiences, and (e) integration of messages with programs to produce maximum effects.

References

Abrams, D. B., Elder, J. P., Carlton, R. A., Lasater, T. M., & Artz, L. M. (1986). Social learning principles for organizational health promotion: An integrated approach. In M. Cataldo & T. Coates (Eds.), *Health and industry: A behavioral medicine perspective* (pp. 28–51). New York: John Wiley.

Albright, C. L., Flora, J. A., & Fortmann, S. P. (in press). Restaurant menu labeling: An environmental strategy for encouraging dietary change. *Preventive Medicine*.

Bandura, A. (1977). *Social learning theory.* Englewood Cliffs, NJ: Prentice-Hall.

Bandura, A. (1986). *Social foundations of thought and action: A social cognitive theory.* Englewood Cliffs, NJ: Prentice-Hall.

Blackburn, H., Luepker, R. V., Kline, F. G., Bracht, N., Carlaw, R., Jacobs, D., Mittlemark, M., Stauffer, L., & Taylor, H. L. (1984). The Minnesota Heart Health Program: A research and demonstration project in cardiovascular disease prevention. In J. D. Matarazzo, S. M. Weiss, J. A. Herd, N. E. Miller, & S. M. Weiss (Eds.), *Behavioral health: A handbook of health enhancement and disease prevention* (pp. 1171–1178). New York: John Wiley.

Botvin, G. J. (1986). Substance abuse prevention research: Recent developments and future directions. *Journal of School Health, 56,* 369–374.

Brooks-Gunn, J., Boyer, C. B., & Hein, K. (1988). Preventing HIV infection and AIDS in children and adolescents: Behavioral research and intervention strategies. *American Psychologist, 43*(11), 958–965.

Centers for Disease Control. (1986). Acquired Immunodeficiency Syndrome (AIDS) among Blacks and Hispanics—United States. *Morbidity and Mortality Weekly Report, 42,* 655–666.

Centers for Disease Control. (1988a). Acquired Immunodeficiency Syndrome (AIDS). *Morbidity and Mortality Weekly Report.*

Centers for Disease Control. (1988b). Guidelines for effective school education to prevent the spread of AIDS. *Morbidity and Mortality Weekly Report, 37*(Suppl. 2), 1–13.

DiClemente, R. J., Boyer, C. B., & Morales, E. S. (1988). Minorities and AIDS: Knowledge, attitudes, and misconceptions among Black and Latino adolescents. *American Journal of Public Health, 78*, 55–57.

DiClemente, R. J., Zorn, J., & Temoshok, L. (1986). Adolescents and AIDS: A survey of knowledge, attitudes, and beliefs about AIDS in San Francisco. *American Journal of Public Health, 76*, 1443–1445.

Dryfoos, J. G., & Klerman, L. V. (1988). School-based clinics: Their role in helping students meet the 1990 objectives. *Health Education Quarterly, 15*, 71–80.

Edwards, L., Steinman, M., Arnold, K., & Hakanson, E. (1980). Adolescent pregnancy prevention services in high school clinics. *Family Planning Perspectives, 12*, 6–15.

Evans, R. I., Roxelle, R. M., Mittlemark, M. B., Hansen, W. B., Bane, A., & Havis, J. (1974). Deterring the onset of smoking in children: Knowledge of immediate physiological effects and coping with peer pressure, media pressure, and parent modeling. *Journal of Applied Social Psychology, 8*, 126–135.

Farquhar, J. W., Fortmann, S. P., Maccoby, N., Haskell, W. L., Williams, P. T., Flora, J. A., Taylor, C. B., Brown, B. W., Jr., Solomon, D. S., & Hulley, S. B. (1985). The Stanford Five City Project: Design and methods. *American Journal of Epidemiology, 122*, 331–334.

Farquhar, J. W., Maccoby, N., Wood, P. D., Alexander, J. K., Breitrose, H., Brown, B. W., Haskell, W. L., McAlister, A. L., Meyer, A. J., Nash, J. D., & Stern, M. P. (1977). Community education for cardiovascular health. *Lancet, 1*, 1192–1195.

Flay, B. R. (1985). Psychosocial approaches to smoking prevention: A review of findings. *Health Psychology, 4*(5), 449–488.

Flora, J. A., Maccoby, N., & Farquhar, J. W. (1989). Communication campaigns to prevent cardiovascular disease: The Stanford studies. In R. Rice & C. Atkin (Eds.), *Public communication campaigns* (2nd ed.). Newbury Park, CA: Sage.

Flora, J. A., & Thoresen, C. E. (1988). Reducing the risk of AIDS in adolescents. *American Psychologist, 43*(11), 965–970.

Furstenberg, F. R., Jr., Morgan, P. S., Moore, K. A., & Peterson, J. L. (1987). Race differences in the timing of adolescent intercourse. *American Sociological Review, 52*, 511–518.

Gilchrist, L. D., & Schinke, S. P. (1983). Coping with contraception: Cognitive and behavioral methods with adolescents. *Cognitive Therapy and Research, 7*, 379–388.

Hansen, W. B., Marotte, C. D., & Fielding, J. E. (1988). Evaluation of tobacco and alcohol abuse/prevention curriculum for adolescents. *Health Education Quarterly, 15*, 93–114.

Hayes, C. D. (1987). *Risking the future: Adolescent sexuality, pregnancy and childbearing* (Vol. 1). Washington, DC: National Academy Press.

Hersch, P. (1988, January). Coming of age on city streets. *Psychology Today*, pp. 28–37.

Hofferth, S. L., & Hayes, C. D. (1987). *Risking the future: Adolescent sexuality, pregnancy, and childbearing* (Vol. 2). Washington, DC: National Academy Press.

Hofferth, S. L., Kahn, J., & Baldwin, W. (1987). Premarital sexual activity among United States teenage women over the past three decades. *Family Planning Perspectives, 19*, 46–53.

Institute of Medicine. (1986). *Confronting AIDS: Direction for public health, health care, and research*. Washington, DC: National Academy Press.

Jessor, R. (1982). Critical issues in research on adolescent health promotion. In T. J. Coates, A. C. Petersen, & C. Perry (Eds.), *Promoting adolescent health: A dialogue on research and practice* (pp. 447–465). San Francisco: Academic Press.

Johnston, L. D., Bachman, J. G., & O'Malley, P. M. (1987). *Drug use among American high*

388   Flora and Thoresen

school, college, and other young adults: National trends through 1986. Rockville, MD: National Institute on Drug Abuse.

Kegeles, S. M., Adler, N. E., & Irwin, C. E. (1988). Sexually active adolescents and condoms: Changes over one year in knowledge, attitudes and use. *American Journal of Public Health, 78,* 460–461.

King, A. C., Flora, J. A., Fortmann, S. P., & Taylor, C. B. (1987). Smoker's challenge: Immediate and long term findings of a community smoking cessation contest. *American Journal of Public Health, 77,* 1340–1341.

King, A. C., Saylor, K. E., Foster, S., Killen, J. D., Telch, M. J., Farquhar, J. W., & Flora, J. A. (1988). Promoting dietary change in adolescents: A school-based approach for modifying and maintaining healthful behavior. *American Journal of Preventive Medicine, 4,* 68–72.

Kirby, D. (1984). *Sexuality education: An evaluation of programs and their effects.* Santa Cruz, CA: Network.

Kirby, D. (1985). Sexuality education: A more realistic view of the effects. *Journal of School Health, 55,* 421–424.

Kotler, P., & Zaltman, C. (1971). Social marketing: An approach to planned social change. *Journal of Marketing, 35,* 3–12.

Lasater, T., Abrams, D., Artz, L., Beaudin, P., Cabrera, L., Elder, J., Kinsley, P., Peterson, G., Rodrigues, A., Rosenberg, P., Snow, R., & Carleton, R. (1984). Lay volunteer delivery of a community-based cardiovascular risk factor change program: The Pawtucket experiment. In J. D. Matarazzo, S. M. Weiss, J. A. Herd, N. E. Miller, & S. M. Weiss (Eds.), *Behavioral health: A handbook of health enhancement and disease prevention* (pp. 1166–1170). New York: John Wiley.

Lefebvre, C. R., & Flora, J. A. (in press). Social marketing and public health interventions. *Health Education Quarterly.*

Maccoby, N., Farquhar, J. W., Wood, P., & Alexander, J. K. (1977). Reducing the risk of cardiovascular disease: Effects of a community-based campaign on knowledge and behavior. *Journal of Community Health, 3,* 100–114.

McGuire, W. J. (1964). Inducing resistance to persuasion. In L. Berkowitz (Ed.), *Advances in experimental social psychology* (Vol. 1). New York: Academic Press.

McGuire, W. J. (1981). Theoretical foundations of campaigns. In R. E. Rice & W. J. Paisley (Eds.), *Public communication campaigns.* Beverly Hills, CA: Sage.

Orlandi, M. A, (1986). Community-based substance abuse prevention: a multicultural perspective. *Journal of School Health, 56,* 394–400.

Perry, C. L., Klepp, K. I., & Shultz, J. M. (1988). Primary prevention of cardiovascular disease: Communitywide strategies for youth. *Journal of Consulting and Clinical Psychology, 56,* 358–364.

Remafedi, G. (1987). Homosexual youth: A challenge to contemporary society. *Journal of the American Medical Association, 258*(2), 222–225.

Ray, M. L. (1983). Marketing communication and the hierarchy of effects. In P. Clarke (Ed.), *New models for mass communication research.* Beverly Hills, CA: Sage.

Rogers, E. M. (1983). *Diffusion of innovations* (3rd ed.). New York: Free Press.

Sallis, J. F., Hill, R. D., Taylor, C. B., Flora, J. A., Killen, J. D., Telch, M. J., Girard, J., & Maccoby, N. (1986). Efficacy of self-help behavior modification materials in smoking cessation. *American Journal of Preventive Medicine, 2,* 342–344.

Schinke, S. P. (1984). Preventing teenage pregnancy. In M. Hersen, R. M. Eisler, & P. M. Miller (Eds.), *Progress in behavior modification.* San Francisco: Academic Press.

Schinke, S. P., Blythe, B., & Gilchrist, L. D. (1981). Cognitive behavioral prevention of adolescent pregnancy. *Journal of Counseling Psychology, 28,* 451–454.

Schuster, C. R. (1988). Intravenous drug use and AIDS prevention. *Public Health Reports, 103*, 261–266.

Smith, P. B., Nenney, S. W., & McGill, L. (1986). Health problems and sexual activity of selected inner-city, middle school students. *Journal of Adolescent Health Care, 56*, 263–266.

Sorensen, R. C. (1973). *Adolescent sexuality in contemporary America.* New York: World.

Strunin, L., & Hingson, R. (1987). Acquired Immunodeficiency Syndrome and adolescents: Knowledge, beliefs, attitudes, and behaviors. *Pediatrics, 79*, 825–828.

Telch, M. J., Killen, J. D., McAlister, A. L., Perry, C. L., & Maccoby, N. (1982). Long-term follow-up of a pilot project on smoking prevention with adolescents. *Journal of Behavioral Medicine, 5*, 1–8.

Thoresen, C. E. (1984). Overview of strategies for health enhancement. In J. D. Matarazzo, S. M. Weiss, J. A. Herd, N. E. Miller, & S. M. Weiss (Eds.), *Behavioral health: A handbook of health enhancement and disease prevention.* New York: John Wiley.

U.S. Congress, Office of Technology Assessment. (1988). *How effective is AIDS education?* (Staff paper). Washington, DC: Government Printing Office.

Vincent, M. L., Clearie, A. F., & Schlucheter, M. D. (1987). Reducing adolescent pregnancy through school and community-based education. *Journal of the American Medical Association, 257*, 320–321.

Zabin, L. S., Hirsch, M., Smith, E., Street, R., & Hardy, J. (1986). Evaluation of a pregnancy prevention program for urban teenagers. *Family Planning Perspectives, 18*, 119–126.

Zelnik, M. (1983). Sexual activity among adolescents: Perspectives of a decade. In E. R. McAnarey (Ed.), *Premature adolescent pregnancy and parenthood.* New York: Grune & Stratton.

Zelnik, M., & Kanter, J. (1980). Sexual activity, contraceptive use and pregnancy among metropolitan-area teenagers: 1971–1979. *Family Planning Perspectives, 12*, 230–237.

Zelnik, M., & Kim, Y. (1982). Sex education and its association with teenage sexual activity, pregnancy and contraceptive use. *Family Planning Perspectives, 14*, 117–126.

23

The National Institute on Alcohol Abuse and Alcoholism's AIDS-Related Activities

Daniela Seminara

Acquired Immunodeficiency Syndrome is a serious medical disorder caused by human immunodeficiency virus. The Department of Health and Human Services has recognized AIDS as a national and international health problem of unprecedented proportions. It is estimated that approximately 1.5 million Americans are currently infected with the AIDS virus, and that 20% to 30% of these individuals will develop AIDS in the next five years. Epidemiological surveillance has identified a range of risk factors that determine susceptibility to HIV. However, more information is needed on factors that may accelerate the clinical expression of AIDS.

A potential risk factor not adequately studied in the literature, in spite of its well-known adverse effects on the immune system and association with drug abuse and other high-risk behaviors, is alcohol abuse. The National Institute on Alcohol Abuse and Alcoholism (NIAAA) is interested in supporting research on the relationship between alcohol and AIDS. To encourage a greater emphasis on AIDS-related alcohol research, NIAAA issued, in September 1988, a special announcement soliciting the submission of applications from investigators in the clinical, epidemiological, and biomedical sciences fields interested in the study of the relationship between alcohol and AIDS.

The current NIAAA AIDS-related research program addresses the topics listed below.

(1) The epidemiology of alcohol use and alcoholism among AIDS patients, seropositive individuals, and populations at high risk for HIV infection: Little is currently known about the incidence and prevalence of seroconversion to HIV positivity among alcoholics and alcohol abusers. NIAAA will support epidemiological studies on the role of alco-

390

hol consumption as a risk factor for seroconversion and its role in the clinical course of the disease after HIV infection.

(2) The effect of alcohol on the biological and molecular mechanisms underlying (a) the risk for acquisition of HIV infection in exposed individuals, (b) the progression from HIV infection to clinical AIDS, and (c) the development of opportunistic infections and pathologic conditions such as Kaposi's sarcoma: The in vitro similarities between the immune dysfunction caused by excessive alcohol consumption and those observed after HIV infection are significant. The T-lymphocyte system seems to be affected extensively by alcohol as well as by HIV. It is possible that alcohol consumption, in combination with HIV infection, may produce additive adverse effects and contribute to the accelerated development of AIDS and the severity of the observed immune dysfunction. In addition, alcohol is likely to play a role as a contributing factor in the pathogenesis of infectious disease, and more studies are needed to understand the mechanism underlying its immunocompromising effect.

(3) The role of alcohol as a mediator of risk-taking behaviors specifically related to unsafe sexual practices and IV drug use, and development of prevention strategies to reduce such behaviors: Effective vaccines to prevent the spread of AIDS and/or effective treatment for this disease may not be available for many years. In the interim, it is necessary to confront the issue of prevention through research directed at behavioral change, including modification of unsafe sexual practices and behaviors associated with intravenous drug use. A review of the literature suggests a number of potential avenues of inquiry. Studies of gay men indicate that users and abusers of alcohol and other drugs during sexual activity constitute a hard-core group that is particularly resistant to adopting and maintaining safe sex techniques. Unprotected sexual activity among the heterosexual community may also be associated with or aggravated by alcohol and drug use.

It has been hypothesized that alcohol may have a direct impact on exposure to HIV (and its transfer) through the mechanism of disinhibition—that is, a disregard for social norms, moral obligations, and behavioral restraint. Alternatively, the relationship between alcohol and AIDS may be indirect, through such processes as selection, attribution, and environmental facilitation. Excess drinking also may be deliberately undertaken as an excuse for behavior that could not otherwise be explained or rationalized, such as indiscriminate sex.

NIAAA will support research designed to explore linkages between alcohol use or abuse and behavior that increases the risk of AIDS and to develop methods and techniques to understand, prevent, and/or change high-risk sexual and drug-abusing behaviors and to sustain the changed behavior over time.

24

Overview of the AIDS Program of the National Institute on Drug Abuse

Charles R. Schuster

The mission of the National Institute on Drug Abuse (NIDA) is to enhance knowledge that will reduce the incidence and prevalence of illicit drug use and associated morbidity and mortality. To achieve this goal, NIDA supports extramural research and research training through the funding of grants and contracts, conducts intramural research at the Addiction Research Center, and disseminates research findings to practitioners in the drug abuse field through NIDA-supported conferences and publications. NIDA also exerts a leadership role by establishing research priorities in line with scientific developments and national trends in drug abuse, and making policy recommendations, based on knowledge derived from research findings, to the executive and legislative branches of government. Furthermore, the staff of NIDA work closely with their colleagues in sister Public Health Service agencies to foster research that is both broad and comprehensive. NIDA's activities in the AIDS area are reflective of these research and leadership functions.

The overall goal of the AIDS program of NIDA is to reduce transmission of HIV infection associated with drug abuse. NIDA's national research program will expand the knowledge base to make possible a better understanding of the nature and extent of AIDS risk behaviors and the progression of HIV disease associated with drug abuse. The current research program emphasizes five elements:

- drug abuse treatment and prevention as HIV control measures
- alternative HIV control measures
- other AIDS/drug abuse research

392

• surveillance
• technology transfer and communication

Drug Abuse Treatment and Prevention as HIV Control Measures

One strategy for the prevention of HIV transmission among drug abusers is drug abuse treatment. NIDA-funded research indicates that to overcome drug dependence, abusers often require repeated and prolonged drug abuse treatment. Evaluation studies of the major treatment modalities—drug detoxification, methadone maintenance, drug-free counseling offered in an outpatient setting, and drug-free counseling offered in a residential setting—have shown decreased drug use for clients in treatment. This decrease, however, has been greatest for those receiving methadone maintenance. Seroprevalence studies have found lower seroprevalence rates among those in treatment compared to those not in treatment and among those with longer histories of treatment. Although treatment is associated with decreased drug use and seropositivity for those who remain under care, a large percentage of admissions drop out in the early stages of the treatment process. Furthermore, drug abuse treatment currently lacks the capacity to care for the estimated 1.1–1.3 million intravenous drug abusers who need treatment.

These issues are being addressed through NIDA-funded research and research demonstration programs. Ongoing research focuses on deficiencies in existing treatment approaches that contribute to poor program performance, illicit drug use during treatment, dropout from treatment and relapse to illicit drug use following treatment, and the development of new and improved methods for the treatment of intravenous drug abuse. This last area of research has taken on new significance as reports from field studies indicate that intravenous use of cocaine alone or in combination with heroin has become more widespread. Both behavioral and pharmacological strategies are needed for treatment, including bringing drug abuse treatment into primary health care systems so that not only the dependency problem is addressed but also other associated medical care problems.

Alternative HIV Control Measures

Evidence from NIDA-funded research indicates that knowledge alone does not alter risk behaviors for a significant portion of drug abusers. Therefore, to be effective, prevention should include multiple approaches ranging from mass medical information dissemination to specific group and individual behavior change strategies. NIDA supports research that examines the impact of intervention approaches representing the full gamut of strategies for drug abusers in a number of settings.

Community outreach demonstration programs are a major component of NIDA's AIDS research activities. At present, projects are being funded in 53 cities in areas of high seroprevalence or with large numbers of intravenous drug abusers. The purpose of these projects is to test various models of getting information to the hard-to-reach intravenous drug abusers who are not in treatment and to their equally hard-to-reach sexual partners. The interventions include outreach as well as more focused behavior change strategies. The primary message of these projects is for addicts to get into drug abuse treatment and to stop using drugs. If they are not able or willing to enter treatment, the message is to avoid sharing injection equipment and to adopt other measures that reduce the risk of AIDS. It is anticipated that over 40,000 at-risk individuals will be reached through this program. Outreach is being conducted through hospital emergency rooms, jails, housing projects, health clinics, and the streets. Information is collected at baseline and at six-month follow-up on HIV serostatus, drug use practices and patterns, health problems, sexual practices, and other issues related to access to a variety of sources of information on HIV disease. These data are collected from all sites and processed at a central location. At the local level, individual investigators will assess interventions unique to their own programs.

Other AIDS/Drug Abuse Research

NIDA is supporting a wide variety of research to improve our understanding of factors related to the spread of HIV infection among intravenous drug abusers and their sexual partners and children. These include studies on the epidemiology and natural history of HIV infection among intravenous drug abusers, their sexual partners, and children; on the role of abused drugs as possible cofactors to HIV infection and the onset of AIDS; on the role of drug use practices in the spread of AIDS and HIV infection; on basic behavioral and genetic factors that contribute to the development of intravenous drug abuse; on strategies for the elimination of intravenous drug abuse; on the development and evaluation of behavior change strategies for controlling the spread of HIV infection; and on the effects of drugs and pharmacological agents used in the treatment of drug abuse on immune function.

Surveillance

In addition to natural history studies, NIDA has established a surveillance system in eight cities to monitor the prevalence of HIV infection among intravenous drug abusers. At present, the system surveys new admissions to methadone detoxification and maintenance treatment programs. Data are collected through personal interviews on drug use practices and patterns as well as sexual activities. In addition, HIV testing and counseling are provided. The data are collected in six-month waves. In early 1989, Wave 3 data are being processed.

Technology Transfer and Communication

NIDA's current involvement in public education includes communication of recent findings of research to drug abuse authorities, treatment personnel, and the general public through the electronic and print media. A national hotline telephone service is maintained by NIDA (1–800–662-HELP), which provides information on the availability of drug abuse treatment services and issues.

Training and technical assistance are provided to drug abuse authorities and treatment personnel so they may deal more effectively with the social, psychological, and medical problems associated with HIV-affected persons. This training includes counseling strategies that can be used by treatment personnel with both HIV positive and negative clients as well as those who have AIDS or who are family members of those with AIDS.

Conclusion

The interface of drug abuse issues and HIV disease constitutes a significant public health problem. Concern is not limited to the spread of the virus throughout the population of drug abusers but extends to their sexual partners, children, and other segments of the non-drug-abusing population who are potentially at risk.

In a short period of time, NIDA has organized a research plan to address the need to control the HIV epidemic within the drug-abusing populating. Funding for this activity has only recently been sufficient to begin a concerted effort in this area. During the next several months, the results of these activities will be forthcoming. Plans are currently being made to build on these findings and to develop new initiatives in the area of HIV infection and AIDS.

25

The National Institute of Mental Health

Lewis L. Judd

Preventing the spread of HIV infection is a public health imperative. Since there is no vaccine for AIDS at the present time, preventing or changing high-risk behavior and maintaining that change are the only available strategies to control the epidemic.

Research on the primary prevention of AIDS through changing high-risk behaviors is a priority in the National Institute of Mental Health (NIMH) AIDS research program. For this reason, NIMH was pleased to provide support for the 1988 Vermont Conference on the Primary Prevention of Psychopathology, with its focus on AIDS prevention.

NIMH, because of its historical interest and expertise in the behavioral sciences, has been involved with the behavioral and mental health aspects of AIDS since 1983. Over the last several years, there has been an increasing emphasis on AIDS prevention research to develop new and more effective models to curb the spread of AIDS. The current NIMH AIDS program consists of extramural research and research training programs, intramural research, a health and mental health care provider training program, and research development activities. In addition to research on behavior change and prevention, NIMH AIDS research focuses on central nervous system effects of HIV infection, behavioral neuroimmunology, clinical research on HIV-related mental disorders, and mental health services research on HIV infection and the severely mentally ill.

The Public Health Service (PHS) and several other groups have recently highlighted critical prevention research needs for AIDS and have provided strikingly consistent recommendations for increasing prevention research. The Charlottesville Report from the Second PHS AIDS Prevention and Control Meeting outlines important research objectives in behavior change and the evaluation of AIDS prevention programs. The Presidential Commission on the HIV Epidemic recommends that NIMH support research to fill gaps in knowledge in the areas of risk behaviors and behavior change.

One of the major recommendations of the Institute of Medicine (IOM) report *Confronting AIDS: Update 1988* calls for the beginning of substantial, long-term, and comprehensive programs of research in the biomedical and social sciences intended to prevent HIV infection and to treat the diseases caused by it. In addition, the National Research Council report, *AIDS: Sexual Behavior and Intravenous Drug Use*, identifies a broad range of new research needed to design, implement, and evaluate better interventions in the future to control the spread of HIV.

NIMH is encouraging additional research on risk-reduction behavior change through a program announcement on "Research on Behavior Change and Prevention Strategies to Reduce Transmission of Human Immunodeficiency Virus (HIV)" in collaboration with other Alcohol, Drug Abuse and Mental Health Administration (ADAMHA) institutes, several institutes of the National Institutes of Health (NIH), and the Centers for Disease Control (CDC). At the present time, NIMH is supporting AIDS prevention projects through individual research grants and through four NIMH-supported AIDS research centers. Collaborations across projects are encouraged to address common research problems, to share strategies and assessments, and to maximize findings. These efforts are providing important information about the determinants, rates, and changes of risk behaviors in different population groups. Interventions are being mounted and evaluated to determine effective strategies for reducing risks for HIV infection. Some of these findings are among those included in this volume.

The NIMH AIDS research program will continue to place a priority on AIDS prevention research, especially epidemiological and intervention studies. Some of the research needs are highlighted in the papers presented at the Vermont conference: the development of theoretical models of health-related behavior to better understand risk-taking behaviors; examination of those factors that maintain high-risk behaviors; application of specific models to all specific targeted populations, including minority and low-income individuals; and the development and evaluation of strategies for motivating behavior change in large populations.

The Vermont Conference enabled researchers, clinicians, educators, and community workers to share information on the prevention of HIV infection and to consider the most promising strategies for future preventive interventions. Meeting the extraordinary challenges of preventing additional HIV infection will require the ongoing efforts and collaboration of a broad range of individuals, groups, and private and public agencies. The Vermont Conference and the chapters in this volume represent one step toward the common goal— preventing AIDS.

Name Index

Abramowitz, S., 247
Abrams, D. B., 379
Abramson, P. R., 298
Adler, N. E., 68, 376
Ajzen, I., 94, 95, 122, 144, 247, 273
Akabas, S. H., 132, 319
Akins, C., 342
Albee, G. W., 17-20
Albright, C. L., 385
Alexander, P., 314
Allen, J. R., 54, 61, 76
Allen, R. L., 273-274
Allen, W. R., 314
Altman, F., 13
Amaro, H., 311, 318
Ames, M. A., 364
Anderson, J. E., 270
Anderson, R. E., 226
Aoki, B., 208, 290-307
Arnold, K., 381
Artz, L. M., 379
Aumann, J., 332
Ayer, W. A., 362

Bacchetti, A. M., 49
Bachen, C. M., 274
Bachman, J. G., 377
Bailey, C., 254
Bakeman, R., 311, 330
Baldwin, J. D., 252, 321
Baldwin, J. I., 252, 321
Baldwin, W., 314, 375
Bales, F., 273
Ball, J. C., 332
Bandura, A., 124, 128-140, 247, 299, 382-384
Bar Hillel, M., 185-186
Barre-Sinoussi, F., 72

Bauman, L. J., 151, 155
Beach, L. R., 113, 144-145, 169
Bearden, W. O., 273
Beck, A. T., 229
Beck-Sague, C., 266
Becker, M. H., 68, 111-112, 114, 117, 144-145, 148, 160, 210, 244-245, 247, 266, 302, 317, 321
Behn, R. D., 176
Bell, A., 242-243, 253
Bellack, A. S., 229, 231
Bentkover, J., 178
Berkanovic, E., 113
Berkman, L., 254
Berry, G. L., 312
Beschner, G., 342
Beyth-Marom, R., 186, 196
Bielby, W. T., 273-274
Birren, J., 253
Blackburn H., 383
Blackshaw, L., 194
Blanker, A. J., 331-332
Bloom, D. E., 86
Blumstein, P., 288
Blythe, B., 380
Bodecker, T., 245
Bodenheimer, H., 113
Bogard, L., 273
Bolognesi, D. P., 79
Bond, L. A., 14
Borcherding, K., 147
Borger, P., 333
Boruch, R. S., 365
Bowman, P., 274
Boyer, C. B., 319, 329, 376, 378
Brandt, A. M., 317, 320
Bransfield, T. L., 135, 225-239

Brock, B., 113-114
Brooks, C. H., 366
Brooks-Gunn, J., 376
Brown, J., 211
Budescu, D. V., 149, 181
Buede, D., 169, 176
Bullington, B., 331-332
Bullough, V., 253
Buning, E. C., 138
Burchard, J., 14
Burgos, N. M., 319
Burns, B., 364
Bye, L. L., 242-258

Calnan, M., 113
Campbell, F. L., 144, 169
Campbell, K., 79
Carliner, G., 86
Carlton, R. A., 379
Carr, J. E., 216
Carrier, J. M., 319
Carroll, G., 74
Carroll, L., 321
Carter, W., 113, 116
Casavantes, E. J., 330-331
Casey, J. T., 189
Castro, K. G., 269
Catania, J. A., 208, 242-258
Cates, W., 245
Caumartin, S., 209-223
Chaisson, R. E., 49, 58, 329
Chambers, C. D., 332
Charap, M. H., 67
Chase, J., 76
Checker, A., 12-13
Chein, I., 332
Chen, J. Y., 237
Cheng, Y. T., 329
Chilman, C. S., 320
Chin, J., 49-50, 64, 68
Christ, G., 237
Christon, L., 275
Clearie, A., 258
Cleary, P., 116, 143-144
Clumeck, N., 225
Coates, T. J., 68, 133, 151, 226, 232, 237, 242-258, 367
Cochran, S. D., 53, 58, 208, 264-269, 309-324
Cockerham, W. 113
Cohen, S., 13

Cohen, H., 329
Cole, W., 147
Cole, L., 249
Cole, G. A., 147
Coleman, S., 298
Combs, B., 146-147, 183, 195
Combs, S., 188
Comstock, G., 273
Condelli, L., 254
Cook, F. L., 148
Coombs, C., 169, 187
Covello, V. T., 146, 178
Covi, L., 214
Crider, R. A., 331-332
Cummings, K. M., 112, 114, 148
Curran, J. W., 50, 54, 58-59, 61-62 64, 274, 310-311, 365-366

Darden, D. K., 275
Darden, W. R., 275
Darrow, W., 245
Davidshofer, I. O., 175
Davidson, T., 331
Davis, R. A., 273
Davis, S. M., 319
Dawes, R. M., 169, 177, 180, 187, 191
De Jong, W. M., 139, 253
Delongis, A., 211
D'Eramo, J., 253
Derby, S. L., 175
Derefinko, A. J., 362
Derogatis, L., 214
Des Jarlais, D. C., 137, 139, 329, 340
Desmond, D. P., 332
Desmond, S., 321
Deucher, N., 365
DeVellis, B., 124
DeVellis, R., 229
DeVos, G., 297
DiClemente, R. J., 319, 321, 378
Dohrenwend, B. P., 211
Dohrenwend, B. S., 211
Dolcini, P., 244
Dolinski, D., 160
Doll, L., 245
Dornbush, R., 255
Douvan, E., 256
Drabek, T. E., 148
Dryfoos, J. G., 381
Dunn, A. J., 84

Durand, R. M., 273

Ebbesen, E. B., 131
Echenberg, D., 366
Eddy, D. M., 186
Edgar, T., 133
Edwards, L., 381
Edwards, W., 144, 169, 176, 181
Eisenstaedt, A. S., 55
Eisenstaedt, R. S., 67
Eisler, R. M., 229, 231
Ekstrand, M. L., 242-258, 367
Elder, J. P., 379
Eller, M., 209-223
Ellis, L., 364
Emmons, C., 118-119, 254
Engleman, E. G., 79
Eraker, S., 114
Erbaugh, J., 229
Ericsson, K. A., 190, 194
Eshleman, S., 209-223
Evans, R. I., 382
Everaerd, W., 255

Fairchild, M., 274
Farber, N., 113
Farley, R., 314
Farmer, R., 74
Farquhar, J. W., 138, 383-384
Fauci, A. S., 79-80
Feather, N. T., 178, 180
Feingold, A. R., 67
Feldman, D. A., 329
Fetzer, B. K., 142, 150, 152
Fielding, J. E., 143, 382
Fineberg, H. V., 184-185
Fischer, E., 247, 254
Fischer, G., 183-184
Fischhoff, B., 92, 142, 145-147, 168-201,
    248
Fischl, M. A., 225
Fishbein, I., 144
Fishbein, M., 92-109, 247-248, 273
Fiske, S. T., 182
Fitzgibbon, M., 361-362
Flick, L. H., 314
Flora, J. A., 257, 349-350, 374-386
Flores, L., 298
Folkman, S., 216
Folks, T. M., 80

Forsyth, B., 149
Fortmann, S. P., 384-385
Fowley, M., 366
Francis, D. P., 61, 64
Franscisc, D. P., 61
Freeman, K., 67
Freimuth, V. S., 133
Friedland, G. H., 64, 309, 311
Friedman, A. E., 209
Friedman, S. R., 139, 329, 340
Fulton, J., 113
Furby, L., 187-188, 195-196
Furstenberg, F. F., 148, 376

Gagnon, J., 129
Gallo, R., 72
Gary, L. E., 312
Gaskin, J. M., 84
Gee, G., 87
Geis, G., 332
Gettys, C. F., 189, 195
Getzen, T. E., 55, 67
Gfoerer, J. C., 331-332
Gibbs, J. T., 314-315
Gibson, D., 252
Gibson, W. C., 155
Gilchrist, L. D., 135-136, 255, 380
Gilner, F., 255
Goh, W. C., 79
Goitein, B., 145
Goldberg, W., 275
Goldsmith, D. S., 340
Goldstein, A. L., 81-84
Gonda, M. A., 76
Gordon, J., 124
Gorsuch, R. L., 229
Gottlieb, M. S., 209
Grady, K., 113
Grady, P. I., 319
Graham-Tomasi, R., 114
Grant, I., 367
Graves, S. B., 274
Green, J., 74
Greenblatt, R., 243, 257
Greene, J., 114
Griffen, D., 76
Grimson, M., 75
Gromski, W., 160
Gross, A., 247, 252, 254
Guinan, M. E., 309-310, 354

Guten, S., 114
Guthrie, D., 313
Gutmann, M., 111
Guydish, J. R., 242-258

Haefner, D. P., 112-113, 157
Haid, M., 366
Hakanson, E., 381
Hakmiller, K. L., 152
Hall, N. R., 21, 72-87
Hallal, J., 113
Hammer, J. S., 364
Hammond, S. L., 133
Hansen, H., 211
Hansen, W. B., 156, 382
Hardy, A. M., 54, 309-310, 366
Hardy, J. 381
Harel, Y., 113
Harris, D., 114
Harris, M. B., 319
Harrison, A. O., 315
Hart, D. V., 298
Haseltine, W. A., 76, 79
Hasher, L., 181
Hawthorne, V., 114
Hayashi, T., 290
Hayes, C. D., 375-376
Healy, D. L., 81
Hearst, N., 21, 47-69
Heerwagen, J. H., 216
Hein, K., 376
Hensen, W. B., 143
Hernandez, M., 332
Hersch, P., 376-377
Hersen, M., 229, 231
Hershey, J. C., 188
Hill, R., 270
Hingson, R., 378
Hintzman, D., 181
Hirsh, M., 381
Hoch, S. J., 158, 195
Hoff, C., 244-246
Hoff, R., 57
Hofferth, S. L., 314, 375-376
Holmes, K. K., 320
Hood, H. V., 135, 225-239
Hopkins, S. A., 329
Horstman, W., 133, 151, 226, 244
Howard, G. S., 359
Howard, J. G., 274, 333

Howe, H., 113
Hoxie, J. A., 80
Hughes, R. G., 147
Hulley, S. B., 21, 47-69
Humphrey, H. H., 37

Inciardi, I. J., 331
Inui, T., 113
Irwin, C. E., 68, 376
Irwin, J., 331
Issel, C. J., 76
Izard, C. E., 251

Ja, D. Y., 290-307
Jackson, R. E., 311
Jacobs, R., 253
Jaffe, H. W., 61, 226, 245
Janis, I. L., 144, 178
Janz, N. K., 111-113, 145, 148, 160, 247
Jerin, M., 114
Jervis, R., 168
Jette, A., 112
Job, R., 252
Joffe, J. M., 14
John, R. S., 147
Johnson, B. B., 146
Johnson, D., 187
Johnson, E. R., 273-274
Johnson, L. D., 377
Johnson, R., 254
Johnson, V., 33, 73
Jones, J. M., 12, 13
Jordan, V. E., 270
Jorquez, J. S., 208, 329-342, 345-346
Joseph, J. G., 68, 92, 111-124, 151, 208-223,
   244-245, 248, 254, 262, 317, 367
Juarez, R., 319
Judd, L. L., 397-399
Jue, S., 298

Kahn, E., 310
Kahn, J. R., 255, 314, 375
Kahneman, D., 147, 158, 182, 186, 188,
   191
Kalechstein, A., 321
Kalish, R., 297
Kamler, J. A., 142, 150, 152
Kanki, P. J., 76
Kanter, J., 375
Kaplan, H., 254

Kardin, M., 290
Kasl, S. V., 211
Kazdin, A. E., 136
Keeney, R. L., 175
Kegeles, F. S., 157
Kegeles, S. M., 68, 113, 242-258, 376, 378
Keidan, J., 321
Kelly, J. A., 135, 208, 225-239
Kessler, M., 14
Kessler, R. C., 209-223
Kiedaisch, J., 14
Killen, J. D., 382
Kilpatrick, J., 86-87
Kim, Y., 380
King, A. C., 384
King, J., 113
Kingsley, I., 236
Kingsley, L., 245
Kinsey, A., 28
Kirby, D., 37-38, 380
Kirby, M., 32
Kirscht, J. P., 92, 107, 111-124, 157, 209-223, 248
Kitano, K. J., 302-303
Kitchen, L. W., 76
Klar, Y., 145
Klein, R. S., 64, 309, 311
Klepp, K. I., 383
Klerman, L. V., 381
Klotz, M. L., 155
Kolodny, R. E., 73, 255
Koo, L. C., 297
Koop, C. E., 274, 317
Kotler, P., 384
Kramer, P., 113
Kraus, S., 266
Krauss, E., 188
Kruglanski, A. W., 145
Kuhl, J., 145
Kukulka, G., 321
Kulik, J. A., 142, 150
Kulka, R., 256
Kunreuther, H., 148

Landrum, S., 266
Lane, H. C., 80
Langer, J., 183
Langlie, J., 114
Langlois, A. J., 79
Langone, J., 321

Larson, D. B., 361, 364
Larson, E. B., 147
Larwood, L., 142, 150
Lasater, T. M., 379, 383
Laudenslager, M. L., 129
Laurence, L., 80
Layman, M., 146-147, 183
Lazarus, R. S., 211, 216
Leavitt, F., 113
Lebow, R. N., 168
LeClaire, G. M., 39-43
Lefebvre, C. R., 384
Letourneau, E., 366
Leventhal, H., 111, 144
Levin, N., 114
Levine, A., 254
Levinson, R. A., 135, 315
Levy, J. A., 226
Lichtenstein, S., 146-147, 175, 183, 185, 188-189, 195
Lichtman, R. R., 152
Lifson, J. D., 79
Link, R. N., 67
Linville, P., 183-185, 188, 196
Lipman, R., 214
Long, J., 331
Longue, J. N., 211
Low, T. L. K., 83
Lumb, J. R., 311, 330
Lund, A., 113
Lushema, R. E., 229
Lyerly, H. K., 79
Lyons, J. S., 361-362, 364, 366
Lyter, D., 245

McAlister, A. L., 382
McCarthy, M., 362
McCarthy M., 361
Maccoby, N., 138, 382
McCray, E., 311
McDermott, L., 249
McGill, L., 375
McGillis, J. P., 81-82
McGrath, M. S., 79
MacGregor, D., 142
McGuigan, K., 254
McGuire, W. J., 131, 382-384
McKusick, L., 133, 151, 226, 232, 237, 244, 247, 252
McMullen, P., 247, 252, 254

Maddux, J., 115-116, 144, 332
Mahler, H. I. M., 142, 150
Maier, S. F., 129
Maile, M. C., 148
Maiman, L. A., 144, 247, 321
Malotte, C. K., 143, 156
Mamlin, J., 114
Mann, J. M., 38, 49-50, 68
Manning, C. A., 189
Mantell, J. E., 132, 136, 319
Margolick, J. B., 79
Marin, B. V., 319
Marin, G., 319
Marlatt, A., 124
Marmor, M. J., 310
Marotte, C. D., 382
Marquis, L., 61
Martin, E., 188, 196
Martin, J. L., 210, 226, 245
Marx, J. L., 355
Maslach, C., 131
Mason, P. J., 274, 311
Masters, W. H., 33, 73
Mata, A. G., 208, 329-342, 345, 346
Matthews, T. J., 79
Maxey, L., 87
Mayer, L., 80
Mays, V. M., 12-13, 53, 58, 208, 264-277,
    311-314, 316, 321, 323-324
Mechanic, D., 252
Medina, M., 332
Melick, M. E., 211
Mendelson, M., 229
Mesagno, F., 237
Mewborn, C. R., 160
Middlestadt, S. E., 92-109, 248
Miller, D., 74
Miller, N. E., 13
Miller, P. M., 229
Mitchell, T. R., 145
Mitchell-Kernan, C., 315-316
Mitnick, L., 13
Miyake, A., 83
Mo, B., 290-307
Mock, J., 229
Montagnier, L., 72
Montelaro, R. C., 76
Montgomery, H., 194
Montgomery, S., 121
Moore, D. S., 319

Moore, J. W., 322, 330-331
Moore, K. A., 376
Morales, A., 208, 330, 332
Morales, E. S., 319, 345-347, 378
Moreshead, W. V., 84
Moretti, R. J., 362
Morgan, J. R., 376
Morgan, M., 187, 195
Morgan, W. M., 365-366
Morin, S. F., 208, 232, 244
Morse, S., 245
Moss, A. R., 58, 329
Moss, S., 113
Mumpower, J., 178
Munns, J. G., 332
Murphy, A. H., 195-196
Musillo, C., 322

Nakamura, J., 290
Narayan, O., 76
Nathanson, C., 254
Navia, B. A., 369
Naylor, P. H., 83
Nelson, V. R., 44-46
Nenney, S. W., 375
Newman, R., 31
Newmeyer, J. A., 329
Ngin, C. P., 290-307
Nicklin, O., 366
Nisbett, R., 146, 175, 186
Nisbett, R. E., 190

O'Donnell, C., 321-322
O'Donnell, L., 321-322
O'Grady, M. P., 21, 22, 72-87
Ohnuki-Tierney, E., 296
Olsen, E., 147
Olson, R. A., 311
O'Malley, P. M., 245, 377
Onishi, R., 58, 329
Ornez, W., 332
Orrego, A., 76
Osberg, T. M., 158
Osborn, J. E., 21-38, 69, 91
Osmond, D., 49
Ostrow, D. G., 211, 252

Padian, N. S., 61, 184
Padilla, E. R., 319
Palsson, P. A., 75

Panygris, F. D., 144
Pappaioanou, M., 269
Parducci, A., 187
Parekh, B., 76
Parish, K. L., 311
Pavich, E. G., 319
Peplau, L. A., 321
Perez, Y. I. D., 319
Perloff, L. S., 142, 150, 152
Perry, C. L., 382, 383
Perry, M., 14
Peterman, T. A., 61
Peters, S. D., 313
Peterson, J. L., 376
Phair, J. P., 361, 363, 367
Piot, P., 49, 55, 61, 64
Pirie, P., 113
Pleck, J. H., 321-322
Pliske, R. M., 189
Poindexter, P. M., 274
Polit-O'Hara, D., 255
Pollack, L., 246, 249
Pollack, R., 253-255
Poma, P. O., 319-320
Poulton, E. C., 184, 187
Poussaint, A. F., 315
Powell, M. L., 84
Price, J. H., 321
Price, R. W., 81, 369
Prodzinski, J., 113

Quadland, M., 253
Qualls, S., 249
Quinn, J., 315
Quinn, T. C., 62

Raiffa, H., 176
Ramos, J., 12-13, 208, 328
Rapoport, A., 149
Rauch, K., 366
Ray, M. L., 384
Read, S., 188, 195
Reagan, N., 275
Rebar, R. W., 83
Redfield, R. R., 225, 268
Reeder, S., 113
Remafedi, G., 376
Reyes, G. R., 79
Reynaldo, C., 245
Reynolds, D. K., 297

Rice, D. P., 366
Rich, K. C., 365
Richardson, D., 311
Richardson, J., 254
Rippetoe, P., 116
Roberts, D. F., 274
Roberts, N., 161
Roberts, V., 269
Robey, W. G., 76
Robinson, I., 270
Rodriguez, R., 311, 318, 330
Rogers, E. M., 247, 254-255, 384
Rogers, M. F., 330
Rogers, R., 115-116
Rogers, R. W., 144, 160
Rokeach, M., 188
Ronis, D., 113
Rosen, C. A., 76, 79
Rosenblum, M., 367
Rosenstock, I. M., 107, 112, 124, 157
Ross, L., 146, 175, 186
Rothbart, G., 274
Russ, J., 216
Ryan, S. M., 129

Safer, M., 144
St. Lawrence, J. S., 135, 225-239
Sallis, J. F., 136, 384
Samuel, M., 291, 330
Sandman, P. M., 155, 161
Sarin, P. S., 83
Sattath, S., 177
Schasre, R., 333
Schecter, G., 291
Schinke, S. P., 132, 135-136, 255, 319, 380
Schlucheter, M. D., 258, 381
Schneider, S. F., 12, 349, 351-356
Schoemaker, P. J. H., 145, 188
Schott, J., 254
Schuman, R., 253
Schuster, C. R., 377, 392-396
Schwartz, S. P., 147
Scitovsky, A. A., 366
Scott, J. W., 316
Scott, N. R., 332
Sechrest, L., 298
Selik, R. M., 269
Selnes, O. A., 367
Seminara, D., 390-391
Shapira, Z., 145

Shapiro, E., 315
Shattis, W., 253
Shelov, S. P., 67
Sheridan, E. P., 361-362, 367
Sheridan, K., 349-350, 358-372
Shilts, R., 315
Shortell, S., 147
Shrauger, J. S., 158
Shultz, J. M., 383
Sidtis, J. J., 369
Siegel, K., 151, 155, 237
Sigurdsson, B.,
Simon, H. A., 194
Simon, W., 129, 254
Skogan, W. G., 148, 383
Sloan, G., 274
Sloboda, W., 13
Slovic, P., 146-147, 175, 177, 183, 185, 188-189, 195
Small, E. C., 315, 381
Small, R. W., 255
Smith, M. C., 266
Smith, P. B., 375
Smith, T. W., 272
Smith, W. S. 330
Snarey, J., 321-322
Sodroski, J. G., 76, 79
Solnick, R., 253
Solomon, D. S., 138
Solomon, M., 253
Sorensen, R. C., 376
Sotheran, J. L., 340
Spaeth, J., 113
Spielberger, C. D., 229
Stall, R., 232, 244-246, 252
Stein, B. S., 79
Stein, J., 168
Steinman, M., 381
Stewart, C., 332
Stockard, R., 274
Stone, G. C., 142, 150, 152
Stoneburner, R. L., 61
Strecher, V., 114, 124
Street, R., 381
Stroman, C. A., 274
Strunin, L., 378
Sue, S., 299
Sun, D. K., 83
Sutton, S. R., 144
Svenson, O., 142, 145, 150, 154, 183, 194

Swartz, P., 288

Tafoya, T., 208, 280-289
Tal, M., 209-223
Tanner, J., 113
Tanner, W., 253
Taylor, C. B., 384
Taylor, S. E., 152, 182, 211
Teel, J. E., 273
Telch, M. J., 382
Telesky, M., 113
Temoshok, L., 321, 378
Thaler, R., 177, 191
Thorensen, C. E., 257, 349-350, 374-386
Thornton, A. H., 83
Townes, B. D., 144, 169
Tucker, M. B., 315-316
Tullman, G., 255
Turner, C. F., 188, 196
Tversky, A., 147, 158, 169, 177, 182, 186, 188, 191
Tyler, T. R., 148

Uhlenhuth, E., 214

Vahouny, G. V., 81-82
Valdiserri, R., 245-246
Van Brussel, G. H. A., 138
Vance, C. S., 210
Van Santen, G., 138
Vaughan, E., 147
Vaupel, J. W., 176
Veroff, J., 256
Vincent, M. L., 258, 381
Visotsky, H. M., 364
Vitaliano, P. P., 216
Volkman, D. J., 80
Von Roenn, B. A., 366
Von Winterfeldt, D., 147, 169, 176, 181

Wagatsuma, H., 297
Wallsten, T. S., 149, 181
Wallston, B. S., 144, 229
Wallston, K. A., 144, 229
Ward, C. H., 229
Warren, D. I., 275
Watkins, Admiral, 31, 36, 38
Watson, S., 169, 176
Watters, J. K., 132, 137, 329
Webb, F., 13

Weinberg, M., 242-243
Weinberger, M., 114
Weinhold, K. J., 79
Weinstein, N. D., 92, 142-163, 183, 248, 253, 312, 314
Wells, R. V., 270
Wherley, N., 332
White, P. E., 147
Whitley, P. N., 31
Wiley, J. A., 226, 232, 244, 252
Wilkeson, A. G., 315, 319
Williams, W. W., 330
Wills, T. A., 152, 157
Wilson, T.D., 190
Winer, D., 247
Winkelstein, W., 60, 244-246, 291, 330
Winkler, R., 195-196
Withey, G. A., 147
Wofsy, C. B., 54
Wolk, C., 113
Wong-Staal, F., 78

Wood, J. V., 152, 157
Worth, D., 311, 318, 330
Wortman, C. B., 209-223
Wyrtele, S., 116
Wyatt, G. E., 313-314

Yanagihara, E., 290
Yim, M., 290
York, B., 14

Zabin L. S., 381
Zacks, R. T., 181
Zagury, D., 79
Zaltman, C., 384
Zawisza, E., 160
Zelnik, M., 375-376, 380
Zenilman, J., 245
Zimbardo, P. G., 131
Zimmerman, R., 111
Zorn, J., 321, 378
Zwick, R., 149

Subject Index

Acquired Immunodeficiency Syndrome (AIDS); alcohol and, 287, 332, 352, 390, 398; as biopsychosocial phenomenon, 351, 358, 366-367; case studies, 44-46; costs of, 36, 86-87, 133, 365-367; decision-making about, 168-201; definition of, 48; dementia complex, 41-43, 81-85, 369; distribution of, 29-34, 49-55, 225-226. see also Epidemiology; diversity of population, 207-208; information about, see Education programs; incubation period, 33, 69; knowledge explosion, 369; medico-social political contexts, 363-365; mental health leadership roles, 363-371; mortality rates, 49, 182-183, 243, 282; outcomes, 370-371; research benefits, 86-87; risk knowledge test, 233, 237; risk reduction model, 247-258; service delivery systems, 365-367, See also specific programs; stigma of, 40, 45, 94, 133, 215, 363; survival rates, 265; vaccine, 24-26; See also Human immunodeficiency Virus (HIV) infection; Risk assessment; Transmission, HIV

Addict(s), see Intravenous (IV) drug users;

Addiction Research Center, 392;

Adolescents, 352; black, 313-314, 315; CVD in, 383-385; level of intervention, 379; prevention and, 320-324, 374-386; research and, 354; risk factors, 136, 270, 330-334, 377-378; socio-economic factors, 270, 378;

Adrenocorticotrophic hormone (ACTH), 82-84

Africa, and AIDS, 26-27, 55, 61

Age, HIV and, 51-52, 336, 375, 378

AIDS Program, Center for Infectious Disease, 265

AIDS Project Los Angeles, 303-304

AIDS-related complex (ARC), 58

AIDS: Sexual Behavior and Intravenous Drug Use (NRC), 398

Alaskan natives, 281-282, 284-285

Alcohol, AIDS and, 287, 332, 352, 390-391, 398

Alcohol, Drug Abuse, and Mental Health; Administration (ADAMHA), 352, 398

Aleuts, 282

Ambulatory care, 367

Amphetamines, 331

Amyl nitrite, 331

Anal intercourse, 59, 225-226, 230; behavioral change and, 119-122, 244-246; incidence of, 243; risk perception and, 252

Anemias, hemolytic, 75

Angel dust, see PCP

Antibodies, neutralizing, 76

Antibody test, see Screening, HIV

Anxiety, 216, 223, 299

Arthritis, 75

Asia, HIV and, 27

Asian AIDS Project, 291, 303-304

Asian AIDS Task Force, 305

Asian-Americans, 264; AIDS by age, 292; distinct ethnic groups of, 293; health behavioral change models for, 299; immigration by, 295; norms of, 294-299; prevention and, 291, 303-305; transmission categories, 292;

Asian Health services, 303-304

Asian Pacific Lesbians and Gays, 305

Asian Pacific Planning Council, 305

Assertiveness training, 228-229, 231-233
Association for People Living with AIDS (APLWA), 46
Attitudes, 273; beliefs and, 103; changing, 91-163; studies on, 68;
Autoimmune processes, 79
AZT, see Zidovudine

Barbiturates, 331
Barrios, see Mexican-Americans
Bars, 227
Bartenders Against AIDS, 243
Beck Depression Inventory, 229
Behavior, AIDS-related; alcohol and, 287, 332, 352, 390-391, 398; cultural differences in, see specific group; external variables, 106-108; health behavior model, 112-114; health belief predictors, 117-122; identification of, 97-98; impact of AIDS on, 81-85; motivation for, 143-144; normative beliefs and, 103; prediction of, 99-101, 111-124; research in, 91-163, 393-394, 398; self-identity and, 315; self-monitored, 234-236; sociosexual contexts, 248; volitional control, 100-101. See also Behavior change;
Behavioral scientists, role of, 358-372
Behavior change aversive emotions and, 252; benefits of, 118-122, 144; cognitive structural, 102-109; goals for, 96-97, 99-100; interventions and, 47; NIDA research on, 393-394; NIMH research on, 398; perceived risk and, 321; psychological costs of, 209-223; recidivism and, 210, 212, 244; risk reduction model, 242-258; risk susceptibility and, 142-163; self-directed, 130; skills needed for, 230; social support for, 136-139; stages of, 249-250; women and, 309-324. See also specific models
Belief systems, 91-163; adolescents and, 321; attitude and, 103; clarifying, 186-187; group differences in, 112, 296-299, 318; health belief model, 111-124; measures of, 122-123; risk susceptibility and, 142-163; subjective norm and normative, 103-106
Berdache, 287-288
Biopsychosocial multidisciplinary approaches, 366-367

Bisexuals, 29-30, 225; Asian, 298; behavioral changes in, 209-223; Blacks, 266-267; mental health and, 364; Native Americans, 288
Blacks; AIDS/HIV rates, 46, 53, 58, 264, 377-378; bisexuals, 266-267; cultural differences, 313-315; early sexual activity, 376-378; gay men, 265-266; heterosexual transmission, 268-269, 315-318; IV drug abuse and, 30-31, 377-378; perception of AIDS risk, 312-313; prevention and, 264-267, 312-318; religion and, 271-273; underclass economics and, 276-277
Bleach, and needle sharing, 66, 132, 346
Blood products, and HIV infections, 62, 311; AIDS rates, 53-54; imports of, 21, 26; tests of, see Screening programs
Board of Ethical and Social Responsibility, 11-12
Body fluids, HIV and, 59, 64, 230
Brain, AIDS and, 41-43, 72-87, 369, 397
Brazil, 27

California State Office of AIDS, 243
CAMP production, 82
Cardiovascular disease, community-based approach and, 383
Caribbean countries, AIDS rates in, 32
Case studies, 39-43
Catastrophic care fund, 289
Celibacy, 131, 246, 314, 322
Cells, viral penetration of, 79
Center for Population Options, 376
Centers for Disease Control (CDC); behavior change and, 209-210; city surveys, 35; contracts of, 359; gay men's disease rates and, 225-226; minority disease rates and, 264, 268, 276, 292, 318, 377-378; prevention and, 352; projections of, 24, 29-34, 57-58; research by, 398; women's disease rates and, 310
Central nervous system, HIV and, 72-87, 397
Chancroid, 55
Charlottesville Report, Public Health Service, 397
Chicago Multicenter AIDS Cohort Study, 209, 212, 245-246
Chicanos, see Mexican-Americans

Children, 352; AIDS incidence, 52, 31, 57, 62-63, 311, 378, 394; ethnic data, 27, 269, 284, 330; prevention and, 381-382. *See also* Adolescents; Infants; Women
Chinatown Health Clinic, New York, 303
Chinese, cultural roots of, 291, 294-296. *See also* Asian-Americans
Chlamydia, 55
Circumcision, 61
Clinical Investigator Award, 353
Cocaine, 31, 331, 336, 345
Cognitive models, 102-109, 111-124, 131, 248
Cognitive social learning theory, 384
Cognitive structural change, behavior and, 102-109
Cognitive theory, 94-108, 131
Communication-behavior change model, 384
Communication Technologies, 244, 256
Community-based intervention, 94, 138, 227-239, 248, 257-258, 346-347, 384. *See also specific projects*
Community outreach demonstration programs, 394
Compliance, research on, 111-124
Condoms; decisions on, 170-171, 316; education in use of, 230, 234; enjoyment and, 253; natural vs. latex, 62; teen's use of, 376, 378; women and, 137, 316, 322
Confidentiality, 37, 170-171, 228, 363
Confronting AIDS, 1986 (IOM), 197
Confronting AIDS: Update 1988 (IOM), 398
Control, and change, 276
Coping and Change Study, 117-122, 209, 212
Coping skills, self-perceptions of, 128-140
Coping strategies, 215-217, 220, 255, 369
Corticosterone, 82
Cosmopolitan, 73-74
Cost-benefit analysis, 144, 366
Crack, 31, 331, 336, 345
Cumulative risk, decision making and, 185
Current Population Survey (1985), 270
Cytolysis, mechanism of, 77
Cytomegalovirus, 77

Decision making models, 247-248; errors in, 178, 180-193; evaluation, 176-177; framing, 187-189; frequence estimates, 181-185; nonoptimality, 191-193; numerical estimates, 184-185; process and, 193-197; quantitative suboptimality in, 181, 189; risk reduction model and, 247-248; risk taking vs., 175-176; subjective optimization, 178-189; trial and error, 192
Decision theory, 168-201; criticism of, 173-175; decision tree, 178; distinctions missing from, 191; expectation rule, 177; language of, 173, 192-193;
Dementia complex, 41-43, 81-85, 369
Denial, 40, 157, 211, 217, 220, 302, 354
Deoxyribonuleic acid (DNA), 75-80
Depression, 40-41, 81, 216, 223, 299
Designer drugs, 331
Diffusion theory, 247
Discrimination, 40, 45, 94, 133, 215, 338, 363
Disinhibition, 391
Division of Community Pyschology, 356
Do-not-resuscitate (DNR) order, 370
Dread risks, 147
Drug abuse, 287, 330-334; NIDA and, 392-396; polydrug use, 336; treatment for, 31-32. *See also* Intravenous (IV) drug abuse
Drug trials, 59, 265, 367

Education programs, 26, 30; behavioral scientists and, 367; classroom and group approaches, 379-380; combining information, 186-187; community-mediated programs, 94, 138; eroticized materials, 210; ethnic-specific, 243, 303-305, 307, 342; federal monies for, 359; opposition to, 131; outreach, 226; practitioner projects, 349, 355, 359-363; protocols for information, 199; television and, 273-275; women and, 319
Efficacy measure, behavior change and, 117-118
ELISA test, 55, 212
Emotions theory, sexual enjoyment and, 251-253
Epidemic psychology, 247

Epidemiology, 21-22; alcoholism and, 390; female to male cases, 310; international, 26-28, 47-69. *See also* Centers for Disease Control

Epstein-Barr virus, 77

Eskimos, 282

Ethnic groups, research and, 354. *See also specific groups*

Expectancy-value theories, 144

Expectation rule, 177

Fear, 144

Framing, decision making and, 187-189

Gangs, heroin use by, 331

Gay Asian Pacific Alliance, 305

Gay men, 53-54; alcohol and, 391; Asian, 298; behavioral changes in, 209-223; Black, 265-266; care giving by, 371; group intervention project for, 225-239; health belief model and, 111-124; Hispanic/Latino, 265-266, 338; HIV infection rates, 56; mental health and, 364; Native American, 287; risk factors, 29-30, 59-60, 119, 225-226, 243-246; stigma of, 40, 45, 94, 133, 215, 338, 363. *See also* Bisexual men; *specific programs*

Gay Men's Health Crisis, 365

Gender; distribution by, 52-53; Native American concepts of, 287-288. *See also* Gay men; Women;

Gonorrhea, 139, 243, 285

Group intervention, gay men and, 225-239

Haitians, 32, 55

Harm, perceptions of susceptibility to, 142-163

Hawaii, Department of Health Services, 303

Hazard response, 142-163

Health belief models, 107, 145, 247; cultural norms and, 302-303; gay men and, 111-124

Health care delivery systems, 93, 365-367

Health education, *see* Education programs

Health Locus of Control Inventory, 229

Health Resources and Service Administration (HRSA), 359

Health threat, 117

Help-seeking behavior, 224-225, 242-258

Hemophiliacs, 58, 114, 284, 311, 368, 371

Hepatitis B virus, 77

Heroin, 30-31, 332-339

Herpes simplex virus, 77, 321

Heterosexuals; Asian, 298, 305, 306; HIV and, 26-27, 33-34, 52-55, 59-60, 63; Hispanic, 319-320; history taking with, 363; prevention and, 65-66; risk estimates by, 184; women, 268-269, 309-311

Hierarchy of effects model, 384

High-risk groups; decision-making and, 91-163; optimistic bias, 154-160; reasoned action theory and, 108; self-rating by, 154-156; risk history survey, 228-229. *See also* Behavior; Risk assessment

Hispanics/Latinos, 272-273; access to health care, 364; AIDS and, 264, 265; cultural differences, 319; gay men, 265-266; IV drug users, 30-31, 267-268, 329-342, 345-347, 377-378; prevention and, 340; subpopulations, 318; women, 268-269, 309, 311, 338

HIV, *see* Human Immunodeficiency Virus infection

Home care, 36

Homophobia, 210, 223, 288, 322, 338

Homosexuals, *see* Gay men; Lesbians

Hopkins Symptom Checklist (HSCL), 214

Hospice care, 36, 43, 366-367

Hospices, 43

Housing, 363

Howard Brown Memorial Clinic, 365

Human Immunodeficiency Virus (HIV) infection; alcohol and, 390; antibody test, 55, 212; asymptomatic, 34-38, 355; behavioral risk factors, 59-64; CNS effects, 72-87, 352, 369; clinical training in, 363; distribution of, 55-58; health belief model and, 117; high risk groups, 53-55; incubation interval, 26-27; in vitro, 78; migration and, 269-271; non-human primates and, 76; numbers of infected, 26-27, 246, 390; outcomes, 370; pathogenesis, 25-26; perceived self-efficacy in, 128-140; process, 76-77; prognosis, 58-59; psychological profile, 368; reinfection, 66; related mental disorders, 353; research, 351-356; screening for, *see* Screening programs;

susceptibility to, 73; thymosin alpha 1 and, 83-84; women and, 309-324
Human rights, 38
Human T-cell leukemia/lymphoma (HTLV-I), 290

Illusion, 211
Immigration, 295, 296, 318
Immune system, HIV and, 72-87
Immunotransmitters, role of, 81-85
Incidence rates, see Epidemiology; *specific populations*
Indian Child Welfare Act (1977), 282
Indian Health Services (IHS), 283
Indian Reorganization Act (1934), 281
Infants; AIDS rates, 53; HIV screening of, 35; mortality rates, 282; perinatal HIV spread, 57, 62-63, 378, 394
Information, see Education
Inguinal lesions, 61
Inhalants, 331, 336, 345
Institute of Medicine (IOM), 24, 197, 209, 398
Insurance coverage, 363
Intentions, behavior and, 95, 99-102, 106
Interferon, 82
Interleukin I, 77
Interventions; adolescents and, 374, 381-382; cognitive-behavioral research, 354; community-based, 381-382; professional vs. volunteer, 365, 369; research on, 349. See also Prevention programs; *specific models, programs*
Intravenous (IV) drug abusers, 287; AIDS rates and, 53-54; Black, 267-268; families of, 342; Hispanic, 267-268; HIV and, 56, 62; mental health and, 364; Native American, 284; NIDA and, 392-396; norms, 137; prevention and, 65-66; self-directed change in, 130-136; teens, 376-377; treatment of, 341; U.S., 30-33; women, 310

Jack off (J.O.) clubs, 246
Japan, blood imports, 26
Japanese-Americans, 291, 294-295. See also Asian-Americans
Japanese Community Youth Council AIDS;
Advisory Committee, 305

Kinsey Institute, 283
Koreans, 291. See also Asian-Americans

Latinos, see Hispanics/Latinos
Learned helplessness, 299-300
Lentiviruses, 75-76
Lesbian minorities, 287, 338
Life events, literature of, 211
Living wills, 370
LSD, 331, 336, 345
Lymphoadenopathy virus (LAV), 72

Mao-cerbaic avium intracellulare (MAI), 42-43
Marijuana, 330-334
Mass media, 92, 132, 149, 243, 273-276, 306, 395
Mastery-modeling approach, 136
Memorability, biases in, 182
Mental health practitioners, role of, 358-372
Mexican-Americans, IV drug use by, 329-342, 345-347. See also Hispanics/Latinos
Migration, 269-271
Military, HIV infection rates, 34-35, 56-57
Modeling, 134-136
Molecular biology, 352
Monocytes, HIV and, 73, 85
Monogamy, 131, 246
Mortality rates; estimating, 182-183; median survival, 49; Native American infants, 282; San Francisco and, 243
Mosquitoes, 297
Motivations, risk-relevant behaviors and, 143-144
Motor impairment, 81
Multicenter AIDS Cohort Study, 369
Multicultural approaches, 289

National Academy of Science (NAS), 24
National Cancer Institute (NCI), 209
National Center for Health Statistics (NCHS), 186, 196
National Center for Nursing Research (NCNR), 353
National Heart, Lung and Blood Institute (NHLBI), 353
National Institute on Aging (NIA), 353
National Institute on Alcohol and Alcohol Abuse (NIAAA), 350, 390-391

National Institute of Allergy and Infectious Diseases (NIAID), 209
National Institute of Child Health and Human Development (NICHD), 353
National Institute of Drug Abuse (NIDA), 353, 392-396
National Institute of Mental Health (NIMH), 209, 212, 350, 355, 359, 397-399
National Institute of Neurological Diseases and Stroke (NINDS), 353
National Institutes of Health (NIH), 352, 398
National Research Council (NRC), 197, 398
National Survey of Black Americans, 274
Native Americans; AIDS and, 264, 280-289; infant mortality rates, 282; Religious Freedom Act (1978), 281
Navajo Nation Department of Health, 283
Needle sharing, 30, 62, 329-342, 345-347; exchange programs, 31-32, 137-138; sterilization and, 65, 132, 137
Networks; barrio-oriented, 331, 335-337, 339, 342, 346; change and, 284; diffusion theory and, 384; family, 288, 294-295
Neurobiology, 41-43, 84, 352. See also Central nervous system
Neuroendocrine system, 84
Neurovirology, 352
New York City hospital model, 365
Newcastle disease virus, 84
Newcomer Health Services, 304
Nonoptimality, in decision making, 191-193
Nonoxynol-9, 62
Norepinephrine, 83
Norms, 263, 301, 331-346; change process and, 254; intention and 101-102; redefinition of, 226; safe sex and, 317, 320
Northwest AIDS Foundation, 283
Northwestern University Medical School, 360

Office of Technology Assessment (OTA), 379
Opium, 331
Opportunisitic infections, see by name
Optimism, and risk judgements, 149-154
Optimistic bias, origins and correlates of, 156-160

Optimizing models, 180
Oral sex, 322
Outpatient care, 36, 41
Outreach, 394. See also Community-based intervention

Pacific Islanders, 293
Parasitic infections, 243
Pasteur Institute, 72
PCP (angel dust), 331, 336, 345
Peer pressure, 263, 302, 346, 382
Peer support, 210. See also Networks
Peptides, 84, 85
Perceived harm, 144-145
Perceived risk, 117, 160-163, 321
Perceived self-efficacy, 128-140
Perceived sexual enjoyment, 242-258
Perinatal transmission, 57, 62-63, 311, 315, 378
Pinto subculture, 331
Pregnancy; adolescent, 315; prevention programs, 381-382
Physician Scientist Award, 353
Pilipino AIDS Advisory Task Force, 305
Pilipinos, 291, 294-295. See also Asian-Americans
Pregnancy, 315, 381-382. See also Perinatal transmission
Presidential Commission on the HIV Epidemic, 36, 398
Prevention, 64-67; Asians and, 297; behavioral scientists and, 367; Blacks and, 317; community-mediated approach, 138; cultural context of, 31, 271-277; drug abuse and, 393; estimating effectiveness of, 187; external variables, 106-108; Hispanics/Latinos and, 318-320, 345-346; impediments to psychosocial models, 139-140; international, 47-69; lack of services, 345-346; modeling principles, 134-136; multicomponent behavioral indexes, 114; multifactorial approaches, 237; NIMH and, 398; perceived self-efficacy and, 128-140; primary models, 91-163; research needs, 397; school-based, 380-383; seeking help and, 255-257; socio-economic changes and, 271; smoking, 382-383; target populations, 338; treatment, 345-346;

women and, 309-324. *See also specific populations, programs*
Print media, 275, 395
Probability theory, 187, 196
Project ARIES, 227-239
Prostitution, 65, 288
Protection-motivation theory, 115-116
Provirus, 75
Pseudo-AIDS syndrome, 74
Psychologists; community, 356; gay-sensitive, 213; research and training agenda for, 349, 351-356; role of, 358-372
Psychoneuroimmunology, 352, 354
Psychosocial variables, 217
Public Health Service (PHS), 397. *See also* Centers for Disease Control
Puerto Ricans, 318. *See also* Hispanics/ Latinos
Pulmonary disease, 75

Quarantines, 211

Race, AIDS distribution by, 53. *See also specific group*
Radio media, 275
Radon testing, decision theory and, 178-179
Range-frequency effect, 187
Reasoned action theory, 93-109, 144, 248, 301-302
Referrals, 369
Religious Freedom Act (1978), 281
Reporting, 29, 210-211, 265. *See also* Centers for Disease Control
Research on Behavior Change and Prevention Strategies to Reduce Transmission of HIV, 352
Research programs, national, 352; multidisciplinary, 355; NIAAA, 390-391; NIDA, 392; NIMH, 397; psychological, 349
Research Scientist Development Award, 353
Research theories, 91-163
Retrovirus, 72, 74-80
Risk assessment, 63; comparative vs. absolute risk, 161-162; cumulative risk and, 185; epidemics and, 23-38; objective risk factors and, 154-156; optimistic bias, 149-154; perceived risk, 117, 124, 148. *See also* Decision making
Risk factors, *see* Behavior

Risk history survey, 228-229
Risk Index (RI), 213
Risk reduction behavior, *see* Behavior change
Risk reduction model, 242-258
The Road to H: Narcotics, Delinquency and Social Policy, 332
Role playing, 135, 228, 233
Roots (Haley), 274
Runaways, 378

Safe sex, 92, 97; alcohol and, 391; assertiveness skills and, 228; gay men and, 230; homophobia and, 210; hot messages, 253; instruction in, 132; lying and, 323; norms and, 139, 320; sexually-transmitted diseases and, 321; socials, 346; videos and, 243. *See also* Condoms
San Francisco, AIDS cases in, 243
San Francisco AIDS Foundation, 87, 256
San Francisco Behavior Cohort, 244
San Francisco Department of Health, 291
San Francisco General Hospital, 291, 365
San Francisco HIV Antibody Counseling and Testing Program, 293
San Francisco Men's Health Study, 244, 291
School-based prevention programs, 380-383
Scientist Development Award for Clinicians, 353
Screening programs, HIV, 34-36; behaviors and, 112-114; confidentiality of, 37, 170-172, 228, 363; mandatory, 133, 210; testing decision, 169-171, 180; tests for, 55, 212
Seattle AIDS information Project, 284
Self-efficacy theory, 115, 247, 299-300
Self-esteem, self-perception and, 157
Self-guidance, 128
Self-management strategies, 231
Self-motivation, 128
Self-perception, and optimistic bias, 149-154
Self-protective behavior, 137, 160-163
Self-regulatory skills, 129-130
Sex-ratio imbalance, 315-318
Sexual history, 363
Sexual intercourse, 23; age and, 375-376; anonymous partners, 119, 243; extramarital, 316; risk factors, 37, 59-64. *See*

also Anal intercourse; Behavior; Heterosexuals; Safe sex; *specific groups*
Sexuality, functions of, 314-315
Sexually transmitted disease (STD); clinics and, 359; immortality and, 317; native groups and, 285; single women and, 320; teens and, 376
Shanti Project, 364
Shooting galleries, 339
Smoking prevention programs, 382-383
Social group influence, *see* Networks
Social inoculation, 382
Social marketing principles, 384
Social modeling, 134-136
Social network diffusion theory, 384
Social networks, *see* Networks
Social stigma, *see* Discrimination
Social support, *see* Networks; *specific programs*
Social workers, role of, 358-372
Spermicidal cream, 62, 66
Stanford Five City Project, 383-384
Stanford perceived self-efficacy study, 128-140
Stanford Three Community Study, 384
State-Trait Anxiety Inventory, 229
Steroidogenesis, thymosin-induced, 82-84
Stop AIDS Project, 226, 243, 256, 304, 346
Subjective expected-utility theories, 144
Subjective norms, beliefs and, 103-106
Subjective optimization, in decision making, 178-189
Surgeon General's report, 169, 171
Surveillance systems; NIDA, 395; uniform format, 289. *See also* Centers for Disease Control; Reporting
Surveys, ambiguity in, 196
Susceptibility beliefs, 247
Syphilis, 139, 243, 285

T-cell function, 77-80, 391
T-cell leukemia (ATL), 290
Tecato subculture, 331
Television, 132, 273-275
Testing, *see* Screening programs
Thailand, 27
Threat, perceptions of, 142-163
Thymosins, 82
Training, professional, 349, 355, 360-363, 395
Transfusions, *see* Blood products

Transmission, 64, 392; behaviorial aspects of, 23; cultural context of, 271-277, 378; heterosexual, 268, 310; means of, 73; perinatal, 52, 57, 62-63, 313, 330, 378, 394; probability judgements, 184-185; social factors, 137
Trinidad, 290
Turberculosis, AIDS and, 291

Uncertainty, role of, 116
Understanding AIDS (U.S. Surgeon General), 169, 171
Unemployment, of Blacks, 315
United States, AIDS/HIV rates, 27, 30-33, 49-51, 55-56, 59, 244, 291, 310
U.S. Congress, 379
U.S. Department of Health and Human Services (DHHS), 390
University of Michigan, 209

Vaccines, 24-26, 69, 91
Vaginal intercourse, *see* Sexual intercourse; Women
Values, 187-188, 195, 359. *See also* specific group
Venereal disease, *see* Sexually transmitted disease
Vermont Conference on Psychological Approaches to the Prevention of AIDS, 358
Videotapes, modeling and, 134-136
Viral DNA, 77-80
Viral RNA, 75, 77-80. *See also* Human Immunodeficiency Virus (HIV) infection
Volunteer movements, 364-365. *See also* *specific programs*
Vulnerability, self-perceptions of, 148-160

Western Blot test, 55, 212
Women; Black, 268, 275; Hispanic/Latina, 318-320; HIV seroprevalence, 57; IV drug abuse and, 333, 365; media use by, 275; Native American, 285-286; prevention issues, 320, 324; prostitutes, 65, 288; research and, 354; risk factors for, 53-55. *See also* Perinatal transmission

World Health Organization (WHO), 47

Zidovudine (AZT), 59, 367

Contributors

George W. Albee, Ph.D., Professor of Psychology at the University of Vermont, is President of the Vermont Conference on the Primary Prevention of Psychopathology and General Editor (with Justin M. Joffe) of the series of volumes published by VCPPP. He is a Past President of the American Psychological Association (1969–1970). He was Chair of the Board of Social and Ethical Responsibility in Psychology (BSERP) when the conference on prevention of AIDS was proposed.

Bart Aoki, Ph.D., is the Clinical Director of the Asian Youth Substance Abuse Project in San Francisco. He also serves as a Clinical Psychologist for the Asian American Recovery Services, Inc., and St. Mary's Hospital Medical Center. He is the founding Co-Chair of the Asian AIDS Task Force, a 200-member advocacy and education group responsible for providing AIDS education and services to the Asian community.

Albert Bandura, Ph.D., is a David Starr Jordan Professor of Social Sciences in Psychology at Stanford University. He is a proponent of social cognitive theory, which accords a central role to cognitive, vicarious, self-regulatory, and self-reflective processes in sociocognitive functioning. Programs of self-directed change of health habits draw heavily on self-regulatory mechanisms. His recent book, *Social Foundations of Thought and Action: A Social Cognitive Theory*, provides the conceptual framework and analyzes the large body of knowledge bearing on this theory. He is a Past President of the American Psychological Association and the recipient of its Distinguished Scientific Contributions Award.

Ted L. Brasfield, Ph.D., is a Research Assistant in the Division of Psychology at the University of Mississippi Medical Center. Before joining the AIDS Behavioral Research Team at the medical center, he worked as a respiratory therapy technician and received his training in this field at the North Mississippi Medical Center. For the past three years, he has focused his professional attention on community-based AIDS prevention research and on training volunteers in the AIDS prevention/ services area. He is an author of journal articles and numerous scientific papers on AIDS risk-reduction intervention research. In addition to his research activities at the medical center, he is a coordinator for volunteer training in the AIDS Buddy Program of the Mississippi PWA Project.

Larry Bye, Ph.D., is a social marketing expert who has played a leading role in the design and evaluation of HIV disease prevention programs in California. He has conducted a number of major AIDS-related knowledge, attitude, and behavior studies, and has worked with the various departments in the Centers for Disease Control on the development and evaluation of AIDS risk-reduction programs. He has authored a number of articles on AIDS prevention for national and international health publications, and has given presentations at numerous AIDS-related conferences, including three of the International Conferences on AIDS (Atlanta, 1985; Paris, 1986; and Stockholm, 1988). He was a Co-Founder of the Stop AIDS Project, Inc., and is currently the President of Communication Technologies.

Joseph A. Catania, Ph.D., is a Research Psychologist with the Center for AIDS Prevention Studies and Division of General Internal Medicine at the University of California, San Francisco. He is currently involved in research on the predictors of sexual behavior among gay men, adolescent heterosexual women, adult heterosexual ethnic minorities, and the elderly. His past work on human sexuality has concerned methodological issues in assessing sexual behavior and the intervention evaluation.

417

He is a member of the NIMH-NIDA AIDS Multicenter work group on psychosexual assessment and a methodological consultant to the Canadian government in the area of sexual behavior and AIDS.

Susan Caumartin, M.A., is a doctoral student in health behavior and health education in the School of Public Health at the University of Michigan. She is a Research Assistant on the Coping and Change Study and is particularly interested in the interrelationships among psychological functioning, behavior, and health status.

Thomas J. Coates, Ph.D., is Associate Professor of Medicine, Director of the Behavioral Medicine Unit, and Co-Director of the Center for AIDS Prevention Studies at the University of California, San Francisco. His research has been directed primarily at chronic disease prevention. He has focused more directly on AIDS since 1983, with a special emphasis on primary and secondary prevention strategies. These studies have included predictors of changes in high-risk behaviors in a variety of populations, predictors of progression of HIV disease, and the development and evaluation of intervention strategies. He also has extensive clinical experience in the area. He has consulted with the U.S. Office of Technology Assessment and the U.S. General Accounting Office, and is a member of the National Academy of Sciences Committee on AIDS Research and the Behavioral, Social, and Statistical Sciences. He also serves on the AIDS Policy Subcommittee of the National Mental Health Advisory Council of the National Institute of Mental Health.

Susan D. Cochran, Ph.D., received her A.B. in anthropology and her Ph.D. in clinical psychology from the University of California, Los Angeles. She completed two years of postdoctoral training in gynecologic oncology as an American Cancer Society Post-Doctoral Fellow in the Department of Psychiatry, UCLA School of Medicine. She is currently an Associate Professor in the Department of Psychology, California State University, Northridge, and codirects the Black Community AIDS Research and Education Project at UCLA. She has been involved in AIDS-related research and clinical practice since 1984. As a health psychologist, she has had a long-standing interest in the application of social psychology theories to such areas as sexual behavior, personal identity, interpersonal relationship choices, and medication compliance.

Maria Ekstrand received her Ph.D. in clinical psychology from Auburn University in 1986. Following a clinical internship at the University of Mississippi Medical Center, she did a postdoctoral fellowship in health psychology at the University of California, San Francisco. She is currently working as Assistant Research Psychologist at the Center for AIDS Prevention Studies at UCSF, where she is a fellow of the American Foundation for AIDS Research. This work focuses on the study of psychosocial risk factors for HIV infection, disease progression, and risky sex relapse among gay and bisexual men. She is also directing an NICHHD grant on biopsychosocial predictors of adolescent sexual behavior at the San Francisco Youth Guidance Center.

Michael Eller is the Research Associate for the Coping and Change Study at the Howard Brown Memorial Clinic in Chicago. In that capacity he is responsible for the ongoing field study and relations to the participants. It is his enthusiasm, skill, and dedication that makes this research possible.

Suzann Eshleman, M.A., Senior Research Associate at the University of Michigan, received graduate training at Cornell University in human development and family studies. Since 1983, she has contributed to a variety of research projects focused on the interrelationship of health, environmental, and social processes. She has been a member of the Coping and Change Study since 1987 and is most concerned with the development of appropriate computer methodologies for the analysis of complex data sets.

Baruch Fischhoff, Ph.D., is Professor of Social and Decision Sciences and Professor of Engineering and Public Policy at Carnegie Mellon University. An experimental psychologist by training, his research focuses on human judgment and decision making. This has included studies of risk perception and communication, as well as of the appropriateness of formal methods of decision making (e.g., cost-benefit analysis, risk analysis) for setting social policy. His current projects concern adolescent decision making (with Lita Furby and Marilyn Jacobs) and explaining technological hazards to lay audiences (with an interdisciplinary group of psychologists, economists, and engineers). The latter project has included several studies of how alternative presentation formats can affect perceptions of the risk of AIDS (performed with Patty Linville and Gregory Fischer).

Martin Fishbein, Ph.D., is a Professor of Psychology and Research Professor at the Institute for Communications Research at the University of Illinois at Urbana-Champaign. In addition, he is Coordinator for the UIUC AIDS Research Network. His research interests include attitude theory and measurement, attitude change, and the relations among beliefs, attitudes, intentions, and behaviors.

June A. Flora, Ph.D., is an Assistant Professor of Communication and Associate Director, Stanford Center for Research in Disease Prevention at Stanford University. She received her Ph.D. in educational psychology from Arizona State University in 1976. She also completed a clinical psychology internship at the University of Washington Medical School and a two-year postdoctoral fellowship in cardiovascular disease epidemiology and disease prevention at Stanford. For the past seven years, she has directed the educational intervention of the Stanford Five City Project (FCP), which focuses on determining the effects of media-based interventions on health behavior. She has recently published several articles and chapters on the learning and communication outcomes of the FCP, and the role of mass media in health promotion. She is currently investigating the application of intervention and formative research methods derived from the FCP to other health areas, such as AIDS.

Joseph R. Guydish, Ph.D., completed doctoral training in clinical psychology at Washington State University in 1987. While an intern at the Langley Porter Psychiatric Institute, and later as a Postdoctoral Fellow in the Department of Psychiatry at the University of California, San Francisco, he specialized in the area of behavioral medicine. During this time, he worked extensively with HIV-affected patients in clinical practice, and developed research interests in HIV-related risk behavior change. He is currently a Visiting Post-Graduate Scholar in the Center for AIDS Prevention Studies, UCSF, researching risk behavior in heterosexual and intravenous drug-using populations.

Nicholas R.S. Hall, Ph.D., received his undergraduate training in experimental psychology, his Ph.D. in neuroscience, and his postdoctoral training in tumor immunology. He now directs the Division of Psychoimmunology at the University of South Florida School of Medicine, where he holds joint appointments in the Departments of Psychiatry and Microbiology. Research programs within this division range from studies of immunologic correlates of psychiatric illness to molecular events underlying the effects of immune system peptides upon neurotransmitter release. His work with AIDS has focused upon localization of HIV components within the brain and their ability to activate the pituitary-adrenal axis.

Norman Hearst, M.D., M.P.H., is an Assistant Clinical Professor of Family Medicine and of Epidemiology at the University of California, San Francisco. He is Adjunct Director of the Center for AIDS Prevention Studies, which provides AIDS research training to scientists from developing countries. He has published articles on the natural history of HIV disease, and on AIDS prevention. His other research interests include the physical and mental health problems of Vietnam veterans.

Harold V. Hood was formerly a Research Assistant at the University of Mississippi Medical Center and is currently an AIDS Patient Care Coordinator with the Hillsborough County (Florida) Health Department and the Florida Department of Health and Rehabilitation Services. He received his B.A. degree from Belhaven College. His areas of interest include the adaptation of marketing principles to community-based AIDS prevention efforts, risk reduction, and community services for persons with HIV conditions. He is author of a number of research publications and professional presentations in these areas.

Stephen B. Hulley, M.D., M.P.H., is Professor of Epidemiology, Medicine, and Health Policy, Vice Chairman of the Department of Epidemiology, and Director of the Prevention Sciences Center in the School of Medicine, University of California, San Francisco. He was educated at Harvard Medical School and the University of California, Berkeley, School of Public Health. He has spent the past 20 years studying diet, smoking, and other risk behaviors that cause coronary heart disease, and developing and testing preventive interventions. In the past 5 years he has turned his attention to the AIDS epidemic, and as Principal Investigator and Director of the UCSF Center for AIDS Prevention Studies he is involved in numerous studies of the behaviors responsible for the spread of AIDS, and of public health approaches to controlling the epidemic.

Davis Y. Ja, Ph.D., is currently the Executive Director for the Asian American Recovery Services, Inc. He is responsible for the formation of education programs for the Asian AIDS Project. He is also the main advocate for the Asian community on AIDS education issues. He recently completed two needs assessment projects focused on attitudes and behaviors toward AIDS in the Chinese and Pilipino gay communities.

Jaime S. Jorquez, D.S.W., is an Assistant Professor at the Arizona State University School of Social Work, in the Center for Hispanic Research.

Jill G. Joseph, Ph.D., is an Assistant Professor of Epidemiology at the University of Michigan School of Public Health. Since 1980, she has been conducting research on biobehavioral and psychosocial aspects of the AIDS epidemic and HIV transmission. Educated at Stanford University and the University of California at Berkeley, she received her Ph.D. in epidemiology in 1980.

Lewis L. Judd, M.D., was appointed as Director, National Institute of Mental Health, in January 1988. Previously, he served 10 years as Chairman of the Department of Psychiatry in the School of Medicine at the University of California, San Diego. He is an expert in the field of clinical psychopharmacology and biological psychiatry, and has published widely in the research literature on psychopharmacology, depression, manic depression, and schizophrenia. He brings to the directorship a broad and rich experience with the Institute over the years, both as a grantee and from his service on many scientific review and advisory committees, including the Institute's own Board of Scientific Councilors. He is on the editorial boards of many distinguished scientific journals and recently published and edited a book, *The Basic Science Foundations of Clinical Psychiatry*.

Susan M. Kegeles, Ph.D., is a Research Psychologist at the Center for AIDS Prevention Studies at the University of California, San Francisco. She is a health psychologist and applies social psychology and decision-making theory to the areas of sexuality, risk-taking behavior, and reproductive health. Her current research interests involve understanding the determinants of AIDS risk behavior and developing interventions to help people in changing activities that put them at risk for HIV infection.

Jeffrey A. Kelly, Ph.D., is Professor of Psychiatry (Psychology) and Chief of the Division of Psychology at the University of Mississippi Medical Center. He received his undergraduate degree from Case Western Reserve University and his Ph.D. in clinical psychology from the University of Kentucky. He is a Past President of the Mississippi Psychological Association, a Fellow in Division 12 of the American Psychological Association, and serves on the editorial boards of numerous scientific journals. He is the author of several journal articles, book chapters, and books, primarily in the behavior therapy area. For the past several years, his research efforts have been focused primarily on the application of behavioral interventions for AIDS risk reduction. He also directs an AIDS/HIV psychology clinic at the medical center and, with Janet St. Lawrence, is the author of *The AIDS Health Crisis: Psychological and Social Interventions*.

Ronald C. Kessler, Ph.D., is a Professor of Sociology and Research Scientist in the Survey Research Center at the University of Michigan. He received his doctorate in 1975, and has focused on investigation of stress events and psychological functioning in diverse populations. He is particularly concerned with development of appropriate methodologies for longitudinal studies and has been working in the area of AIDS since 1984.

John P. Kirscht, Ph.D., is a Professor of Health Behavior and Health Education, School of Public Health, University of Michigan. He has worked primarily in the area of health-related prevention, with emphasis on understanding the components of changing risky behaviors within the framework of cognitive theories.

G. M. "Missy" LeClaire went to colleges in both Maryland and Virginia. Missy, as she is known to all, previously worked as an accounting and office administrator for several large firms. Since her husband's death she has become very active in the AIDS education movement. She has made over 150 radio appearances, including broadcasts on Radio Free Europe. She has also appeared on both national and local television to discuss AIDS. In addition, she travels extensively, giving freely of her time, lecturing on AIDS. Though extremely busy, she also serves on the Board of Directors for the National Association for People with AIDS (NAPWA) and is an officer in Lifelink, an active AIDS organization in the Washington, D.C. area.

Alberto G. Mata, Jr., Ph.D., is a Postdoctoral Fellow at the University of Texas Health Science Center, Center for Health Promotion, and an Assistant Professor at Arizona State University, School of Social Work, in the Center for Hispanic Research.

Vickie M. Mays, Ph.D., received her B.A. in psychology and philosophy from Loyola University of Chicago and completed her doctoral studies in clinical psychology at the University of Massachusetts, Amherst. She has also pursued advance training in psychiatric epidemiology and survey research methodology both as an NIMH New Investigator Research Award recipient with the UCLA Epidemiology Catchment Area Project and as a Postdoctoral Fellow at the University of Michigan's Institute of Social Research in the Program for Research on Black Americans. Since 1984 she has been involved in AIDS-related clinical practice, education, community-based consultations, and research. She is currently an Associate Professor of Psychology at the University of California, Los Angeles, where she is the Director of the Black Community AIDS Research and Education Project. She is also a National Center for Health Service Research Fellow at the RAND Corporation, where she is pursuing an

M.S.Ph. in health services research and epidemiology in conjunction with UCLA's School of Public Health.

Susan E. Middlestadt, Ph.D., is an Assistant Professor of Advertising in the College of Communications at the University of Illinois at Urbana-Champaign. Her research interests include research methods, communications and persuasion, the analysis of behavior and behavior change with specific emphasis on the development and evaluation of health communications.

Bertha Mo, Ph.D., M.P.H., is a graduate of the University of California, Berkeley. She is the Co-Chair of the Asian AIDS Task Force in San Francisco and has been active in educating the Asian community about AIDS. She also serves as a consultant for various national AIDS information and education agencies, including the Office of Minority Health, Organization of Chinese Americans, and the Centers for Disease Control. She is currently the Director of Consultation, Education and Information for the City of San Francisco Department of Public Health, Mental Health Division.

Edward S. Morales, Ph.D., is a clinical and consulting psychologist and was one of the founders and directors of the UCSF-AIDS Health Project, and of the Center for AIDS Prevention Studies-Multicultural Inquiry and Research on AIDS. He also was one of the founders of the Multicultural Alliance for the Prevention of AIDS, one of the first minority AIDS prevention programs funded. He has extensive clinical and research experience in the field of substance abuse and was Clinical Director of the Bayview Hunter's Point Methadone Program. In 1987 he completed a seven-year term on the San Francisco Citizen's Alcoholism Advisory Board, where he was Chair of the Program Committee. His clinical and research experience also includes specializing in issues concerning ethnic minorities, gays and lesbians, and multiple minorities. He is currently a Research Associate of the Center for AIDS Prevention Studies, Coordinator of Program Development for Bayview Hunter's Point Foundation, President of Psychodynamics, Inc., an evaluation and consulting firm, and in private practice.

Stephen F. Morin, Ph.D., is Legislative Assistant for Health Policy to Congresswoman Nancy Pelosi (D-California). He is a Past Chair of the Board of Social and Ethical Responsibility for Psychology and current Chair of the APA Task Force on Psychology and AIDS. He is the immediate Past President of the California State Psychological Association.

Van R. Nelson, raised and educated in the East, now makes Seattle his home. He is the Founder and Director of the Association of People Living with AIDS (APLWA), Seattle, Washington. As a Black man diagnosed with HIV infection, he discovered a lack of services, understanding, and support for the ethnic minority community. More important, as he began to access services he found them culturally inappropriate to HIV-infected individuals of color. He tried to develop ethnic minority outreach through established organizations and service providers. These avenues were unable, both financially and psychologically, to support his ethnic minority outreach efforts. To better provide support services to the HIV-infected ethnic minority community, he became a member of the National Association of People with AIDS (NAPWA); soon afterward, he established APLWA and a NAPWA coalition in Seattle for people of color. NAPWA was one of the first national organizations to make sweeping changes in its structure by expanding support to better represent the needs of people of color and the physically challenged. He is currently on NAPWA's board and has become an articulate speaker/writer/activist. He also directs the activities of his local coalition and continues to devote most of his energies to the national and local levels.

Chiang Peng Ngin, M.P.H., received his master's degree in public health from the University of California, Berkeley, with concentrations in epidemiology and biostatistics. He serves as the Program Coordinator for the Asian AIDS Project, the first Asian AIDS education project in the country. His research interests include AIDS education and debunking myths surrounding AIDS in the Asian communities. Prior to joining the Asian AIDS Project, he taught in the Asian American Studies Department at UC Berkeley and served as a consultant to the Asian American Health Forum.

Maureen P. O'Grady has an undergraduate degree in experimental psychology from St. Joseph's University (Philadelphia, 1980). After obtaining an M.A. in psychobiology at the University of California, Santa Barbara, in 1983, she continued her studies at the same institution, where she received a Ph.D. in neuroendocrinology in 1986. She then moved on to George Washington University, where she did her postdoctoral training in behavioral immunology. She is now an Assistant Professor at the University of South Florida School of Medicine, where she has a joint appointment in the Department of Psychiatry and Behavioral Medicine and the Department of Medical Microbiology and Immunology. Her primary research interest is in the developmental aspects of the interactions among brain, behavior, and the immune system.

June E. Osborn, M.D., is trained as a pediatrician and as a virologist, and served on the faculty of the University of Wisconsin Medical School for 18 years, where she was Professor of Medical Microbiology and Professor of Pediatrics. In 1984, she became the Dean of the School of Public Health at the University of Michigan as well as Professor of Epidemiology, and Professor of Pediatrics and Communicable Diseases at the University of Michigan Medical School. She has served as an adviser to the federal government, private foundations, and the World Health Organization in a number of capacities relating to the AIDS epidemic. She is a member of the WHO Global Commission on AIDS, and has written widely on topics relating to AIDS epidemic policies at the national and international levels.

Juan Ramos, Ph.D., is Deputy Director for Prevention and Special Projects at the National Institute of Mental Health, where he has been since 1968. His areas of interests include prevention, refugee mental health, and AIDS. He has been active in the definition, design, and establishment of community-based mechanisms specific to AIDS issues based on combined shared goals reflecting community needs, strengths, and concerns of the committed leadership. His keen interests in the mechanism of community-level concerns and the impact they have on addressing the problem of AIDS continue to be important to the research efforts of the Institute.

Janet S. St. Lawrence is Associate Professor of Psychology at Jackson State University and Clinical Associate Professor of Psychiatry (Psychology) at the University of Mississippi Medical Center. She received her undergraduate degree from Boston University and her Ph.D. in clinical psychology from Nova University. She was the recipient of the 1985 President's New Researcher Award from the Association for the Advancement of Behavior Therapy and has served on the editorial board of *Behavior Therapy*. She is the author of approximately 60 articles in the behavior therapy field, with her work most recently focusing on AIDS primary prevention, attitudes concerning AIDS, and psychological therapy for persons with HIV conditions. With Jeffrey A. Kelly, she is the author of *The AIDS Health Crisis: Psychological and Social Interventions*.

Stanley F. Schneider, Ph.D., is Associate Director for Research Training and Research

Career Development in the Division of Basic Sciences at NIMH. For most of his career at NIMH he has been involved with programs for the training of psychologists and others. His interest in and involvement with the AIDS program at NIMH came about as a result of the Institute's major reorganization in 1985, when his colleague, Ellen Stover, piqued his curiosity and invited him to join her. She had been the only person working on AIDS at the time. A brief look at the problem was enough to convince him that this was a critically important task, one that has occupied him since then. It is his opinion that AIDS provides psychologists with extraordinary opportunities for research that may make a difference and for training that necessarily will involve several other disciplines, with the breadth and perspective this can bring.

Charles R. Schuster, Ph.D., is an internationally recognized researcher on the psychopharmacology of drugs of abuse. He received a doctoral degree in psychology from the University of Maryland in 1962, where he developed a widely used animal model of self-administration of drugs that has been critical to the prediction of the abuse liability of drugs and the identification of underlying behavioral and biochemical processes in drug abuse. Formerly Professor of Psychology, Director of the Drug Abuse Research Center, and Acting Chairman of Psychiatry at the University of Chicago, he assumed the Directorship of the National Institute on Drug Abuse in 1986. At NIDA, he directs both an intramural and an extramural research program to identify the nature and extent of the drug abuse problem as well as research into its prevention and treatment. He also is called upon to represent NIDA's program to Congress and other branches of government and to advise lawmakers on drug abuse problems. In addition, he has long been active on international policymaking and advisory boards in the area of drug use and abuse.

Daniela Seminara received her Ph.D. cum laude in cell biology from the University of Rome, Italy. After completing her postdoctoral work at the Institute of Human Genetics of the Catholic University Medical School of Rome, she became Associate Professor of Pediatrics in the same university. During her tenure there, she conducted clinical research related to biochemical and immunological aspects of several inborn metabolic diseases. From 1979 to 1982 she was a Visiting Fellow at the National Institutes of Health, studying the metabolic and immunological derangements in sphyngolipidosis in an in vitro macrophage model. In the following years she held a joint appointment as Assistant Professor of Anatomy at Howard University Medical School in Washington, D.C., and Visiting Scientist at NIH, studying the pathogenesis of diabetes development. She joined the National Institute on Alcohol Abuse and Alcoholism in 1987, and, due to her expertise in the areas of biochemistry, cell biology, and immunology and her activities as Program Officer for Alcohol and Immunology, she has recently been appointed AIDS Coordinator for this Institute.

Kathleen Sheridan, Ph.D., J.D., is the Deputy Director of the Comprehensive AIDS Center at the Northwestern University Medical School.

Terry Tafoya, Ph.D., was trained as a traditional Native American storyteller. He is a Taos Pueblo/Warm Springs Indian who uses legends in the form of therapeutic metaphor as a regular part of his clinical practice as a family therapist. He is a Professor of Psychology for the Evergreen State College, in Olympia, Washington, and serves as Clinical Faculty for the University of Washington Medical School. His sex research has concentrated on the relationships of interracial same-sex couples and he is on the summer faculty for the Kinsey Institute for the Study of Sex, Gender and Reproduction in the area of cross-cultural sexuality. He is currently on academic leave to direct the training of the National Native American AIDS Prevention Center in Oakland, California.

Margalit Tal, Ph.D., is the Research Associate to the Coping and Change Study at the University of Michigan. Originally educated in Israel, she received doctoral training at the University of Michigan, focusing on survey studies on the stress-coping process.

Carl E. Thoresen received his Ph.D. in counseling psychology from Stanford University in 1964. After two years on the faculty at Michigan State University, he returned to Stanford in 1967 as a professor. Currently he is serving as Associate Dean for Academic Affairs in the School of Education. His research concerns health- and disease-related problems, including AIDS prevention, coronary-prone behavior pattern (Type A), and chronic stress in children and adolescents. He was awarded a Guggenheim Fellowship in 1973, and served as a Fellow at the Center for Advanced Studies in the Behavioral Sciences in 1984–85. He recently received an honorary Ph.D. from Uppsala University (Sweden) for his work in psychology and health. He has authored several books, journal articles, and book chapters. He currently directs the Ph.D. specialty in health psychology at Stanford and is Director of Research, Meyer Friedman Institute, Mt. Zion Medical Center, San Francisco.

Neil D. Weinstein is Professor of Human Ecology and Psychology at Rutgers, The State University of New Jersey. His research concentrates on the responses of individuals to hazards. This research addresses why people take or fail to take precautions against illnesses such as AIDS, environmental and occupational risks, crime, and natural hazards. His work has included empirical studies of risk perception, especially optimistic biases in perceptions of personal susceptibility, research into ways of explaining risk magnitudes to the public, investigations of public responses to the risk from radon, intervention research to increase self-protective behaviors, and efforts to improve theories of individual precautionary behavior.

Camille B. Wortman, Ph.D., Professor of Psychology at the University of Michigan, has conducted nationally recognized research on adaptation to various stressful circumstances, including bereavement, ill health, and role strain. She received her Ph.D. in social psychology from Duke University in 1972 and has conducted AIDS research since 1984.

NOTES

NOTES

NOTES

NOTES

NOTES

NOTES